Learning Disability Nursing Practice:

Origins, perspectives and practice

Learning Disability Nursing Practice

Origins, perspectives and practice

Edited by

Mark Jukes

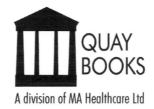

QUAY
BOOKS

A division of MA Healthcare Ltd

Quay Books Division, MA Healthcare Ltd, St Jude's Church, Dulwich Road, London
SE24 0PB

British Library Cataloguing-in-Publication Data
A catalogue record is available for this book

© MA Healthcare Limited 2009
ISBN-10: 1-85642-385-9; ISBN-13: 978-1-85642-385-4

1005968083

Printed by CLE, Huntingdon, Cambridgeshire

Contents

Contributors

Editor

Mark Jukes is Reader in Learning Disabilities, Department of Community Health and Social Work, Birmingham City University, Edgbaston Campus, Birmingham, England

Contributors

Peter Allen is a retired biomedical scientist. Much of his career was spent at St Margaret's Hospital, Walsall. He is a well-known local historian with a particular interest in social history. He can be contacted at 130 Dunsheath, Hollinswood, Telford, Shropshire TF3 2DB, England

Jill Aylott has a PhD in Autism and is Research Lead at the Centre for Professional and Organisation Development, Faculty of Health and Wellbeing, Sheffield Hallam University, Sheffield, England

Owen Barr is Head of School, School of Nursing, University of Ulster, Londonderry, Northern Ireland

Susan Brady is Clinical Lead for Health Facilitation and an Advanced Nurse Practitioner for Learning Disabilities Services in South Birmingham Primary Care Trust, Birmingham, England

Martin Bollard is Senior Lecturer in Learning Disabilities and CiPel Reader, Coventry University, Coventry, England

Catherine Doherty is Epilepsy Specialist Nurse, St. Stephens Centre, South Birmingham Primary Care Trust, Birmingham, England

Carmel Doyle is Lecturer in Intellectual Disabilities, School of Nursing and Midwifery, Trinity College, Dublin, Eire

Dave Ferguson is Consultant Nurse (Mental Health in Learning Disability) and Academic Practitioner, Hampshire Partnership NHS Foundation Trust and University of Southampton, Southampton, England

Tony Gilbert is Deputy Head of School of Social Work and Primary Care, Plymouth University, Plymouth, England

Colin Griffiths is Lecturer in Intellectual Disabilities, School of Nursing and Midwifery, Trinity College, Dublin, Eire

Bob Hallawell is Academic Lead in Learning Disability, Division of Nursing, School of Nursing, Midwifery and Physiotherapy, University of Nottingham, Nottingham, England

Simon Jones is Deputy Service Manager, Bristol Community Learning Difficulty Service, Bristol, England

Anne Kingdon is Consultant Nurse in Learning Disabilities (Forensic), Cheshire and Wirral Partnership NHS Foundation Trust, and Honorary Senior Lecturer, University of Chester, England

Duncan Mitchell is Professor of Health and Disability, Manchester Metropolitan University and Head of Clinical Services, Manchester Learning Disability Partnership, Manchester, England

Ruth Northway is Professor of Learning Disability Nursing, Unit for Development in Intellectual Disabilities, Faculty of Health, Sport and Science, University of Glamorgan, Pontypridd, Wales

Tony Osgood is Lecturer in Intellectual and Developmental Disability, Tizard Centre, University of Canterbury, England

Penny Pritchard is Service Manager, Developmental Neurosciences and Learning Disabilities Directorate, Stonefield House, St. Georges Hospital, South Staffordshire and Shropshire Healthcare NHS Foundation Trust, Stafford, England

Fiona Rich is Senior Lecturer in Learning Disabilities, Department of Community Health and Social Work, Birmingham City University, Birmingham, England

Caron Thomas is Consultant Nurse in Learning Disabilities and Head of Nursing, Learning Disabilities, Developmental Neurosciences and Learning Disabilities Directorate, St. Georges Hospital, South Staffordshire and Shropshire Healthcare NHS Foundation Trust, Stafford, England

Introduction

This book claims to be a first in providing a text that encapsulates not only the origins of nursing in the learning disability field but also contemporary perspectives and areas for specialist nursing practice.

Readers may initially be confused when a book which is entitled *Learning Disability Nursing Practice* commences with three chapters given over to the history of a colony and research into mental deficiency nursing. However, for many readers these chapters will present a rich source of what constitutes a little understood era that promoted segregation, a setting apart from society, as opposed to the now more enlightened approach of citizenship and person-centred practice.

For many students of learning disability nursing, whether working in health or social care settings, their professional and historical roots remain largely hidden or are portrayed negatively through reported scandals and inquiries. This book therefore intentionally covers a significant part of the history of this branch of nursing and traces the beginnings of a unique colony for people known to be mentally deficient, in the context of society, and the creation of social policy which advocated a solution to what was called mental deficiency.

The book is divided into four sections: origins, perspectives, practice, and further perspectives.

Section one (origins) describes Great Barr Colony and explores the conceptions of practice of actual attendants and nurses who worked there. It gives readers an in-depth focus on aspects of work and practice not accounted for in the literature to date.

Section two (perspectives) explores social policy perspectives from the past eras of the workhouse, the colony and the hospital, through to the present age of citizenship. Research in learning disability nursing practice is identified through scoping exercises to identify its current status. The section questions the research and practice developments that have come of age and that constitute a challenge within an evidence-based health and social care world.

Section three (practice) identifies a wide range of specialist areas of nursing practice, including community learning disability nursing, epilepsy, forensics, health facilitation, autism, mental health, challenging behaviour, children's services and working with people with profound and multiple learning disabilities.

Section four (further perspectives) addresses areas of contemporary and future concern, namely, educational curricula for nurses and the importance of inter-professional education and practice development.

Section One: Origins

Chapter 1 by Peter Allen opens with an in-depth account of the history of Great Barr Park Colony, later to be known as St. Margarets Hospital. Its aim is to contextualise the era of the colony and hospital in terms of the social policy that influenced such provisions for people who, over time, and through the nomenclature of perjorative labels, were deemed as being mentally defective, subnormal or having a mental handicap.

Mark Jukes follows in *Chapter 2* with research that examines the perceptions of practice of attendants and nurses who were trained and worked at Great Barr Park Colony from 1927 up to the formation of the National Health Service in 1948.

In *Chapter 3* Duncan Mitchell concludes the section with an in-depth account of the difficulties in the relationship between mental deficiency and learning disability nursing. The focus is upon the work of the General Nursing Council and how it grappled with the question of whether work in mental deficiency could be described as nursing.

Section Two: Perspectives

Tony Gilbert, in *Chapter 4,* commences this section with an in-depth appraisal of social policy adopting a theme of 'The Four Ages of Learning Disability': the age of the workhouse, the age of the colony, the age of normalisation and the age of citizenship.

Ruth Northway (*Chapter 5*) considers and pursues learning disability research in terms of promoting this essential activity. She generates ideas about how this can be effectively achieved. Recent work is highlighted which places into perspective the current status of research within learning disability nursing practice.

Section Three: Practice

This section commences with *Chapter 6* on the development of community learning disability nursing from its origins to contemporary practice. What is illustrated is an area of work that has been determined and influenced through external events and policies, rather than by internal appraisal and analysis from nurses themselves. Mark Jukes and Simon Jones identify that learning disability nurses have a predominantly health focus, which has the potential impact of promoting change and inclusion for people with learning disabilities and their families.

Susan Brady in *Chapter 7* continues the theme of health in this section on learning disability nursing practices. She provides an in-depth analysis into her work and research as a strategic health facilitator in Birmingham. Susan's research focuses on the adoption of an electronic health screening template by general practitioners, with the ultimate aim of improving health screening for people with an intellectual disability.

Epilepsy and learning disability are almost synonymous by virtue of their co-existence in this population. In *Chapter 8* Fiona Rich and Catherine Doherty present an extensive and comprehensive overview of epilepsy, and also consider the role of the learning disability nurse as a specialist practitioner.

In *Chapter 9* Colin Griffiths and Carmel Doyle explore key areas for assessment and health planning which are essential to apply when relating and working with people who have a profound and multiple learning disability. With an increase of the incidence in learning disability, the involvement of specialist nurses in this area is also bound to be a focus for increased intervention.

Dave Ferguson (*Chapter 10*) explores the dual diagnosis of mental health problems and learning disability. Although contemporary mental health services for people should have its roots in mainstream services, Dave explores the contribution specialist services and the learning disability nurse can provide in educating mainstream providers, family and paid carers.

In *Chapter 11* Tony Osgood provides an overview of one of the most difficult to define and ultimately contentious areas of practice within the field of learning disability nursing – challenging behaviour. Tony provides a rich account of some of the critical issues associated with challenging behaviour that a nurse will encounter in professional practice.

Anne Kingdon follows the theme of specialism in *Chapter 12*, and in this case an emergent area within learning disability nursing practice, that of forensics. The role of the nurse in this area of practice is still in its infancy in terms of community-based provision. The purpose of this chapter is to explore the context and practices of forensic learning disability nursing.

Jill Aylott (*Chapter 13*) provides us with an illuminating account of her work with people who have the diagnosis of an autistic spectrum condition. In particular, Jill shares her research into developing a communication and sensory profile. This is an invaluable resource allowing the learning disability nurse to gain further insight and to develop skills with people who have a different perspective on communication.

Owen Barr has extensive experience as a practitioner and researcher into the needs of children with learning disabilities and the effects their problems have on their families. In particular, in *Chapter 14*, Owen examines how policy and services are planned and the role of professionals in services, with the ultimate goal of promoting equal choice and value.

Section Four: Further perspectives

A new range of demands within health and social care presents new ways of delivering services to clients – which includes nurse education.

In *Chapter 15* Bob Hallawell illuminates some of these challenges specifically within pre-registration nursing curricula in an era of citizenship and person-centred approaches. There have been recent Nursing and Midwifery Council consultations over whether learning disability remains as a discrete field of practice, as do other specialties, or whether it is destined to remain a square peg in a round hole.

Martin Bollard (*Chapter 16*) explores the ubiquitous area of inter-professional education. Collaboration between the professions is not a new concept, but how to provide inter-professional learning is still embryonic for many higher educational establishments. Martin pursues how this may be achieved, highlighting how people with a learning disability can be at the centre of such programmes.

In the final chapter (*Chapter 17*) Caron Thomas and Penny Pritchard outline how practice development for learning disability nurses can sustain and promote their practice. This can be achieved through having a person-centred and carer focus and being involved in research, education and practice-based learning which ensures an evidence-based approach to practice.

This text gives an original and invaluable perspective into the origins and contemporary practices of learning disability nursing. The reader can examine the past and present formulations into what constitutes learning disability nursing practice across the parameters of health and social care.

Mark Jukes
Birmingham City University

Acknowledgements

I would like to extend my thanks to the attendants and nurses who participated in the research reported in *Chapter 2*, some of whom are no longer with us, who willingly and enthusiastically shared the experiences of their previous lives. Talking with them gave me great insight and I was humbled by the gift they offered.

I would also like to thank all the contributors to this text who are extremely active in promoting person-centred practices in their work with people, families, carers, and students across a broad spectrum of care.

Finally, I would like to thank Margaret for all her patience and support and for being a constant sounding board for my endeavours in promoting quality education and practices with people, families and students within the field of learning disability.

Section One:

Origins

CHAPTER 1

Mental deficiency institutions: Have the obituaries been fair and balanced?

Peter Allen

*Read not to contradict and confute, nor to believe and take for granted...
but to weigh and consider.*

Francis Bacon

Introduction

The 20th century was the Dark Ages for people with learning disabilities: they were incarcerated in institutions akin to prisons, systematically abused by uncaring nurses and denied basic human rights. Falling foul of parents, being a petty criminal or giving birth to an illegitimate child was sufficient reason to be 'put away' for an indefinite period.

If your exposure to the history of this special group of people is largely through the literature generated during and after the 1970s – the 'scandal decade' – you may well subscribe to these views. But such a standpoint is distorted and largely inaccurate.

From a close scrutiny of that period and its aftermath emerged a rash of publications intensely critical of institutions for the learning disabled. One such book looked at the life experiences of eight men and nine women who had spent an average of 47 years in an institution, certified under the Mental Deficiency Act of 1913 (Potts and Fido, 1991). Reading the book makes us uncomfortably aware of the injustices and inhumanity that characterised their lives. But just how much of that can we blame on the inherent shortcomings of institutionalised systems of care?

To be outraged is a perfectly understandable response, but we need to keep in mind we are viewing these accounts with modern eyes. The first half of the 20th century was a period of great social upheaval: despair, privation and dehumanisation was commonplace among the ordinary working classes. The most vulnerable sections of this social stratum suffered disproportionately.

Any studies based on edited interviews have well-recognised methodological shortcomings. These vignettes of life in an institution would be immensely more valuable if we were able to compare them with the life experiences of an age-matched control group brought up in the community. Those mental defectives[1] classified as 'feeble-minded'[2] under the Mental Deficiency Act and 'controlled' by statutory supervision, mostly in their own homes, are obvious candidates. Their education would probably have been through the Special School system; at the age of 16 they would leave and try to procure employment in a harsh world. How did they fare during the years of the Depression and after? Was their quality of life superior to that of their institutionalised peers? How were they affected by ignorance and prejudice? We have not been told.

Although such comparative studies are absent in the literature, the many UK and USA longitudinal and follow-up studies applicable to feeble-minded defectives in open society offer some insights (Tizard, 1958). During the Second World War thousands of UK and USA high-grade defectives living in the community were drafted into the army to perform the more menial tasks. Three of the many studies listed by Tizard examined their performance: a high degree of failure was reported with around half being discharged as unsuitable. Their life experiences in the community were far from positive.

A thorough review of the literature by Cobb (1969) concluded that '…as compared with a non-retarded control group, the retarded show a higher incidence of marital, civic and occupational failure, especially in the early stages.' A more recent analysis arrives at much the same conclusion: '…various follow-up studies of such key indicators of adult adjustment as employment, relationships, criminality, and adult mental health do not give cause for optimism' (O'Brien, 2001). The evidence suggests our missing control group in the community would also have given Potts and Fido (1991) a constellation of depressing life experiences.

Current perceptions of the institutional era are profoundly downbeat, which is saddening. This negativity has been exacerbated by a few miscreants who disgraced the nursing profession around the 1970s. Their actions cast a shadow over ordinary hard-working nurses who considered nursing in an institutional setting as a supremely rewarding experience. Large numbers devoted the whole of their working lives to the care of the learning disabled;

---

[1] *The history of learning disability is littered with changes in nomenclature. The terms used in this chapter will be seen to fluctuate according to the time period under discussion. Many of the older terms are now only used pejoratively*

[2] *The term 'feeble-minded' was in use from the middle of the 19th century (Brady, 1864; Duncan and Millard, 1866) to distinguish more able mental defectives, largely regarded at the time as lazy or wicked, from idiots and imbeciles.*

it was not uncommon for three generations of a family to follow each other into a nursing career. Whatever the inadequacies of the institutional system, it is beyond debate that generations of caring, highly-motivated professionals gave care and succour to the learning disabled equal in measure to anything on offer in this more 'enlightened' age.

A balanced appraisal of the era of mental deficiency institutions requires you to take a close look at why and how these establishments were set up, how they functioned on a day-to-day basis, and their response to change. You will look in vain in the academic literature for such an overall view. This vacuum may partially be filled by this warts-and-all historical summary, in essence a complete life-cycle, of Great Barr Park Colony (Barr Colony), the fourth largest such establishment for mental defectives in England. Like so many of its ilk, it was in turn spawned and destroyed by the same agent – social pressure.

Barr Colony, known as St Margaret's Hospital after 1948, was established on the old Great Barr Hall Estate, a location in the West Midlands near to what is now Junction 7 of the M6. Walsall and West Bromwich, two large towns central to its evolution, are situated close by. It has the distinction of being the first large mental deficiency colony to be approved by the Board of Control under the Mental Deficiency Act of 1913.

The evolution of mental deficiency colonies

Why was the Mental Deficiency Act of 1913 received with so much enthusiasm? Why were so many mental defectives taken out of society? How was it possible for impoverished Poor Law Unions to acquire landed estates? To answer these and other questions we need to examine the social dynamics then in play.

Overcrowding and intermixing in Poor Law establishments

From Elizabethan times up until the passage of the Poor Law Amendment Act in 1834, provision for the poor was administered at parish level. The system had many critics; assistance was often meted out in a haphazard manner and abuse was rife both by relievers and relieved. The new Act formed parishes into unions with their neighbours, abolished out-relief, and required those in need to surrender their liberty and enter purpose-built residential workhouses. Diet and conditions were standardised nationally by central Government edict and rigidly applied at local level by Poor Law Guardians, elected from the ratepayers. It was envisaged that a Draconian regime would discourage the unemployed able-bodied, those mostly in receipt of relief at that time, from pursuing a life of indolence on the local rates.

By the early part of the 20th century, very much against expectation, some 85% of persons receiving assistance were suffering from physical, mental or 'moral' disability. Poor Law institutions were increasingly becoming choked with the aged and infirm, abandoned and orphaned children, mental defectives, consumptives and other disadvantaged classes.

In 1905, a Royal Commission was appointed to enquire into the workings of the Poor Law system. Many far-reaching proposals were incorporated in their report (Royal Commission on the Poor Laws and Relief of Distress, 1909). In particular, the Royal Commission strongly favoured the removal of all children from workhouses. With the recommendations of the report in mind, Poor Law institutions throughout the land were inspired to seek ways of segregating the various classes according to their individual needs.

So what was the plight of local mental defectives before the Mental Deficiency Act changed the scene irrevocably? Alas, appropriate records for Walsall and West Bromwich Poor Law Unions do not survive in sufficient volume for the question to be answered authoritatively. But there is much to be gleaned from local newspapers – particularly the lengthy reports of weekly meetings of the guardians. Such information was eagerly devoured, after all guardians were spending local money and ratepayers were their severest critics.

This is the picture at the turn of the century. For ordinary working-class families, leading a hand-to-mouth existence, the added burden of a dependent mental defective was financially crippling. Unless able to hold down some kind of lowly employment, and so contribute towards their own upkeep, relatives of these unfortunates must, of necessity, place them in the hands of the Poor Law authorities. Within the workhouse they would perform the most menial domestic tasks or, if their disability was more profound, live out a wretched life in the imbecile wards of the infirmary. As a last resort those who were particularly troublesome would be sent away to the county asylum at Burntwood, certified under the lunacy laws. Guardians were no spendthrifts and they loathed having to pay the high maintenance charges so incurred.

Less costly arrangements were occasionally entered into with fellow unions possessing the necessary expertise and resources to handle special groups. In 1913, to relieve overcrowding, West Bromwich Guardians had 26 imbeciles boarded out with Stourbridge Union, with the facility to send double that number if they so desired (*Midland Chronicle*, 1913).

Defectives in middle-class families fared a little better than their impecunious fellows. For the privileged few the Midland Counties Idiot Asylum had been established at Knowle in the late 1860s. It offered residential care for around 60 patients and was the only asylum of its type in the whole of the five counties making up the central Midlands. Demand far outstripped resources and 'candidates' were elected to the asylum at the annual meeting of subscribers – that for 1897 was held in Walsall with the Mayor presiding (*Walsall Observer*, 1897). Friends of a patient were required to contribute towards their maintenance with any shortfall made up from voluntary subscriptions and income from investments.

Revealing statistics for the year 1914 are available for both local unions. Under new classification which had just been instituted, West Bromwich Guardians reckoned there were 340 persons in the union's institutions who could be identified as mentally defective, or 47% of the persons then being maintained (*Midland Chronicle*, 1914). Practically the whole of the remainder were chargeable through sickness, accident or bodily infirmity.

At Walsall the situation was less acute. Out of a total of 570 souls in the workhouse 40 were certified imbeciles, 21 uncertified epileptics and 24 feeble-minded: all would have been dependent mental defectives residing in the infirmary. The workhouse was also home to 118 paupers over the age of 70 (*Walsall Observer*, 1914b).

The majority of these defectives were transferred to Barr Colony as soon as it was up and running. Their quality of life would be improved dramatically by that short trip from the workhouse and there would have been no dissent.

Growing interest in the affairs of the feeble-minded

It was not until late in the 19th century that the first piece of legislation devoted exclusively to mental defectives was enacted. Until then they had been inextricably linked with the mentally ill. The Idiots Act (1886) empowered local authorities to build institutions specifically for the 'care, education and training of idiots and imbeciles' and guaranteed a capitation grant similar to that given for pauper lunatics. The potential of the Act was never fully exploited: when superseded by the epochal Mental Deficiency Act 25 years later only eight new institutions had been established in the whole of England and Wales.

Towards the close of the 19th century, a number of factors led to a growing interest in the affairs of society's casualties. Compulsory education for all children was introduced by the Education Act (1870), and dull and backward children became an inescapable educational problem. Many would previously have been camouflaged in a less-demanding society. At the same time, new knowledge of heredity and the eugenics movement associated with Francis Galton gave rise to acute and, with hindsight, exaggerated fears of racial degeneration.

Concern was firmly focused on 'the frightening fertility of the feeble-minded'. This was a newly-defined class of mental defective not so severely impaired as idiots and imbeciles, but numerically greater and requiring 'care, supervision, and control for their own protection or the protection of others'.

In the wake of this near-hysteria, a Royal Commission on the Care and Control of the Feeble-Minded was appointed in 1904. Available evidence was reviewed and enquiries made into the incidence of mental defect. The Royal Commission estimated there were nearly 150 000 mental defectives who had not been certified under the existing lunacy laws. Of these, just over a third were under Poor Law supervision in workhouses, cheek-by-jowl with the destitute, but normal, poor. Another third were receiving no care or supervision at all; and the remainder were either children at school or inmates in prisons, inebriate reformatories and similar institutions.

Evidence given to the Royal Commission by A F Tredgold (1870–1952), then one of the foremost authorities on mental deficiency in England, is especially illuminating. His monumental textbook on the subject was required reading for over 60 years (Tredgold, 1908). It was his opinion that 'In 90% of patients suffering from mental deficiency the condition is the result of a morbid state of the ancestors' (Hearnshaw, 1964). Environmental factors were discounted or regarded as being of only minor importance.

The Royal Commission seriously considered the social implications of mental deficiency, particularly with reference to drunkenness and illegitimacy. They concluded in their multi-volume report (Royal Commission on the Care and Control of the Feeble-Minded, 1908), that the provision of suitable institutions, especially for female mental defectives of child-bearing age, was an urgent necessity.

Opinion in the country was also on the side of statutory control. The view of minor officialdom is epitomised in the following resolution sent to all Poor Law Boards in 1911 by Halifax Town Council. It was widely recognised that Boards of Guardians acting in unison could sway a social issue and such lobbying was commonplace. We know that Walsall Guardians gave their whole-hearted support to the resolution (*Walsall Advertiser*, 1911):

> *In the belief that the absence of control of the adult feeble-minded is a contributory factor of great importance in relation to crime, to immorality, and to the problem of unemployment, and believing furthermore that this lack of control goes to the great fecundity of the feeble-minded, and seriously reduces the mean average of the health, the intelligence, the morality, and the physique of the race, this Council earnestly begs His Majesty's Government to place in the hands of some authority, subject to special safeguards as may be thought advisable, the permanent control of these unfortunates.*

The debate was fuelled by data 'revealed' by cacogenics, the then fashionable science of racial degeneration. The deliberations of these doom-and-gloom merchants were widely published: the American studies of the Jukes and Kallikak families are typical (Dugdale, 1877; Goddard, 1912).

The main recommendations of the Royal Commission were accepted by the Government of the day and embodied in the Mental Deficiency Act of 1913. In essence, the Act outlined the circumstances which rendered defectives 'subject to be dealt with' – the pivotal clause of the new Act – and prescribed a form of procedure for them to be 'sent to or placed in an institution for defectives or placed under guardianship'. Local authorities were expected to provide these institutions and to appoint suitable officers whose duties covered 'supervision, protection and control'. They were further obliged to 'ascertain', certify and detain mental defectives in their area coming within the scope of the Act.

It is on record that there was little opposition to the original Bill when it was being debated in Parliament. On the contrary, there was an urgent desire for such legislation from all quarters. This is evidenced by the considerable furore unleashed when the Bill was delayed in its passage. When a holdup was announced in November 1912 it brought forth a vigorous protest in the form of a round-robin from no fewer than 28 prominent politicians, educationalists, medics, academics and men-of-letters, including presidents of such prestigious bodies as the Royal Society, the Royal College of Physicians and the Royal College of Surgeons. Even the Archbishop of Canterbury and the Lord Mayor of Birmingham were signatories (*The Times*, 1912). Their appeal to the Government and Members of Parliament was strongly worded:

> *All we would venture to urge is that the House should avert, and rapidly avert, the calamity of allowing the present neglect of the mentally defective to continue, for this neglect is causing untold suffering to thousands of feeble-minded individuals who, because it is impossible under the existing law to train them and care for them, become inebriates, prostitutes, criminals, and paupers. These persons leave behind them a new generation of mentally and physically degenerate children, not only continuing but increasing, the numbers who must be supported at the expense of the community.*

Note the reference to the 'untold suffering' of the feeble-minded and the desire 'to train them and care for them'. There was genuine concern to improve their lot: removal from society was considered necessary for the remedial process to be successful.

The decline of landed estates

The decline of the English country house at the end of the 19th century was a significant factor in the proliferation of mental deficiency colonies and other institutions. Several decades of political and economic turmoil had taken their toll, particularly the agricultural depression fuelled by the influx of cheap corn from America. The coup de grâce was the introduction of death duties in 1894. Small landed estates were coming on the market in increasing numbers and could usually be acquired cheaply. For cash-strapped authorities they were a godsend: plenty of building land, a 'big house' for administrative purposes, and an affordable price-tag.

Great Barr Hall, equidistant from Walsall and Birmingham, was such an estate in decline. It had been the principal residence of the Scott family of Great Barr, a middle-rank nobility, until a failure of male heirs. Under testamentary instructions the estate was put up for auction in 1911 – at precisely the time the West Bromwich Poor Law Union was looking to increase its accommodation facilities. It was inevitable the guardians would take an interest.

Great Barr Hall has an enviable history. Although today in advanced decay it remains a building of international importance for its associations with the Lunar Society of Birmingham. The Hall was the favourite meeting place of these harbingers of the industrial revolution. The landscape is also valued for having been worked on by William Shenstone and later Humphry Repton, landscape designers of the first rank.

The importance of the Lunar Society of Birmingham in world history cannot be over-emphasised. They have been described as '…the most remarkable group of thinkers and inventors in the 18th century – which had a more potent effect upon civilisation than that of any other society in history' (Pearson, 1930). Testimonials do not come more effusive than this.

The working of the Mental Deficiency Act

Confusion and misunderstanding frequently surrounds this monumental piece of legislation. It therefore seems appropriate to present a short summary of the sections dealing with classification and certification – the italics are mine to stress pivotal words and phrases. A number of books offered practitioners detailed guidance on the procedures to be followed under the Mental Deficiency Act and later amending Acts (Shrubsall and Williams, 1932).

Note that only after a person had been confirmed as mentally defective could they be dealt with under the Act. Stories of people being 'put away' solely at the whim or caprice of a parent or magistrate are inaccurate.

The Mental Deficiency Act in outline

Under the Act mental defectives were classified into four categories:

- **Idiots**: Persons so deeply defective in mind from birth or from an early age as to be unable to guard themselves against common physical dangers.
- **Imbeciles**: Persons in whose case there exists from birth or from an early age mental defectiveness not amounting to idiocy, yet so pronounced that they are incapable of managing themselves or their affairs.
- **Feeble-minded**: Persons in whose case there exists from birth or from an early age mental defectiveness not amounting to imbecility, yet so pronounced that they require care, supervision and control for their own protection or for the protection of others.
- **Moral defectives**: Persons who from an early age display some permanent mental defect coupled with strong vicious or criminal propensities on which punishment has had little or no deterrent effect.

Having defined mental defectiveness, the Act lists the circumstances that render a defective 'subject to be dealt with':

A person who is a defective may be dealt with under the Act by being sent to or placed in an institution for defectives or placed under guardianship:

- at the instance of his/her parent or guardian OR
- if, *in addition to being a defective*, he/she is a person:
  - who is found neglected, abandoned, or without visible means of support, or cruelly treated; or
  - who is found guilty of any criminal offence...; or
  - who is undergoing imprisonment or penal servitude, or is undergoing detention...by order of a court...; or
  - who is an habitual drunkard...; or
  - (who has been ascertained to be incapable by reason of mental defect of receiving benefit or further benefit in special schools or classes...);
  - who is in receipt of poor relief at the time of giving birth to an illegitimate child or when pregnant of such a child.

The law required, in all cases, that a petition for an Order to place a defective in an institution or under guardianship was accompanied by medical certificates signed by two qualified medical practitioners, one of whom was approved for the purpose by the Board of Control, the body charged with the general superintendence of matters relating to the supervision, protection and control of defectives. In most cases the additional signature of a judicial authority would be required, after such inquiry as was thought fit. There were severe penalties for anyone obtaining a certificate by supplying incorrect information.

Doctors were left largely to their own judgement as to what constituted a diagnosis of mental defectiveness. Lack of training, prejudice, imprecise criteria, and the absence of standardised psychometric testing led to a climate of arbitrariness. In fairness, most tried their best under difficult circumstances.

Orders expired at the end of one year unless extended. If the Board of Control, after consideration of special reports (from Statutory Visitors or the medical officer of the institution), considered that continuance of the order was required in the interests of the defective, the order remained in force for a further period of one year and then for successive periods of five years.

Little use was made of guardianship – the placing of a defective under the control of an appointed person in a home setting. That person could be a parent or other relative, an employer or someone not connected with the defective. This was much to the dismay of the Board of Control, who favoured its use, particularly in the case of children. If the placement failed, transfer to a certified institution was a simple matter of a variation of the original order.

Supervision, voluntary and statutory, was the simplest form of control under the Act. No judicial order was required and it merely consisted in the visitation and general oversight of the defective in his or her own home by the local authority, usually through a special officer. Local authorities were required to provide suitable training or occupation: for low-grades, unable to profit by instruction in special schools, this was usually done by means of occupation centres.

Local response to the Mental Deficiency Act

Walsall Council appointed its first Mental Deficiency Act Committee immediately the Act came into force in April 1914. It consisted of nine members: six from the council and three Poor Law Guardians. Even though the new Act legislated for a complete break with Poor Law Unions, the resources and experience of this body proved indispensable.

In the fullness of time, with the approval of the Board of Control, statutory committees throughout the land began to appoint voluntary associations to care for mental defectives. In Walsall the Civic Guild of Help, affiliated to the National Association of Guilds of Help, was so appointed in 1921. Similar work was undertaken by voluntary bodies in West Bromwich.

Guild members took their new duties very seriously and a sub-committee (three reverend gentlemen and five women – all volunteers) was quickly set up. The first priority was to form a register of mental defectives in the borough: within three years they had collected 172 names by assiduous enquiry. It was largely through excessive zeal that Walsall came to have twice as many registered defectives per thousand of the population as any other borough in the country.

Alas, as in all institutions at this time, there were a few distraught individuals at Barr Colony who, either through underlying mental illness or an inability to accept the loss of freedom, chose to take their own lives.

The Great Barr scheme

Around 1910, West Bromwich Poor Law Guardians were becoming increasingly concerned with the overcrowding in the infirmary, nursery and mental deficiency departments. As one of the largest Poor Law Unions in the Midlands, serving a population of nearly 200 000, their problems were particularly acute. A committee was urgently set up under the Chairman, Mr A L Wells, to advise on possible solutions. Mr Wells was a farmer: his fellow guardians included a draper, ironmonger, ironfounder and grocer.

Great Barr Hall Estate was then on the market. Wells put forward a proposal that its purchase would enable the guardians to carry out in full the recommendations embodied in the Royal Commission report. Such a bold suggestion, certain to be a burden on the rates, would have fallen flat a few years earlier. Public opinion had moved on and the proposition found favour among fellow guardians.

The principal lot of 557 acres, comprising Great Barr Hall and park (including two large lakes, six lodges and Park Farm) was snapped up by West Bromwich Guardians for a modest £28 000. The Local Government Board had sanctioned up to £40 000 for its purchase.

How poignant that, way back in 1836, the first chairman of Walsall Poor Law Guardians was Sir Edward Dolman Scott, late owner of this ancient pile. Paupers would soon be enjoying their own kind of privilege within these walls.

West Bromwich and Walsall Unions join forces

It had not escaped the notice of the West Bromwich Guardians that their colleagues in Walsall were also considering extra provisions for the poor. Without hesitation Walsall Guardians agreed to join the scheme and share capital costs. Following the Reports of the Royal Commission on the Poor Laws, strong rumours were abroad that the combination of Poor Law Unions for certain purposes, particularly provisions for children and epileptics and the feeble-minded, was about to be made compulsory. Better to combine voluntarily with a union close at hand than have a foreign scheme foisted on them.

There was precedence for this close collaboration. The two unions had set up the District Schools at Wigmore as early as 1870. In a residential setting, children chargeable to the two unions had received a good education for over a generation. Admittedly, the regime was harsh and restrictive, but it was considered by all as far superior to languishing within the confines of the adult workhouse. Even though discipline was strict, with the freedom to roam and visit relatives severely curtailed, the inmates were probably better off overall than some local children.

As soon as the estate had been acquired the removal of children and infants from the two workhouses was given top priority. Great Barr Hall had been badly neglected over the years and months were spent preparing it for its new role. New and up-to-date sanitary appliances were fitted throughout and hot water installed. The bedrooms and dressing rooms on the first floor were turned into dormitories. Several rooms were set aside for isolation purposes and staff accommodation. Some of the outbuildings at the rear were converted into a hand laundry. When taken over the estate had no mains water, metalled roads, gas, electricity or telephone. Untreated sewage was discharged directly into the lower pool.

The formal order setting up a Joint Committee was issued by the Local Government Board in October, 1912, just in time for the official opening of Great Barr Hall for the reception of its first pauper residents. The refurbished building was opened with considerable pomp and ceremony. The band of the District Schools at Wigmore was brought in to play sweet music for the dignitaries and souvenir pamphlets, drawn up by the Clerk to the West Bromwich Guardians, were freely distributed (Walsall and West Bromwich Unions (WWBU), 1912). No opportunity was passed by to publicise proposals for the future of the estate and to give the historical associations of the Hall.

The first children, a contingent of 25, were received into the Hall on 25 November, 1912. Within a few weeks the accommodation for 100 children and 20 mothers had been taken up. The youngsters thrived in their new surroundings and after just nine months the matron was able to report to the Committee that gains in height and weight were well above average. But there was no way of shedding the Poor Law mantle: mothers were only permitted to visit their offspring once in every three months.

There were initial difficulties in attracting staff to the new institution. Attempts to obtain a sister from among the nurses at Birmingham Children's Hospital met with no success. Nurses in the employ of Poor Law authorities were considered lesser beings.

At Barr the medical care of the children was for many years in the very capable hands of an eminent consultant physician, Dr J M Smellie, later appointed Professor of Paediatrics at Birmingham University. In contrast, a mile away at Hamstead village the vicar was obliged to start a Medical Service Club to provide medical and surgical treatment for those poor mining families not covered by the State Health Insurance Acts. Members had to scrape together a few pennies each week to ensure elementary health cover for their children and themselves (SPHPM, 1933).

The inter-war years

When the Mental Deficiency Act came into effect in April 1914, it was the expectation that local authorities would make provisions for farm and industrial colonies for the training and employment of mental defectives. Instead, local authorities made heavy use of a clause in the Act which allowed them to delegate responsibilities back to the guardians. The Board of Control was initially very reluctant to allow this to happen. However, the advent of the First World War created unfavourable financial conditions and the Board was obliged to modify its views. Ten years after the Act came into being 169 local authorities had been allowed to take this retrograde step, resulting in a third of all detained defectives remaining within the Poor Law system. The remainder were cared for in a miscellaneous collection of institutions, hospitals and training colonies run by local authorities, philanthropic bodies, and the Board of Control itself (Board of Control, 1924).

Ways of carrying out the obligations laid down in the Mental Deficiency Act of 1913 were being regularly explored at county level. It was widely rumoured that a single county institution dealing with cases for the whole of Staffordshire was favoured. It was imperative that this element of the Great Barr Scheme was expedited with all good speed. It made good economic sense to do so rather than wait for the county to intervene and impose a more expensive system over which it would have no control.

There were other financial advantages accruing from such a scheme. Mental defectives chargeable on the local rates were spread far and wide in sanatoria, boarding-out facilities, convalescent homes and institutions for the feeble-minded. By collecting them together under one mantle they could be dealt with in homes provided by the guardians at much less expense.

Around this time many joint ventures were entered into with the pooled resources of two or more proximate Poor Law Unions. It turned out that only three schemes were of sufficient size and sophistication to survive into the post-1948 NHS era: Prudhoe Hospital in Northumberland (Day, 2000), nearby Monyhull Hospital (Hutchings, 1998) and Barr Colony/St Margaret's Hospital.

First in the country

Some 12 months after the inauguration of the Great Barr Scheme and with the infants and children now more suitably accommodated, the guardians were able to look to the needs of the mentally defective.

A Birmingham architect, Gerald McMichael, was instructed to prepare plans. The Local Government Board initially approved four homes for 225 patients – 45 men, 40 women, 70 boys, and 70 girls.

It was the first large-scale scheme of its kind approved by the new Board of Control. Guardians from the two Poor Law Unions assembled in May 1914 for the ceremonial cutting of the first sod (*Walsall Observer*, 1914a). They were well aware the scheme was breaking new ground in more than one sense and they '...thought it probable it would become the pattern scheme for the whole country'. But the thoughts of those present, like many of their fellow countrymen, must have been on the storm clouds gathering over Europe. Three short months later Britain was at war with Germany.

Building work gets under way

Because of the intervention of the First World War national energies were diverted elsewhere. Progress on the scheme was slow and the price of building materials rocketed. It was almost impossible to obtain certain items and local builders were forced to borrow from each other. Able-bodied construction workers were equally hard to come by.

The first two buildings, single and double-storey blocks for boys and men, were completed by September 1917. They were roofed with Buttermere slates and faced with York stone screeds – a real extravagance at the time. Permission was then sought from the Board of Control for their certification. Acting as agents for the guardians, application was made by West Bromwich Council for approval under the much-abused convenience of Section 37 of the Mental Deficiency Act.

The trials and tribulations of a burgeoning colony

The early days of the fledgling colony were dogged by problems. Despite advertising widely the clerk was unable to obtain male attendants for the new blocks. He was left with just two alternatives: attempt to obtain suitable candidates through the Labour Exchange or, very much as a last resort, advertise for female attendants. Permanent support services had yet to be built and meals were prepared in a temporary wooden kitchen. Laundry was contracted out to a Walsall firm.

After a period of administrative chaos the Joint Committee appointed a new matron who was to serve their requirements particularly well. Miss E Hailey, from nearby Monyhull Colony, was certainly the best qualified of the applicants for the post. During the previous three years she had been First Assistant Matron at Monyhull and before that Matron of the Hayes Cottage Hospital. Her training in nursing children and her considerable administrative experience helped see the colony through its formative years. She was appointed in July 1918 at a salary of £110 per annum, with rations, uniform and furnished apartments (Walsall Local History Centre (WLHC), 1918).

Matron Hailey would have total day-to-day control over all that took place in both the colony and a children's hospital of 120 beds which, until closed down in 1932, served the medical needs of 'normal' Poor Law children from Walsall and West Bromwich. Only the workmen on the estate were outside her jurisdiction. Everything came within her purview, from checking the quality of the steam coal to the issuing of fishing permits. Incidentally, a day's fishing in 1919 in the colony lakes would set you back 10 shillings – three days pay for a probationer male attendant on £56 per annum.

Matron Hailey retired in April 1932, after nearly 14 years service. She was presented with a suitably-inscribed wireless set.

Pomp and ceremony

The remaining two blocks were finished in May 1918, but not brought into use until 1921. In 1916, and again in 1918, newly-completed buildings were offered unsuccessfully to the War Office for the use of shell-shocked soldiers. The guardians were greatly peeved to have their show of patriotism rebuffed on two occasions.

Owing to the exigencies of wartime the first three blocks were opened without formality. But the guardians were determined to open the fourth with appropriate commemoration. It would also serve as an opportunity to update local ratepayers on this pioneering venture: there had been much criticism of the scheme for the financial burden it imposed on local ratepayers.

Guardians and their friends from West Bromwich and Walsall were ferried in by 'exceedingly comfortable' motor char-a-bancs on that mild autumn afternoon. Fine speeches followed and it was pointed out that the site chosen for the embryo colony was ideal for its purpose, with full advantage being taken of natural amenities (*Midland Chronicle*, 1921):

> *Facing southwards, it commands a lovely view of the portion of the park which lies in the direction of the Handsworth Lodge. The grassy land dips down from the site to the lakes in the valley, the shimmering water, set in a background of stately woodland, forming a charming feature of this picturesque piece of the estate.*

Mr Wells reminded those assembled that the colony was a training establishment, with all the patients being taught useful work. The men and boys were engaged in shoemaking, tailoring, builders' work (including bricklaying and painting), horticulture and agriculture. The whole of the levelling around the building had been done by the patients under the directions of the estate foreman. (*Plate 1*)

Great progress had been made in the shoemaker's shop and patients were now able to make complete boots. During the previous 12 months 223 pairs of boots and slippers had been made and three times that number repaired. The tailor's shop had only recently started up and inmates were already showing aptitude for the work.

The women were engaged in domestic work, in the hand laundry and in knitting socks and vests. In the near future they hoped to be able to provide the various institutions of the two Poor Law Unions with articles of clothing made at the colony.

Major expansion in the mid-1920s

In January 1924, in order to relieve the overload, the Mental Deficiency Act Committee of Walsall Town Council asked the Joint Committee administering the colony to take low-grade as well as high-grade defectives. They agreed, reluctantly, and McMichael was again consulted. Plans were furnished for an additional 342 beds together with ancillary buildings. The new construction, ranged around the original four villas in a pleasing horse-shoe shape, provided matching accommodation for males and females. It was commissioned and in use by September 1929, just before the Poor Law system was disbanded (WWBU, 1929). It brought the accommodation up to 640 beds. The scheme was proudly written up in the architectural press (*Architects' Journal*, 1930; *The Builder*, 1933). (*Plate 2*)

Further pre-War extensions separate the sexes

Just before the Second World War, in response to a continuing need for more beds, a further 11 homes, in a 'dignified phase of Georgian architecture', were erected on land several hundred yards to the north-west of the established colony. It more effectively segregated the sexes and soon became known simply as the 'male side'.

The new buildings, formally opened in May 1938 by the Earl of Harrowby (Walsall and West Bromwich (Barr Colony) Joint Board (WWBJB), 1938), increased the accommodation to 1355 beds. The colony was now the fourth largest in the country and the cost of a bed had been reduced from 42 shillings (£2.10) to 28 shillings (£1.40) a week. According to Walsall's retiring Town

Clerk the colony was '…in size, economy, and efficient administration, the finest in the kingdom' (*Walsall Times*, 1940). The homes were all named after serving members of the Joint Board. New workshops were named the Macmillan Workshops out of respect for the Medical Superintendent.

A considerable amount of site work was done by the colonists themselves under the direction of the clerk of works. This included the making of thousands of concrete blocks, the very extensive rough excavations entailed in the construction of new roads, underground ducts, levelling of ground and formation of terraces. They were also responsible for the garden layout of all the homes.

The philosophy behind mental deficiency colonies

America embraced the notion of training colonies for the feeble-minded many decades before Great Britain. The earliest discussion of such an establishment for central England was in May 1901 at the West Midland Poor Law Conference. Poor Law Guardians were urged to combine resources for such a purpose. It was the catalyst which brought Birmingham, Aston and Kings Norton Boards of Guardians together in a joint scheme (Birmingham Union, 1913). From it sprang nearby Monyhull Colony, opened in April 1908, with initial accommodation for 216 inmates.

The resident Medical Superintendent of Monyhull Colony, Dr A M McCutcheon, wrote one of the few in-depth statements of the philosophy behind training colonies in this country (McCutcheon, 1925). The objects of treating mental defectives in closed institutions were expounded in a long article:

> *(1) To correct their anti-social conduct. (2) To develop their self-respect and ensure their happiness. (3) To teach them various kinds of work for which they are best fitted by reason of their mental and physical condition, and to recover from them some contribution, however small, towards the cost of their maintenance. To lead up to discharge if possible. (4) To prevent the procreation of children, and so to stop the handing on of the blight to successive generations.*

This was best achieved by:

> *…segregation in institutions, preferably of the colony type, whereas sterilisation, which is advocated by some, solves only one of the objects, namely, that of preventing procreation of children. It certainly does not tackle the conduct aspect, nor the work aspect, and it is surprising the number of defectives that one finds trying to carry on jobs with very*

indifferent success. These are the people who drift about from place to place, unable to hold a position for any length of time, and this surely constitutes a distinct menace to our industrial position in the world.

Some account of the occupational 'treatment' at Monyhull may be of interest:

We are always told that ordinary people do not benefit from idleness, but it is astounding how quickly defectives go downhill mentally and physically if they are not kept suitably occupied. It is regrettable that, in a number of institutions where defectives are housed, one can see them ranged round the walls at almost any hour of the day, doing nothing except getting into trouble and making a nuisance of themselves, and at the same time deteriorating generally. We have therefore made it a rule that everyone, man woman or child, each working day, goes out to some definite occupation... Thus each home is emptied during the day of all but the sick and those engaged in domestic duties. The patients get a change of surroundings, of faces, and to a certain extent of staff, and this seems to keep them much more contented and happy.

From the outset Barr Colony was run on similar general principles. From 1929 it was under the direction of the much-respected Dr D M MacMillan, the first resident Medical Superintendent. He was in post until 1952 and was largely responsible for the colony's reputation as one of the finest in the country. At times he was greatly concerned with both the non-suitability of many of the inmates and the danger of becoming swamped with cases of the 'low-grade unimprovable type'. His views were vividly expressed in a report to the Joint Committee in September 1929 (WLHC, 1929):

There are many patients in the colony suffering from varying degrees of mental decay – a very different thing from mental deficiency – quite a number are suffering from senile changes. These patients defeat the object of a colony and add to the nursing difficulties. They conduce to dreariness, idleness and monotony instead of the busy, happy corporate life of a modern mental defective institution. Whilst I have every sympathy with the aged and infirm, and appreciate very highly how well cared for these are here, I respectfully submit that they are not suitable cases for a progressive institution for the mentally defective.

The Board of Control made similar noises. In a letter to the Joint Board they suggested that the question of removing old and senile cases to a more appropriate institution, and replacing them in the colony with younger patients capable of being trained, should be brought before the Walsall and West Bromwich Town Councils.

The considerable costs of running a training colony were partially eased by entering into formal agreements with local authorities and Poor Law Unions without adequate facilities of their own. The Joint Committee contracted to take a number of defectives, on agreed terms, for a fixed period of 21 years (WLHC, 1920). Birmingham City Council was the first to negotiate such an agreement. From August 1920 they had the facility for the reception and maintenance of up to 100 defectives, as and when the need arose.

Over the years formal arrangements were made for the reception of defectives from Coventry, Wolverhampton, Smethwick, Nottinghamshire, Worcestershire and Derbyshire. Each agreement contained a clause specifically excluding 'dangerous criminals or defectives who were bed-ridden or whose infirmities rendered them incapable of being employed or trained at an industrial colony'. Contracting bodies could be asked to remove any defectives who became a burden through physical or mental incapacity.

Such arrangements have left their mark. The policy of resettlement in the community led to the repatriation of many long-stay residents to distant localities to which they no longer had any affiliation.

One-way traffic

In 1937, the running of the colony was given unusual prominence in a series of telling debates at meetings of Walsall Town Council and their Mental Welfare Committee. Issues were repeatedly aired over a period of several months, revealing valuable information on the workings of the Mental Deficiency Act in a local setting. The Act had then been up and running for nearly a quarter of a century.

The protracted debate started with comments made during a Walsall Town Council meeting to discuss the quarterly report of the Joint Board (*Walsall Observer*, 1937). Councillor Tibbits commented that Walsall had twice as many defectives per thousand under institutional treatment as any other borough in the country. On the other hand they had only 2% on licence (Leave of Absence on Licence), whereas the Board of Control recommended up to 10%. It was his belief that the town's Mental Welfare Committee used only institutional treatment to deal with defectives.

Councillor Tibbits noted that holiday leave was freely granted to all suitable patients and they were returned to their parents for Christmas and Bank Holidays. They were even allowed to go to the pictures. It was his belief that if patients were fit to return home periodically, they were fit to be returned to communal life and to take their proper place in the world. Barr Colony should be a training centre, not a concentration camp.

Continued vituperative attacks by Councillor Tibbitts prompted members of the colony staff to send a letter to the editor of one of the local newspapers (*Walsall Times*, 1937a). They were incensed at what they saw as unwarranted criticism:

> *People seem to think that all that has to be done is to have patients here for a short while and then release them completely cured... We who have worked in other institutions know that these people are the recipients of far more freedom than many under the same circumstances and this freedom is the result of Dr MacMillan's efforts. We respect Dr MacMillan...and know that he is irreproachable in his treatment and management... We know from experience that this colony is one of the best conducted and happiest in the country. Walsall might well glory in the possession of such an institution. So they should. Who should know better than ourselves?*

Interesting statistics came out in a reply prepared by the Walsall Mental Welfare Committee in May 1937 (*Walsall Times*, 1937b). They condemned Councillor Tibbits' criticisms of their work as 'astoundingly incorrect'. In Walsall there were 654 defectives on the books: 228 were under voluntary supervision, 142 under statutory supervision, 24 under guardianship, and 260 (including six on licence) under institutional treatment. About one in six was under 16 years of age. Of the 654 reported defectives, 420 were ascertained as being 'subject to be dealt with' under the Mental Deficiency Acts. This last statistic debunks the myth that those 'subject to be dealt with' were invariably institutionalised: nearly 40% of this group remained in the community.

Seventy three of the 394 under voluntary or statutory supervision or under guardianship, principally children, attended the Occupation Centre. Apart from six guardianship cases living out of Walsall, the whole of the 394 cases referred to were living in their own homes in Walsall.

The Mental Welfare Committee confirmed the statistic that Walsall had twice as many defectives as any other borough in the country, but insisted this was simply that mental welfare work in Walsall was in a specially advanced state. This was due to two main causes: firstly, the pioneer work done by the Walsall Civic Guild of Help over many years, mostly in ascertaining and reporting the whereabouts of defectives, and secondly to the existence, in the shape of Barr Colony, of one of the few adequate institutions for mental defectives in the country.

In the same newspaper report Councillor Tibbits was roundly condemned for turning down an invitation to become a member of the same Mental Welfare Committee he had damned so thoroughly.

The Joint Board felt that criticisms of training were entirely misconceived and were based on an inadequate knowledge of the work of the colony. They prepared a detailed 10-page report to answer critics (WWBJB, 1937). The report stated that out of 680 patients at the colony, no less than 526 were employed in useful work. Much of the colony's requirements in furniture, clothing and boots were made in the workshops. Other male patients worked on the farm and in the gardens. Some 130 female patients were engaged in laundry and kitchen work, sewing and darning. Other patients were engaged in weaving, poultry-keeping, bricklaying, painting, and mat and rug making.

The question of licence and discharge was fully addressed. Since 1930, 43 patients had been tried on licence: six were finally discharged, two transferred to the books of another authority and seven were returned for various reasons. This was not a record to be proud of but the Medical Superintendent, Dr MacMillan, pointed out a number of mitigating factors. Firstly, the colony had 116 epileptics, an unusually high proportion. In the days before potent medication many would be unsuitable for licence. Secondly, the colony also took all grades and ages of patients on a non-selective basis and suffered from the lack of a suitable hostel as a preliminary to trial on licence.

The situation was to change over the years. By 1947 there were 175 (13%) patients out on licence. Overcrowding and the demands of wartime had considerably relaxed selection criteria.

Being out on licence did not suit everyone. One female returned to the colony at her own request. She found herself lonely and missed the social amenities of the colony (WWBJB, 1941b). Such sentiments ring true to this day. The tales are all too frequent of ex-patients whose lives have been anything but enriched by inappropriate 'community care'.

For some the old place never lost its attraction. In 1943 a number of patients out on licence expressed a desire to return to the colony for their summer vacation (*Walsall Observer*, 1943).

A half-way house between licence and discharge was a long time coming. Daisy Bank Annexe, a large country house set in its own grounds, some three miles from the hospital, was acquired in April 1955 (WLHC, 1955). It served as a hostel for 21 male patients capable of earning a living with only limited supervision. They were employed by outside bodies and paid normal wage rates. Further long-term residential accommodation was built on this site in the 1980s as part of the resettlement programme.

Links with the outside world

Public scrutiny was actively encouraged from early on. Starting in 1933, the colony was thrown open to the general public each year in June or July for a splendid garden fete. This tradition continued right through to closure. Visitors were allowed to inspect some of the homes. In 1939 a staggering 2500 people attended (*Walsall Observer*, 1939). The day would usually conclude with dancing to the strains of the colonists' dance orchestra. Concert parties frequently visited from outside.

A much-anticipated sports day for the colonists was held annually in midsummer. Challenge cups were presented to the best male and female athletes.

The value of youth movements in the training of higher-grade mental defectives was well recognised by those running training colonies. A national conference to deal with matters concerning the Scout Movement among epileptics and the mentally defective was an annual event in the 1930s.

With security in the colony always tight, scouting allowed pent-up youthful exuberance to find expression. Staff and resources were readily available and many colony troops did exceedingly well in competition with their 'normal' peers in the outside world. Barr Park Scouts, affiliated to the Handsworth section of the movement, was formed in November 1928, and flourished well into the 1950s. Attendant A E Leath was appointed from within the colony as its first scoutmaster. The scouts regularly attended rallies at Handsworth Park and carried off the coveted Gough-Calthorpe Shield on a number of occasions. A picked detachment of colony scouts formed part of the Guard of Honour on the occasion of the Prince of Wales' visit to Birmingham in October 1934. The Girl Guides section was equally successful in its ventures.

A creditable football team, entered in the Handsworth League, was formed from among the colonists in the 1930s and performed 'moderately well'. One of the highlights of the 1940/41 season was a charity match on Boxing Day against Hamstead Colliery. Half of the money raised was allocated to the Red Cross – the rest was given to the colony. Hockey and netball matches were organised for the girls.

The demise of the Poor Law system

Following enactment of the Local Government Act (1929), which disbanded the Poor Law system, the colony was vested by the Ministry of Health (successors to the Local Government Board) in the Councils of the County Boroughs of Walsall and West Bromwich. As from 1 April 1930, a Joint Board managed the colony until brought within the National Health Service in July 1948.

The Second World War and after

Members of the Royal Medico-Psychological Association (now the Royal College of Psychiatrists) made an observation visit to the colony on 8 June 1939, just three months before the outbreak of hostilities. It was one of the greatest honours ever paid to Barr Colony and a personal compliment to its Medical Superintendent, Dr D M MacMillan. The visit was at their request and about 40 members (including an ex-President) came from as far afield as Sunderland and Devon. The visitors made an extensive conducted tour of the 36 building blocks of the colony and were given every opportunity to study methods of treatment and administration in use. Dr MacMillan told the assembled psychiatrists: 'This is the greatest day of my life' (*Walsall Times*, 1939).

Life at Barr Colony was severely disrupted by the outbreak of the Second World War. Many of the staff were drafted into the armed forces. Jobs were protected but few returned after demobilisation. The depleted workforce was further burdened by the additional responsibility of providing an emergency medical service hospital of 350 beds for War victims from the existing facilities. Extended leave was granted to about 30 patients to release beds for civilian casualties. The Board of Control intimated that overcrowding would be permissible in the ordinary homes by up to 25%.

Attracting staff to the depleted colony proved particularly difficult. The Medical Superintendent was despairing (WWBJB, 1941a):

I can scarcely get any but elderly men as temporary male attendants, and such is the demand for women in highly paid war work that I cannot get female staff for the various departments, especially domestic and nursing. We have in addition the responsibility of running the EMS wards aggravating our nursing and domestic problems. Rather than solving the domestic servant problems of outsiders, I think we should now help our own by licensing some of these trained patients to ourselves.

Despite the severe staff shortage, repeated applications from a conscientious objector for a post of attendant were turned down.

War conditions and reduced supervision brought persistent absconding. One night two females escaped from their locked home during blackout. On another occasion five females escaped to freedom through a window in the clothing store. In January 1944 two girls absconded and spent several nights in a hut at a nearby army camp. They misconducted themselves with American soldiers for which they received half-a-crown (12.5p) to £1 (WWBJB, 1944).

The men were equally active: on one night six males (all persistent run-a-ways) took advantage of being taken to the shelters in an air raid warning to make good their escape.

During the early years of the war the EMS hospital required 54 staff to deal with the many civilian air-raid victims and military casualties. On one memorable evening they were asked at short notice to admit a convoy of 80 evacuees from London – they coped admirably.

Many of the services were provided by colony personnel who relished the opportunity to make a significant contribution towards the war effort. One charge nurse worked an amazing 110 hours during a particular week which had seen three blitzes.

The EMS functioned on the site for six years during which 3130 civilian and military patients received treatment for a wide variety of surgical and medical conditions (WWBJB, 1946). They left behind a fully-functioning theatre and X-ray facilities which the colony turned to good use.

The colony experienced air-raids at first hand on several occasions. The worst raid was on the night of 30 July 1942, when large numbers of incendiary and explosive bombs rained down on the colony. One inmate died and four others received shrapnel wounds.

Despite severe privation, the recreation, education and employment of the colonists was carried on 'comparatively well', with regular dances, fortnightly cinema shows and the traditional annual sports day and Christmas and New Year festivities.

In October 1942, 11 male colonists were doing daily farm and garden work for neighbouring farmers for which they were paid 11 pence (less than 5p) per hour. Half-a-crown (12.5p) per week was allowed as pocket money – the rest was credited to the Joint Board.

In response to the national call to 'Dig for Victory' a total of 112 acres of the colony parkland were turned over to agriculture. The colony was to become nearly self-sufficient in many commodities. In 1945 the Medical Superintendent could report that 16818 lb of pork, 936 lb of offal and 2873 lb of lamb and mutton had been produced for colony use. A beginning was being made in breeding goats to give an additional supply of milk for tubercular patients. Over 21 tons of millable wheat had been sold (WWBJB, 1945).

Farming activities were carried on until the mid-1950s. In 1954 the Ministry of Health reviewed hospital farming and found that 190 hospitals in England and Wales (mainly mental illness and mental handicap) were farming 40000 acres (Ministry of Health, 1955). They felt that farming was not a suitable activity in a modern health service and brought it to a close.

The advent of the National Health Service

Barr Colony was brought within the National Health Service in July

1948; shortly afterwards it was renamed St Margaret's Hospital. It was now managed by a Hospital Management Committee comprising members nominated by various bodies, with a Chairman appointed by the Regional Hospital Board. The policy of the hospital was governed by the Committee which had the Medical Superintendent and a Group Secretary as advisers.

Chronic staff shortages dogged the post-war period, largely through returning servicemen moving on to other employment. On 31 March 1947 there were 1356 patients and just 73 male and 60 female nurses. Only eight domestics were in service, less than a third of the pre-war figure (WWBJB, 1947). Four of the female homes had to remain closed after wartime use. It is clear the assistance of high-grade defectives was absolutely vital at this time for the colony to function. This unhealthy situation was the same throughout the country. Inevitably, it allowed malpractice by a few to flourish in over-stretched establishments with weak management.

Local and national recruiting campaigns were organised in the summer of 1947. Recruiters were particularly successful in Ireland and the imported nurses, happy with their lot, spread the word back home. A sizeable Irish contingent was a feature of the hospital until its closure.

Nurse training

From 1930 Barr Colony was a recognised training school for the Certificate in Mental Deficiency Nursing of the General Nursing Council and the examination of the Royal Medico-Psychological Association (RMPA). Part of the training included sick nursing, handicrafts and games. Between 1930 and 1950 113 candidates passed the RMPA examination with five gaining distinctions. During the same period 47 candidates passed the Final Examination for the General Nursing Council (GNC) Certificate in Mental Deficiency Nursing (St Margaret's Hospital Management Committee (SMHMC), 1950).

Workshop staff began to take the same examinations in 1940. It marked a new era and delighted the Medical Superintendent (WWBJB, 1940):

> *It has taken me 10 years to get workshop staff to come to our lectures, though I have always contended that it is as essential for all members of the staff who have the care and training of defectives to know as much about the nature of mental deficiency as the men and women in the homes.*

A White Paper in 1946 recommended that the RMPA examinations should cease and that an agreement ought to be reached with the GNC to become the sole examining body. Some believed a better arrangement would be to form a body like the Central Midwife's Board. It was a blow to the

RMPA but the recommendation to fuse with the GNC was largely considered the correct one, as long as there was some give and take. Dr MacMillan had consistently advised the nurses to go in for the GNC examination, although more difficult, as the certificate carried valuable privileges.

Changes brought about by the Mental Health Act (1959)

By mid-century well-controlled studies had failed to reveal expected decrements in national intelligence or wholesale racial degeneration as widely forecast decades earlier. Even with amending Acts the old Mental Deficiency Act had also run its course.

The reforming Mental Health Act of 1959 marked a watershed in attitudes towards the mentally handicapped. The all-inclusive Act reflected a basic change in informed opinion. For the first time legislation was devised with the needs of the mentally handicapped as primary consideration.

St Margaret's Hospital (Barr Colony, rebadged) was looking forward to the new challenges. The Matron was looking for 'young people with education, initiative and drive...who have the courage and determination to join in pioneering this new and hopeful era under the New Mental Health Act' (SMHMC, c.1961).

The 'golden age' at St Margaret's

The 1960s and 1970s are widely regarded as the years when mental handicap institutions were at their nadir. That assessment is largely unjustified, particularly when viewing the record of individual institutions. There was certainly no climate of stagnation at St Margaret's; on the contrary, it was a period of innovation and progressive measures.

St Margaret's Hospital was always respected as a leader in the care of the mentally handicapped. Services were continually under review to ensure best practice – which may surprise the detractors. The appointment of Dr A P Buchan as Medical Superintendent in 1958 ensured the continuance of that pioneering spirit.

One innovation was to set up adult education classes in the evenings, with teachers being brought in from outside the hospital (Duncan, 1958).

Early on Dr Buchan introduced an 'open door' policy throughout the hospital. All the homes, including the refractory ones, were opened. When introduced it met with considerable resistance from nursing staff, but was later recognised as being years ahead of its time (Csucsmi, 1987). The policy resulted in a considerable reduction in patient violence, frustration and absconding.

A Recreational Therapy Department was set up in the 1960s with male and female patients mixing freely for the first time. Activities were geared to the needs of each individual with progression through gradually more demanding activities, all recreational based. This process continued until the resident was able to participate in athletics, football, cricket, field events, drama, musical revues and choir. The various teams were extremely successful in inter-hospital tournaments.

The associated Happy Wanderers Club was the first hospital-based club in the country to become affiliated to Mencap's National Federation of Gateway Clubs. Members participated in inter-club activities in the community and took part in the Special Olympics in the USA and France with great success. The Club also raised money for deaf, blind and under-privileged children – a useful lesson that others in the community require help too.

World's first male matron

In April 1960, Mr Eamonn Connors was appointed the world's first male matron at the hospital. His arrival was greeted with amusement by the national media: more thoughtful articles followed in time (*Nursing Mirror*, 1961; Packer, 1965). He was responsible for the female nurses; male nurses were answerable to Mr W G H Ridley, the Chief Male Nurse. Shortly after Mr Connors' appointment an attractive enamelled badge was presented to all members of the nursing staff. Its motto *non nobis solum* (into the light) accurately reflected the guiding principles of the hospital. The badge was proudly worn by nurses throughout their careers.

In 1962, a League of Friends was formed in the hospital – at its peak it had 300 members from all walks of life. As well as befriending individual patients without relatives they organised outings and social activities to enrich the lives of the patients. In 1971 the League raised money for the provision of a social centre adjoining the assembly hall, where much of the therapeutic and social activities later took place. In 1983, the League raised £12000 to provide 'totally soft play environment' equipment for residents with limited mobility.

In 1963, a unique unit for severely mentally handicapped children (up to the age of four) was set up on James Home, a spacious single-storey building. It was a 'short-term care' scheme which fully involved parents. It aimed to '...preserve the parent–child relationship, while preventing a permanent admission of the child to the hospital' (*Nursing Mirror*, 1963).

In February 1965, St Margaret's Hospital was featured along with Leybourne Grange Hospital, Kent, in a Nursing Mirror feature to recruit male mental handicap nurses (*Nursing Mirror*, 1965).

In 1965, one of the early single-storey colony buildings was home to a pioneering venture, the first of its kind in the country, in which mentally handicapped children, aged between seven and 14, were brought up under the care of a house mother in a family atmosphere.

It is around this time that the School of Nursing became one of the first in the country to provide a preliminary training scheme for student nurses studying mental handicap.

In 1970, a cytogenetics (chromosome analysis) section was set up in the small self-contained pathology laboratory, probably the only specialist facility of its kind in any mental handicap hospital.

A peak of 1487 beds was reached around 1972, making St Margaret's the largest hospital of any speciality in the West Midlands.

The scandal decade

The 1970s marked a decade in which repeated controversy convulsed the nursing profession. It all started with allegations by the *News of the World* of ill-treatment of patients and other irregularities at Ely Hospital. The accusations resulted in a full-scale inquiry and a devastating report (DHSS, 1969). A whole series of further scandals followed in quick succession at other mental handicap hospitals: Farleigh, Coldharbour, South Ockenden and Normansfield. All of them resulted in official inquiries and Government reports.

Secretary of State at the time, Richard Crossman, responded to the Ely scandal by providing additional funding and launching a series of initiatives. All this attention eventually led to the landmark White Paper *Better Services for the Mentally Handicapped* (DHSS, 1971). Among other things the publication recommended existing services should be extended and improved. Its lasting legacy was in advocating an accelerated shift in emphasis from care in hospital to care in the community. A widely disseminated book, *The Politics of Mental Handicap,* is probably the best source for the issues then being aired (Ryan and Thomas, 1980).

The final years

At the beginning of the 1980s there were dramatic changes to the hospital infrastructure. To reflect pre-admission origins residents were assigned to one of four therapeutic teams serving defined areas, namely: Walsall, Sandwell, Wolverhampton and South Staffordshire. Each team was led by a consultant psychiatrist and included nursing staff, social workers and psychologists. The teams involved all staff in a series of programmes dealing with admission, assessment, treatment, training, review and discharge. Outpatient clinics were set up for each defined area.

A *flurry of building activity*

The early 1980s also saw a substantial injection of funds from the Regional Health Authority to further improve facilities for residents. An extensive activity centre was built to provide occupations such as carpentry, pottery, art therapy, sewing and handicrafts. It was all very reminiscent of the activities which colonists engaged in decades before.

The centre contained a fully-equipped flat, comprising kitchen, dining room and bedroom, in which the residents were taught domestic skills. Other facilities included a coffee bar, a shop and a unisex hairdressing salon. The building was officially opened on 10 July 1980 by Sir David Perris MBE JP, Chairman of West Midlands Regional Health Authority.

The National Development Team for People with a Learning Disability (NDT), set up as part of the Department of Health, was invited to the hospital in 1981 to review progress following an earlier visit in 1976, when it severely criticised conditions. Much had been done in the meantime to address matters. The number of patients had been reduced from 1200 to 900, with about 130 patients discharged into the community.

The authorities were understandably taken aback at the 44-page report which described the condition of many bathroom and toilet areas on the homes as 'appalling and an affront to human dignity'. The NDT also condemned the dispersal of children throughout seven adult wards. They advocated a rapid run down in the number of beds used for long-stay children, and to use them almost entirely for short-stay and phased care. Despite these criticisms the NDT did note considerable overall improvement since their last visit.

Building work was under way on four mental handicap units (MHUs) when the NDT made their 1981 inspection. These bungalow-style MHUs, in occupation by the end of 1981, were designed to provide comfortable, modern, long-stay accommodation in a 'family style' setting for 96 adults and children. Residents had their own bedroom or shared with only two or three other people. Each home featured two living rooms, a spacious dining area, bathrooms, laundry room and staff facilities. Residents were encouraged to share the domestic chores (Walsall Area Health Authority (WAHA), 1982).

The NDT were 'disturbed' to be told the Regional Health Authority had sanctioned the project. There was no mincing of words: 'This must contravene Department of Health and Social Security Policy and we feel that, as the necessary finance appeared to be available, this would have been better employed in the provision of community units outside St Margaret's' (Marston, 1981).

A carefully designed shop to high street standards was opened on site in February 1982. 'Peggy's Shop' stocked a wide range of up-to-date fashion clothes, plus footwear and accessories. The facility provided an ideal training opportunity for residents to purchase from an authentic retail outlet. At the same time clothing assistants were employed on each home to ensure personal clothing met individual preferences and was well maintained.

The rehabilitation process gets under way

A full-scale programme of resettlement in the community was under way by 1980. Media comments such as 'liberation day', 'unwilling prisoners' and 'friendless and without relatives' merely reinforced commonly-held stereotypes (Lym, 1980). The remarks were an affront to those involved in implementing a sensitive social programme.

A rehabilitation scheme was centred on two large converted houses (the Pre-Discharge Unit), formerly doctors' accommodation. During the day residents followed gainful employment outside the hospital. Much effort went into acquiring essential skills for a successful transition into the community. Progress monitoring and follow-up was undertaken by a specialised team.

By the summer of 1991 the whole of the male side had been vacated and after an interval of 50 years both sexes were again populating the original colony site.

There was certainly no air of gloom when the hospital celebrated 'Seventy-Five Years of Caring' in 1987. An ambitious programme of 14 events for residents and staff covered the whole of October, including a Civic Reception, reunion of retired staff (some from very early colony days), Jubilee Day, rock concert and Grand Dance. A symposium: Changing Provisions of Care and a Salon Culinaire were attended by colleagues from all over the country.

Plans for a base hospital

In the mid-1980s the West Midlands Regional Health Authority identified St Margaret's as one of four mental handicap hospitals in the region to be developed as a specialised base hospital. It was to provide specialist support facilities to groups of districts on a sub-regional basis for a catchment area of approximately 1.2 million people.

From April 1991, the hospital began to operate as a provider unit directly managed by Walsall Health Authority (WHA, 1990). Provisions were in place to provide for the care of some 300 people through service agreements with 20 of the 22 different Health Authorities within the West Midlands.

The hospital was geared up to providing three broad categories of service to people with a mental handicap:

- Clinical intervention on a short-term basis with the emphasis on treatment and rehabilitation (89 beds).
- Care and treatment for those whose needs could not be adequately met in the community at any given time (156 beds).
- Medium to long-term care for a settled elderly population, who were likely to remain in the hospital (55 beds).

To the astonishment of many an £11 million plan was announced in Spring 1992 to completely shut down the hospital over the next five years (*Express and Star*, 1992). The remaining 283 residents were to be moved to smaller care homes and bungalows in the community. The plan was backed by Walsall, Sandwell and Wolverhampton Health Authorities, the three main stakeholders, and was approved by West Midlands Regional Health Authority. Many of the 600 staff were found jobs in the community caring for former residents: their skills and experience were vital to the success of the plan.

In April 1993, Walsall Community Health Trust (WCHT) was formed. It assumed overall responsibility for the vestigial hospital and for people with learning difficulties and mental health problems within the borough.

St Margaret's was formally closed in March 1997, although a small number of high-dependency residents remained on the estate in the MHUs until 2004. As the last surviving example of a complete mental deficiency colony in England, attempts were made to preserve some of the earlier buildings for posterity (Allen, 2003). Although recognising 'The early date of the colony, its survival almost intact and its increasing rarity as a site type mean that it is indeed confirmed as being of national importance in its own right' (Rutherford, 2003), there was no will among the authorities to preserve a small number of the early buildings for posterity. All buildings have now been razed to the ground. A housing estate of 445 dwellings will soon supplant the old colony site.

Conclusion

The era of institutionalised systems of care does not require defending: it was of its time and can stand on its own record. As originally conceived, training colonies gave purpose and direction to the lives of many mental defectives who were failing in a society which had neither the resources nor the infrastructure to provide community care. These specialised institutions never reached full potential: they were thwarted by chronic underfunding and the unreasonable demands put upon them.

By mid-century large institutions had run their course. Increased affluence and vastly more sophisticated social care systems had opened up new possibilities. Staff at enlightened hospitals, like St Margaret's, acknowledged this climate of optimism and were changing the system step-wise from within. The social commentators of the 1970s and 1980s were witnessing a system in its senescence. Their added input helped create the critical mass which obliged Government to make available long-overdue funding for care in the community.

This chapter will hopefully have provided material for a more reasoned debate on a period of history for which no-one should apologise. It might perhaps persuade some to confront their own prejudices.

Let me leave you with the words of Mr W G H Ridley, Chief Male Nurse in the early 1960s (SMHMC, c.1961):

Within 10 minutes of entering this hospital the visitor is able to sense without any lingering doubt that this is a happy hospital. What is it that creates this almost tangible atmosphere? One often comes across it in unlikely places, even in hospitals with an inheritance of old inconvenient buildings that smack of the past history of 'chilly charity and poor law' to live down. It is certainly not dependent on streamline buildings, expert planning, up-to-the-minute equipment, or vast numbers of staff. But it is the staff themselves who create the happiness; cheerful kindly people, all of them with their various tasks, who serve ungrudgingly whatever the difficulties, convinced that this is a worthwhile job.

Note

An archive of some 340 items relating to Great Barr Park Colony/St Margaret's Hospital is housed at the Local History Centre at Walsall, West Midlands. The deposit comprises nearly 160 minute books of the early committees, covering the whole period from 1912 until 1948; the Medical Superintendent's reports; and a miscellaneous collection of files dealing with contracts, insurance policies, tenancy agreements, etc. The Centre also possesses a bound collection of Annual Reports and Abstracts of Accounts covering the years 1937–45. Walsall and West Bromwich newspapers are another very rich source of information. This author has a large private archive which is shortly to be deposited at the same location. Consult www. greatbarrhall.com for information on the antecedents of the hospital estate

References

Allen P (2003) *Evidence to Support an Application for Upgrade of Existing Registered Landscape at Great Barr Park, Walsall, to Grade II**. April 2003. [Private archive]

Architects' Journal (1930) Great Barr Colony, Staffordshire. Recent Additions for the Accommodation of Mental Defectives. *Architects' Journal* **14 May:** 748–53

Birmingham Union (1913) *Monyhull Colony for the Care of Epileptic and Feeble-Minded Persons. Souvenir of Foundation Stonelaying.* 14 November

Board of Control (Lunacy and Mental Deficiency) (1924) *10th Annual Report.* HMSO, London

Brady C (1864) *The Training of Idiotic and Feeble-Minded Children.* Hodges, Smith, Dublin

Cobb HVZ (1969) *The Predictive Assessment of the Adult Retarded for Social and Vocational Adjustment: A Review of Research. Part 2: Analysis of the Literature.* Vermillion, Department of Psychology, University of South Dakota

Csucsmi H (1987) *Reflections on the Recent Past History of St Margaret's Hospital.* [Private archive]

Day K (2000) *Prudhoe and Northgate Hospitals. A History: 1914–1999.* Morpeth, Northumberland: Prudhoe and Northgate NHS Trust

DHSS (1969) *Report of the Committee of Inquiry into Allegations of Ill-Treatment of Patients and other Irregularities at the Ely Hospital, Cardiff.* Cmnd. 3975. HMSO, London

DHSS (1971) *Better Services for the Mentally Handicapped.* Cmnd. 4683. HMSO, London

Dugdale R (1877) *The Jukes: A Study in Crime, Pauperism, Disease, and Heredity.* Putnam, New York

Duncan AC (1958) Further education for adult defectives: An experiment at Great Barr Park, (near) Birmingham. *Nursing Mirror* **17 Oct**(Suppt): ii–iii

Duncan PM, Millard W (1866) *A Manual for the Classification, Training and Education of the Feeble-minded, Imbecile and Idiotic.* Longmans, Green, London

Express and Star (1992) Health chiefs back hospital shutdown. *Express and Star* **15 April**

Goddard HH (1912) *The Kallikak Family: A Study in the Heredity of Feeblemindedness.* Macmillan, New York

Hearnshaw LS (1964) *A Short History of British Psychology 1840–1940.* Methuen, London: 154

Hutchings D (1998) *Monyhull 1908–1998: A History of Caring.* Brewin Books, Studley, Warwickshire

Lym P (1980) A new life for the unwilling prisoners of St. Margaret's. *Evening Mail* **13 May**

Marston P (1981) Hospital conditions 'are still appalling'. *Evening Mail* **29 Oct**

McCutcheon AM (1925) Institutional treatment of mental defectives, with special reference to occupation. *Journal of Mental Science* **LXXI**(295): 694–70

Midland Chronicle (1913) The boarding out question. Further discussion by the West Bromwich Guardians. *Midland Chronicle*, **10 Oct:** 7

Midland Chronicle (1914) Treatment of mentally defectives. Guardians Clerk's Interesting Report. Assurance regarding Great Barr. *Midland Chronicle* **31 July:** 5

Midland Chronicle (1921) The Great Barr Colony. Opening of the "James" Home. An interesting function. *Midland Chronicle* **28 Oct:** 5

Ministry of Health (1955) *Report of the Ministry of Health for the Year Ended 31 December, 1954*. Cmnd. 9566. HMSO, London

Nursing Mirror (1961) Male Matron at St. Margaret's Hospital, Birmingham. *Nursing Mirror* **3 March:** Includes 5 photographs

Nursing Mirror (1963) Unit for Mental and Physically Handicapped Babies. *Nursing Mirror* **22 March:** x–xI. Includes 6 photographs of the unit

Nursing Mirror (1965) Opportunities for Men: Nursing the Mentally Subnormal. *Nursing Mirror* **12 Feb:** 221–4. Includes 6 photographs

O'Brien G (2001) Adult outcome of childhood learning disability. *Developmental Medicine and Child Neurology* **43**(9): 634–8

Packer E (1965) Muscling in on a Matron's world. *Observer Weekend Review* **5 Sep**

Pearson H (1930) *Doctor Darwin*. Dent and Sons, London and Toronto: vii

Potts M, Fido R (1991) *'A Fit Person to be Removed': Personal Accounts of Life in a Mental Deficiency Institution*. Northcote, Plymouth

Royal Commission on the Care and Control of the Feeble-Minded (1908). *Report of the Royal Commission on the Care and Control of the Feeble-Minded*. HMSO, London. This monumental work of eight folio volumes includes 13 folding plans of infirmaries, workhouses, etc., and 20 photographic illustrations of American institutions visited by the Commission

Royal Commission on the Poor Laws and Relief of Distress (1909). *Report*. Cmnd. 4499. HMSO, London

Rutherford S (2003) *Great Barr Park – St Margaret's Hospital Site:*

Report for English Heritage Parks and Gardens Register Team. 13 June

Ryan J, Thomas F (1980) *The Politics of Mental Handicap.* Penguin Books, Harmondsworth, Middlesex

Shrubsall FC, Williams AC (1932) *Mental Deficiency Practice: The Procedure for the Ascertainment and Disposal of the Mentally Defective.* University of London Press, London. An extensive selection of specimen forms is included

SMHMC (c.1950). *Make Nursing Your Career at St Margaret's Hospital.* c.1950. [Private archive]

SMHMC (c.1961) *Into the Light.* c.1961. Student nurse recruitment brochure. [Private archive]

SPHPM (1933) The Hamstead Medical Service Club. *St Paul's Hamstead Parish Magazine* **April**

The Builder (1933) Mental Colony, Great Barr Park. *The Builder* **24 Nov:** 833–5

The Times (1912) Mental Deficiency Bill: An appeal to Parliament. *The Times* **28 Nov:** 6

Tizard J (1958) Longitudinal and follow-up studies. In: Clarke A, Clarke A (eds). *Mental Deficiency: The Changing Outlook.* Methuen, London: 422–9

Tredgold AF (1908) *A Text-Book of Mental Deficiency.* Baillière, Tindall and Cox, London: The eleventh edition was published under editors in 1970

WAHA (1982) Official Opening of Aldridge, Beacon Chase and Scott Homes and Peggy's Clothes. *WAHA* **15 March**

Walsall Advertiser (1911) Care of the Feeble-minded. *Walsall Advertiser* **7 Jan:** 7

Walsall Observer (1897) The Midland Counties Idiot Asylum. Annual Meeting at Walsall. *Walsall Observer* **8 May:** 7

Walsall Observer (1914a) Great Barr Hall Scheme. Mental Defective Colony to be established. *Walsall Observer* **16 May**

Walsall Observer (1914b) Guardians and boarded-out children. Extra allowance for clothing. *Walsall Observer* **30 May**

Walsall Observer (1937) Something Wrong? Councillor Cliff Tibbits' Criticisms of the Barr Mental Colony. *Walsall Observer* **13 March**

Walsall Observer (1939) Colony has 2,500 Visitors. Work of the institution revealed at annual fete. *Walsall Observer* **8 July**

Walsall Observer (1943) To Colony For Holiday. Request from former patients of Great Barr Institution. *Walsall Observer* **24 July**

Walsall Times (1937a) Great Barr Colony controversy. Members of staff take up defence. *Walsall Times* **10 April**

Walsall Times (1937b) "Astoundingly incorrect" statement. Mental Welfare Committee Replies to Councillor critic. *Walsall Times* **8 May**

Walsall Times (1939) Learned body at Barr Colony. Visit of Medico-Psychological Association. *Walsall Times* **10 June**

Walsall Times (1940) Administration of Barr Colony. "Finest" in Kingdom. Appreciation of Work of Mr H Lee. *Walsall Times* **27 July**

WHA (1990) *St Margaret's Hospital Prospectus 1991–1992. [December 1990]. An overview of the services provided by the hospital.* [Private archive]

WLHC (1918) Walsall Local History Centre 178/1/33. Walsall and West Bromwich Unions Joint Committee. *Committee Minute Book* **24 July**

WLHC (1920) Walsall Local History Centre 178/2/79. Walsall and West Bromwich Unions Joint Committee. *Agreement as to the Maintenance at Great Barr Park Colony of Persons Certified Under the Mental Deficiency Act 1913.* **18 August**

WLHC (1929) Walsall Local History Centre 274/48. Walsall and West Bromwich Unions Joint Committee. *Medical Officer's Report Book 1929–1932*

WLHC (1955) Walsall Local History Centre 274/39. St Margaret's Hospital Management Committee. *Hostel Sub-Committee Minutes*

WWBJB (1937) *Barr Colony for Mental Defectives. Report ... with reference to certain criticisms of the colony.* WWBJB **22 April**

WWBJB (1938) *Souvenir and Programme of Proceedings on the Occasion of the Opening...of Further Extensions to Great Barr Park Colony.* WWBJB **5 May**

WWBJB (1940). *Medical Superintendent's Report.* WWBJB **26 June**

WWBJB (1941a) *Medical Superintendent's Report.* WWBJB **22 Feb**

WWBJB (1941b) *Medical Superintendent's Report.* WWBJB **21 April**

WWBJB (1944) *Medical Superintendent's Report.* WWBJB **25 Jan**

WWBJB (1945) *Annual Report and Abstract of Accounts for the Year Ended 31 March, 1945.* WWBJB

WWBJB (1946) *Annual Report and Abstract of Accounts for the Year Ended 31st March.* WWBJB

WWBJB (1947) *Annual Report and Abstract of Accounts for the Year Ended 31st March.* WWBJB

WWBU (1912). *Souvenir and Programme of Proceedings on the Occasion of the Opening of Great Barr Hall.* WWBU **23 Oct**

WWBU (1929) *Souvenir and Programme of Proceedings on the Occasion of the Opening…of Extensions to Great Barr Park Colony.* WWBU **26 Sept**

CHAPTER 2

Striving towards ordinariness within a regulatory system

Mark Jukes

Introduction

There is a distinct paucity in the literature about the actual work and lived experiences of attendants and nurses working within the colony type of institution prior to the National Health Service Act (1948) in the United Kingdom. At this time males were called attendants and females, nurses.

As a result of this Act responsibility for colonies was assumed by the National Health Service and they were renamed as hospitals for the mentally deficient.

This chapter presents findings from research the author undertook to examine attendants' and nurses' perceptions of their practices from 1927 to 1948. These attendants and nurses were trained and worked at Great Barr Park Colony.

The research spanned three epochs, 1927–1948, 1948–1970 and 1970–1990, and a total of 30 nurses participated. However, this chapter concentrates on those findings from the period 1927–1948, the golden age of the colony, and on the introduction of the National Health Service.

The focus is on eight attendants' and nurses' views of the colony, their explanation for working and their attitudes to working practices. This takes place within a unique period of social policy and history, where the influence of eugenics had paved the way not only for the Mental Deficiency Act (1913), but also for the creation of new institutions (controlled by local authorities and run on 'colony' lines) to enable the full implementation of the legislation (Chester and Dale, 2007).

The principle aim was to examine and tell the attendants' and nurses' stories with the adoption of a grounded theory methodology (Glaser and Strauss, 1967). In addition to the eight attendants/nurses, a sibling of the first medical superintendent appointed, and who lived at the colony, also participated in the study.

The attendants and nurses, who were exclusively appointed, trained for the Royal Medico-Psychological Association, Mental Deficiency,

RMPA(MD) Qualification. They all worked within Great Barr Park Colony, later to become St. Margarets Hospital, an institution that was recognised as being one of the best colonies in the country providing care and training for people who were classified as being mentally deficient. (*Plate 3*)

Methodology

Grounded theory has its roots in sociology and first came to prominence in the 1960s as a result of co-originator's Anselm Strauss' and Barney Glasers' sociological research on dying in hospitals (Strauss and Corbin, 1990; Charmaz, 2000). Their research work enabled them to craft a method which meant they could generate systematically a substantive theory which was grounded in empirical data.

At the core of grounded theory is the principle that, rather than developing a theory and then systematically seeking out evidence to verify it, researchers set out to gather data and then systematically develop the theory derived directly from their data (Dey, 1999).

It has sometimes been suggested that qualitative research methods produce descriptive studies. In terms of grounded theory, Strauss and Corbin (1990) firmly refute this, stating that grounded theory must not just be descriptive, but should have explanatory power. It has therefore maximum application when it is dealing with qualitative data of the kind gathered from participant observation, or semi-structured or unstructured interviews (Turner, 1981).

Grounded theory constructs and concepts are grounded in the data, and hypotheses are tested as they arise from the research (Field and Morse, 1985). It is based on two qualitative data analysis processes, the first being that the researcher codes all the data, while systematically analysing these codes to verify or prove a given proposition or relationship. The second process involves inspecting the data for properties of categories, the use of field notes or memos to track the analysis, and develops theoretical ideas. However, Glaser and Strauss (1967: 102) suggested more of a hybrid from these traditional two data analysis processes through

An analytic procedure of constant comparison, the explicit coding procedure of the first approach and the style of theory development of the second.

If a researcher approaches a phenomenon with a given set of hypotheses, the research may fail to discover the true nature of the phenomenon as a result of being blinded by the assumptions built into the hypotheses (Hammersley, 1990). Wiener and Wysmans (1990:12) maintain that the concept of grounded theory is not always understood and that theory in this approach means,

> *Identifying the relationship between and among concepts, and presenting a systematic view of the phenomenon being examined, in order to explain what is going on.*

It is this explanatory power and process that is critical in areas, in particular, where little is known, and it stresses the importance of the context in which people function. A justification therefore of why grounded theory has been adopted as a methodology for this study, as an attempt to further understand, and have explanatory power, into what is happening through the lived experiences of attendants and nurses within a colony for the mentally deficient prior to the establishment of the National Health Service in 1948.

Glaser and Strauss (1967) advise that rigid preconceived ideas prevent development of the research, imposing a framework which may block the awareness of major concepts that emerge from the data.

Grounded theory helps health professionals to give up their own model of professional patient care and management, in order to adopt an alternative perspective based on the perceptions and beliefs of staff.

For this they need flexibility and open minds, qualities which are related to the processes involved in the practice of in this case mental deficiency, but also in the furtherance of understanding intellectual/learning disability nursing, which demands a more open and flexible approach.

Since grounded theory evolved and has spread the two co-originators have gone separate ways to produce how grounded theory was to be generated in terms of different perspectives regarding the 'data analysis process', and specifically the procedures used.

Readers are encouraged to read the Walker and Myrick (2006) paper where discussion focuses upon the different data analysis processes involved in coding, from Glaser and Strauss's individual perspectives, and where the major differences attached to issues of emergence and verification are pursued.

Data collection

A number of strategies were employed to identify the hidden population of attendants and nurses. A purposive sampling and snowball methodology of contact was adopted with participants contacting other potential interviewees in an attempt to gain contact with past and present nurses who worked at the colony/hospital. As a supplementary means to this approach a database was identified which contained some past retired and present nurses, and a letter was written to be broadcast on a Birmingham local radio station by a local university academic and radio television historian on a local history programme. The letter invited nurses who worked at the colony/hospital to contact the researcher and this yielded a number of contacts.

The human resources department and the Director of Nursing and Operational Services were contacted, and permission was granted to carry out the research with those members of staff who were still working for the Trust. Ethical approval from the ethics committee was also sought, and approval to carry out the research was granted.

For retired members of staff, contact was made by posting a letter of introduction about the researcher and aims of the research intending to be carried out, with a stamp addressed returnable section agreeing or not agreeing to take part, and whether or not they agreed to be contacted. If a participant agreed to participate a mutually convenient date was arranged for an interview to take place in his or her home.

A semi-structured interview was devised by the researcher, the duration of which was approximately 90 to 120 minutes. The interviews were recorded on a portable tape cassette recorder. Results of the interviews were transcribed and verification was obtained through allowing participants to read their own transcripts and to comment further on the content if they so wished.

Analysis of the transcribed interviews commenced through an analytic process and coded according to the procedure originally laid down by Glaser (1978). The core themes generated through the analysis consisted of the following:

- Pre-entry influences (Family, sport and necessity for work).
- Nature of training ('It was practical training').
- The role of the attendant/ nurse ('It was total care involvement').
- Perceptions of qualities to be a good attendant/nurse ('Patience, humour and to know them').
- Institution as a regulatory system ('Friend to expert, authoritarianism').
- Perceptions on attributes, characteristics the patients had ('You can't dictate to them').
- Institution as a regulatory system ('A place geared for the effective care and training of the mentally deficient – it kind of justified things').
- Institution as a regulatory system ('It was organised living, organised as ordinary life is organised').
- Institution as a regulatory system: Expert militarianism ('Discipline, power and control').
- Those who have the right attitudes ('Positive role models').
- Medical superintendent ('He was keen in nurturing activities'; 'Lord and master').
- Points of change (There was no consultation).

In grounded theory the major category which links all others is known as the core category and, like a thread, this category is woven into the whole study and provides the storyline.

The core category is known as the basic social/psychological process involved in the research and demonstrates the ideas that are most significant to the participants. The core category generated from the research is '*striving towards ordinariness within a regulatory system*'.

Pre-entry influences

The reasons for entering the colony were localised, in that these ranged from, for men, having family connections with the colony, to wanting a job that was 'not the same'.

Nolan (1993:107) has observed from a comparative study that entry into mental health nursing, for some men, was partly motivated by the excellent sporting facilities that were provided.

Attendant A: '*I think first of all because my uncle was involved, he was a nurse at 'B' Asylum. I wanted a job which wasn't the same thing all day sitting down at a desk or within an office, and thirdly I wanted a job where I could play games, sport and be paid for doing it. At the time, mental deficiency was the ideal situation, because you were expected to take part in all these activities with the patients.*'

Others were ending their service with the War and, because of the uncertainty of employment prospects, the colony offered secure full-time work.

Attendant D: *I was in the fire service at the time, full-time, and then towards the end of the War we had to have time off. Nobody wanted all these surplus firemen now the War was over. We had two days off and one on, and that gave us an opportunity to do a part-time job. Well, I knew the charge nurse – the main charge nurse, and he put me on to this upholsterery job, part-time. I am an upholsterer, so I used to go full-time and came out of the fire service.*'

Attendant N: '*I came out of the Air Force in 1947, I had an idea about occupational therapy, and I did apply for a course in Devon. There was a three year waiting list there but adverts were appearing for St Margarets. Well, I thought that was in the same direction, so I applied and that's how I landed a job at St Margarets. I started in 1949.*'

Attendant B: '*Under a sense, circumstances, I wasn't attracted to the work in any way. As a matter of fact I hated the sight of it, but it was just one of those things, and that it was War time and no other work was available, and as I say I had me arm damaged you know, so I couldn't do no manual work and they stuck me down there. The authorities, the doctors ordered it personally.'*

Attendant S: *'I started the same week as the NHS started, July 1948. I had always had a hankering to have something individual for myself, something of my own. We were Irish lads over here on a six month passport. Now I met this girl at a dance at the hostel, and this girl was a student nurse at Great Barr, and her father was a charge nurse, and we started a great romance. She was the one who put it into my head.*

Young women, deemed too young at 17 to train for general nursing work, were attracted to the colony because they could join at a younger age. A further incentive was that it paid more than general nurses once qualified.

Nurse F: *'Well I first started at ... sanatorium TB nursing. My mother and father were against that, really against it, so I had to leave there because my mother and father didn't well, you know, tuberculosis was very prevalent and they were afraid of me catching it and taking it home to my brothers and sisters. So I left there and that's why I started at St. Margarets. I was too young to go into general nursing care because you had to be 18, and I was only just 17 and they accepted me.*

Nurse C: *'I started when I was 17 and a half, it was advertised as a children's hospital, so I went there and had to do 2 years training, and if you left before that 2 years was up you were fined. It was £5, a terrible lot of money in those days, but when qualified you got more pay than in general nursing, although this kind of work was looked down upon then.'*

Nature of training/practice

Training for the RMPA was largely taught through a series of lectures from the medical superintendent, assistant medical officer and the ward sisters for practical nursing skills.

A member of the family of the first medical superintendent comments on this training:

Interviewee U: *'The nurses had their RMPA Certificate. He [the medical superintendent] gave the occasional lecture, but it was mainly the sisters and they had general training where they could get their RMPA and it was very successful. Those that obtained their qualifications were able to become sisters and have charge of the homes and have extra pay.'*

Attendant B: *'Well training was non-existent really, only practical, it was ward training, nothing else you know. We used to go to the lectures after you had been there a couple of years, and so we used to go twice a week for an hour. Most of the training was ... practical training. No books – we had one book the Green Handbook, that was all. You did all the training in your own time. If on nights you would go to a lecture between 9 and 10 and then back again the following night.'*

Attendant A: *'When I started the Certificate was the RMPA Mental Deficiency (MD), because at that time there were two certificates. The RMPA (Mental) and the RMPA (MD). It was a body of examiners based on the RMPA, and the training was under two to three headings. You could either opt for nursing, which is what I did, or you could opt for the occupational side of things. So you could in the end when finishing with your certificate, you would have occupational therapy as part of the end product, so the training was quite different in those days. I opted for nursing – other people for occupational therapy, and that of course involved all sorts of different things like boot making, tailoring and there were exams for those particular subjects as well as the total care of mentally deficient people. So you had examiners in carpentry, examiners in boot making and in occupational therapy. I started in 1939.'*

Attendant D: *'Oh! The doctors that were there, they gave us anatomy and physiology and the sisters the practical side, you know the nursing side. For the RMPA I did...*
[Attendant D shows his certificate, which was already on the dining room table for me to inspect. It included: Section A: Bedside nursing; Section B: Special method of teaching mentally defective children; Section C: The training of mentally defective adults; and Section D: Physical training, drill, dancing, indoor and outdoor amusements. The certificate was dated 31 May 1949.]
As an upholsterer I did Section A because they didn't test me on upholstery because training mentally defective adults would have covered it.'

Attendant S: *'[We had] lectures on types of conditions that patients suffered from and types of behaviour patterns. A general hospital ward sister taught general nursing care. We had a choice of doing the RMPA examinations or becoming a State Registered Nurse. The introduction of the NHS afforded new systems of training under different pension schemes.*
'They insisted on teaching long-winded ideas about the tracts of the nervous

systems, the various centres of the brain. You had to go to the post mortem room to see the pathologist doing post mortems, and he would make a cut in the brain, and would say this is so and so fissure. All this sort of thing. Well! It didn't impress me at all, it meant nothing. I thought the most important things for learning the practice was to know nothing whatever about your classification of patients, to know nothing really about the social policies and all the rest of it [but rather] to actually be introduced to other people and to gradually find out what advantages and disadvantages that we had.'

Attendant N: *'We had a smattering of general training, which a lot of wasn't applicable. We had guidance in regard to behaviour problems, and then of course we put that to practice on the homes, and I think by looking back it was quite valuable, well I think that stands out really.'*

The role of an attendant/nurse

Attendants and nurses were very clear and descriptive about how they perceived there identity and practice and the nature of their work with the people at the colony. This was 'total involvement' a 'total experiencing' and exposure with patients living within the colony.

Attendant A: *'You were expected to take part in all the activities with the patients. You were expected to involve yourself with them. You didn't just go in with the patients and watch them. In fact, I can still make a pair of boots now if it came to a push. I can still lay out a cricket pitch, I can still lay out a football pitch with large circles, that sort of thing you were taught. Handicrafts, I can still crochet, because you were involved – you had to do these things. You just didn't sit back and watch, you had to do them if you were to fulfil your role properly.'*

Mitchell and Smith (2003) cite Frieze Stephens (1933) on the employment of nurses in mental deficiency as being a relatively cheap and multi-skilled group and where:

> *'It would result in effecting a saving not only on maintenance costs but also on capital outlay, for then provision would not have to be made separately for such officers as the kitchen superintendent, laundry mistress, needleroom mistress, handicrafts mistress and their necessary reliefs, all of whom would be members of the nursing staff, while patients would do the work of hired housemaids, sewing maids, and so on.'*

Attendant A: *'There were no occupational therapists as such, the attendant was, and part of his training originally was, the Royal Medico-Psychological Association (RMPA) certificate and part of that was occupation. It was done largely sitting next to 'Charlie' sort of thing I know. But it was part and parcel of his training. He had to know about occupational therapy. So there were no other people in the colony other than the attendants; no OT people, no domestic people.'*

'Domestic work was done by the attendants, the laundry by the laundry manager who did the RMPA qualification like the nurses, but he was concerned with patient occupation. Everybody did the psychiatry part of the RMPA, and then the bits they got after, like occupational and recreational therapy.'

Great Barr Park Colony Institution Rules included Rule 104 which stated: Outdoor exercise should be provided daily,and every patient capable of receiving it should undergo a frequent course of instruction in physical drill.

Attendant T: *'We had quite a lot of games, games were very popular. Outdoor and indoor games. Numerous activities all the time. Some patients were great at darts and playing football.'*

Education of the children was also a role attendants and nurses were required to fulfil as a wider part of their role within the colony.

Institution Rule 101 stated: As far as possible all the older patients shall be taught useful trades, whilst the younger patients shall receive daily instruction in school, especial regard being paid to training for hand and eye.

Stevens (2000) identifies and acknowledges the influence of Margaret McDowell on the Board of Control's thinking about employing educational methods for mentally defective children. Her book, *Simple Beginnings in the Training of Mentally Defective Children*, published in 1930, was also recommended reading in the RMPA nurse training handbook, *Manual for Mental Deficiency Nurses* (RMPA 1931: 428). McDowell (1930:6) states:

'I want to impress the necessity of an honest struggle to learn to see these children as they are, not as we wish them to be. All are different, all worthy of our understanding.'

Not all education however, was confined to the classroom.

Nurse C: *'I used to train the children for concerts, teaching them to dance and all sorts of things. God! it was hard work, 'cause you get some beautifully, but they can have their off day and, "I'm not going to do this", and I used to take their part until they'd got over it – and they'd come back again. It was blummin' hard work, but I put on a concert, it was a concert I made up. I got them doing some dancing, the cancan, all sorts of things we did and bits of poetry.'*

'We had a school for the children as well – they had to go to school. There was a trained teacher, but of course she had to have help. As you can imagine with mentally deficient children and ... erm actually I loved it, very, very hard work.'

Attendant A: *'The school in those days for the children, the school was run by the nursing staff with the headmaster who was a nurse – the charge attendant. It had not at that time come under the education authority, so you had, as an attendant, to go with the children to school, and you had to stay with them at school. You were expected to do some teaching at the school – so it was total involvement.'*

A member of the medical superintendent's family once again provides an insight into the skills and qualities of the nurses during the 1930s.

Interviewee U: *'They got very good nurses, because times were hard for job getting. I mean there was excellent people, people with musical talents among the staff. Good pianists, singers and all the rest of it, and they passed these skills on to the patients. We used to have excellent concerts that the staff taught the patients. Singing and dancing, entertainment and costumes that they made themselves, and the most marvellous entertainments at Christmas. The patients always had a fancy dress party and that was marvellous, the costumes they got up to. The staff helped them and it was really a brilliant affair, the costumes they thought of.'*

Perceptions on qualities to be a good attendant/nurse

The qualities required to be a good attendant/nurse at Great Barr Colony included patience, humour and knowing the residents.

The institution rules on general management included Rule 109. This stated: All attendants shall treat their patients kindly, and shall not speak harshly to them. They shall be responsible for the safety, cleanliness, and general condition of their patients, and for the good order of the homes or workshops. They shall attend to the dressing and undressing of their patients, carefully searching for injuries, bruises, or other marks, and reporting any such at once to the superior officer, who shall forthwith report thereon to the Medical Superintendent. Acts of harshness or violence to patients, dishonesty, intemperance, or disobedience to orders shall render any attendant or servant liable to instant dismissal without notice or equivalent payment.

Perceptions into the qualities required to be a good attendant or nurse were based on how they viewed their role, their interaction with the patients and how needs were addressed.

Attendant A: *'The word nurse should never have been used, because we tend to give a name to something and then to give a set of attributes to that something, and if you talk about nurses, you are talking about people who look after the sick, the physically ill people going into hospital for operations and that sort of thing, but at Great Barr you had 1500 to 1700 patients and sickness was minimal then and they had no more sickness than the average population outside... The name nurse was the wrong name for people then and at that time nurses were known as attendants, you were attendant on the needs of the mentally deficient person, and to me it may not have been a nice name, but it had more meaning to the general public than the word nurse'.*

Nurse C: *'Terrific lot of patience, because you do get abused by some of the patients, and I think you have to have a certain amount of sympathy as you couldn't do the work, and a sense of humour – make fun out of things that didn't look funny at the time that didn't put the patient off how he felt, bring a smile to his face. But you've got to be friends to them I think – they've got to have confidence in you. I have great sympathy for them – I think that's why I was able to stick it all and I also had a senior position. Being as helpful and kind to the patient as you possibly can, and no ill treatment, no injuring the patient in any way. Hitting them was absolutely against all the rules. You do get one or two that can't stand being insulted or hit and they retaliate which is only human nature after all's said and done, it was very hard not to retaliate, very hard... You've got to work with patients and practically live with them to really know if you're good to nursing and looking after them.'*
'There were one or two nurses which I didn't like at all, which I thought could be aggressive.'

Nurse F: *'Well, coming across a nurse that was a bit rough you know, you do get them, when they were feeding, they used to be really rough when using a spoon, and hold their mouths open. Well, I hadn't used to like that. When I used to see them be rough and shout at them, well they weren't supposed to treat them like that you know.'*

Attendant B: *'The first one is a sense of humour, patience and that's it more or less. Once you've got a sense of humour you can laugh things off if you want, which perhaps might upset you normally.'*

Attendant S: *'There was a type of person, in actual fact, there are more of them of the worst type around now are still getting into the care world. They are in actual fact using a similar type of approach in their control, even in smaller homes... They are carrying out the ins and outs of everyday living, but in fact they are looking down. They are looking down on the patients.'*

Attendant N: *'I should say patience above all things for dealing with the type of mentally defective patient, that's the outstanding virtue I imagine.'*

Attendant D: *'I always liked my job, and I always cared for the patients. I looked at my job as a Christian, which gave a different impetus altogether to when I came to work with mental patients. I had a closer relationship, tried to put my Christian faith into my workshop, and they knew I was a Christian and there was no swearing and that language what have you, and they knew I would never stand for it... Religion makes a difference for treating people, makes all the difference. Everybody knew where I stood – discipline but a caring discipline.'*

Institution as a regulatory system

Friend to expert authoritarianism – instilling a caring discipline

Mitchell and Smith (2003) observe within mental deficiency nursing a preoccupation with both care and control, which, combined together, produce a competing purpose for nurses. Mitchell and Smith further posit that the concept of emotional labour provides a means of describing and understanding the often invisible work employed, among others, by those in the caring professions. As a concept it involves using emotions in the work in order to provide security and to produce confidence in others (the patients).

From the following accounts, we can begin to understand from the attendants' and nurses' perspective that relationships with patients in the colony were indeed based upon discipline and control, which from the attendants/nurses' perspective was an imperative as a need to preserve order. There would have been 50 to 60 patients living in the homes without the availability of drugs to assist in the management of unruly behaviour or aggressive conditions.

The RMPA's *Manual for Mental Deficiency Nurses* (1931) was still advocating a custodial approach based upon control, and, according to O'Hara (1967), the charge nurse had become 'a punitive authoritarian figure whose skill was equated in terms of maintaining order'.

However, Dr Jordan, as cited in Hutchings (1998:22–23), from neighbouring Monyhull colony justifies the need for discipline as a means of control:

Our colonists, from the nature of their affliction, stand in more need of personal control and supervision than does the average normal person. All good and successful men and women have been disciplined in their youth, and continue to discipline themselves. Our colonists cannot discipline themselves, but they can learn to obey our few and simple rules, and by doing so, can become, as most of them have become, good, happy and successful colonists.

Attendant N: *'To be friends to a certain extent, but there was a matter of discipline. You see with 60 patients on the ward well, be friendly with them and all that, but of course in a way you had to stand aloof to preserve that discipline, and I think on the high-grade homes that worked out pretty well, just to sort of keep them in their place and keep your place. It was necessary above all else, because of the numbers on the home. The average number I think in those days was somewhere between 60 and 65, but of course they all had companionship with themselves, and a word or two with the staff, and overall it worked out all right.'*

The Mental Deficiency Act (1913) defined four groups of 'defectives subject to be dealt with': Idiots, who were unable to guard themselves against common physical dangers; imbeciles, who were mentally defective to a lesser extent than idiots but 'incapable of managing themselves or their affairs'; feeble-minded persons, who were affected to a lesser extent than imbeciles but still required 'supervision and control for their own protection and the protection of others'; and moral defectives who, in addition to being mentally defective, had 'strong vicious or criminal propensities' and needed attention because of the dangers to others.

The following extracts refer to this latter group of moral defectives (stubborn or unmanageable/hard-to-treat patients), who were accommodated within refractory homes.

Attendant T: *'They had a punishment home as well, where if someone became too difficult to cope with they went to the refractory home – Wills. The regime down on Wills was that the staff were all tough men, young tough men – they had to be tough – because, if one turned their back, someone else had to be watching for him, because someone would come up behind them and break their neck, or whallop them. You see patients were violent in those days... You would have to be on your toes all the time, mentally alert all the time. Couldn't afford to come into work half-dead after the night before or something like that. Just had to be highly alert, if you didn't you'd suffer physically yourself, there was never enough personnel there to cope with it.'*

Attendant A: *'You were the staff, they were the patients, and therefore your control over them was such that it instilled a method of discipline. You were encouraged to be friends, to accept the patient as another human being, who had certain limited abilities and difficulties, and you were expected to help him through those difficulties, and they were definitely encouraged. You were encouraged to take part in everything that they did.'*

Attendant D: *'Patients looked up to staff because they could discipline the patients. It wasn't a harsh discipline, although it had to be a discipline, because you'd got 65 patients in every home. Where there was discipline it was a caring discipline. It's a lot of patients when you've got violent ones, you know – who put the windows through, and you've got the schizophrenia, you've got the "fit" patients, those who have epileptic fits – you had the whole range. You had to know all about these patients, you got to know them personally, and you knew when they were going to have a fit, or would be starting to play up. So where there was discipline it was a caring discipline. There was no doubt about that, and I knew all the head attendants, because I did work for everyone in the colony, so I knew them all.'*

As well as sports and entertainments the staff were involved with work which was very much a focus for structure and organised living within the colony. Keeping the patients occupied and busy was all part of the life of an attendant and nurse at the colony.

Attendant T: *'The head gardener used to have groups of people with him, and with my background I would start and dig with them, and you would supervise as well. There might be someone who's trying to hit someone with a spade. You had to have your eyes open too. You were never on your own, they'd always make sure there was someone with you, with really violent characters. With schizophrenics that wouldn't happen at all. There were always two, or more, there'd be four or five staff. Sometimes, and they'd be out there in the gardens doing work with their spades and forks. Supervision would have to be fairly tight, cause one had only to throw a bit of soil at somebody else accidentally, and all hell would break out. That was reality all in all, no drugs at that time for anybody... The patients did a lot of cleaning on the home, and did a lot of the gardening work outside.'*

Attendant A: *'Of course, among these you had the behaviour problems, those who were really in the colony not so much because of their mental inability, but that they were unable to cope with the demands of society, and they had behaviour problems, these were difficult for us. Refractory wards or where the bad lads were if you know what I mean, they were the most intelligent ones, probably with IQ's which today would not be considered* having a mental deficiency. The lads on these wards, their ability to play games was far better than in most of the homes, so I tended to gravitate to that type of home.'

Attendant T: *'Many of them could knock your head off.'*

Attendant B: *'Some of them had marvellous brains. We had a kid on the punishment ward. He'd only got to look at a key. He'd make you one. You know the locking doors, they'd take the screws out, saw them off and put the heads back. You wouldn't know they'd gone. We had some fun on there.'*

Nurse C: *'I mean there were some patients would slosh you one, whether they liked you or not when they had their moods come on, which we had plenty of didn't we. Doors stripped off, pushed into the side ward, banging and screaming, smashing the windows – plenty of smashing the windows. God! Some of them were wicked, I don't know where they got their language from – obscene language.'*

Nurse F: *'There was no favouritism, I loved them – but you can't afford to do that – I was too silly really, well you weren't supposed to get involved and that is why we used to be changed every three months to work on a different home.'*

Perceptions on patients' attributes and characteristics

Amidst the discipline, power and control which was exercised in order to keep order, the attitudes towards patients was a respectful relationship. They could not be dictated to as this would build resentment. An attempt was made to see patients as individuals and as people not different from the nurses. A family analogy is used and people who demonstrated a wide variety of skills and abilities are identified.

Attendant B: *'You got to know them, I mean you worked with them 12 hours a day, 6 days a week. No question of looking Gary's sister up – you do it, and it was there in front of you. We used to live with them, we could almost forecast what they were going to do the next day. You could point them out, how they were getting upset... There were some you liked, some you disliked. But you were there to attend to them, not form relationships, there was no favouritism, we used to look after them. I used to take the dog for a walk in the park at night, and an ex-patient, who was out on licence, if he was coming up the road, he would see me in the park at the gate while I went out of the park until I got home. He wouldn't budge, he wouldn't speak only "Goodnight gaffer", but he would stand there and watch until I got straight up into the flats. That's the relationship, for what it's worth. Respect I suppose. They were loyal, not too familiar, not too friendly. Favouritism any sort of favouritism – you were finished – you would have to treat them all the same.'*

Attendant B: *'They used to call me "Pop'" most of them. Well as a matter of fact it was more than like a family, you were with them more than you were with your own, kind of thing, because you were 12 hours there and then when you got home you would have your meal then off to bed. You would see more of the patients than your own family, and they used to look to us for guidance kind of thing, any little problem they would come to us. I was more a father figure I should imagine.'*

Attendant A: *I remember these people with great affection, and I still see some of the people today. People will stop in the middle of wherever and say "Hello Mr F", and they would almost stand to attention which is you know a bit off putting, perhaps in many ways, and people will think it's really quite odd. But no, it's a relationship we established in 1938/39 and these people are still going strong, you were the staff – they were the residents, the relationship was probably closer than it is today.'*

Attendant B: *'It was a very broad spectrum I think. You got some of the lowest imbeciles, we used to call them. (You are not allowed to say it now – low grades), to the criminals (high grades). They were all mixed up together. Murderers were in the punishment block.*
'The patients were individuals and had to be treated as such. You couldn't treat any two patients the same. One used to like a bit of sternness and be corrected, but try that with another one! Twenty nine years I was there and I never had a patient strike me, and I worked on all the homes. You can't dictate to them, they resented that.'
'There wasn't mental handicap – it was mental deficiency a vast difference, there wasn't a handicap in any way. Well there was some of them on Lee Home. They were all bed cases, no handicaps, it was mental deficiency.'

Attendant S: *'A few patients had an enormous amount of skills, some of them could have done all sorts of jobs and they had this quality that once they got into a job they got extremely good at it, providing again nobody interfered too much. They had enormous potential for training and development for all sorts of things, games, work, all sorts of jobs and they would be first class employees. I learnt a lot about the abilities of people who were labelled backward, subnormal. That, in actual fact, was the worst possible label you could have put on them – they were not subnormal. They had there own achievement levels, and they had there own potential.'*

Attendant T: *'We knew there were people that were special, that needed special care and special attitudes to them, and so we knew it wasn't normal nursing. It was different and I think we were well prepared for that kind of role. It was because of our own background. We didn't see them as daft or stupid or anything like that. We just saw them as people. Because we were living in there, we didn't see ourselves as very different from them at all. Me and J and people like us, you know, and a few more young people came at that time to do their training. We lived in as students, on the homes, we had a little room at the top of the stairs, it was reserved for the resident nurses. Only the student nurses were living in. So you were there 24 hours a day really, and that was the idea of course that you were there to be called at night. If an emergency occurred when they were desperately unable to cope. It was another pair of hands. They'd send one of the patients up to get you.'*

Boy Scout and Girl Guide Troops were in existence in most colonies where 'from 1937–1955, they were allowed to join local troops at annual camps and were expected to work for their badges like any other children' Brown (1995). At Great Barr Park Colony the Scout Troop in particular excelled in its activities with other troops. (*Plate 4*)

Attendant A: *'They had varied learning difficulties. In those days they varied from what would be called feebleminded, who were quite able, in most cases, to read and write. We had people who could play chess, play draughts, play billiards. They were able to take part in scouting activities. In fact the Scout Troop at Great Barr led by Mr L won the Gough-Calthorpe Shield so many times, that they in the end, didn't enter for it, so to give other people a chance. They had excellent football teams, cricket teams.'*

Interviewee U: *'I remember there were Scout Companies, a Guide Company and the patients had there own sports day. I remember seeing some of the lads doing some kind of Scottish dancing with swords, and they were doing it very, very well indeed. There was a Girl Guide Company which members of the staff ran. There were the concerts where people worked together, and the entertainment that they put on was between the staff and the patients.'*

Attendant D: *'I mean patients then were all sorts. There were absconders and all sorts. Patients needed constant supervision, so I had patients in the workshop when I came full-time. It was unstable otherwise when I was on and off, not there every day.'*

Institution as a regulatory system

Role of the colony

The role of the colony was to be a place geared for the effective care and training of the mentally deficient – it kind of justified things.

The following extract is taken from a speech made by Mr (now Sir) Lawrence Brock, CB, who was Chairman of the Board of Control at the opening of the extensions to Great Barr Park Colony in 1929. It is extracted from the *Walsall Observer*, 28 September, 1929 and was reproduced in the programme of proceedings for the opening of the further extensions to Great Barr Park Colony, 1938, by the Joint Board of West Bromwich and Walsall.

> *The real criterion by which they judged whether a person should be segregated was whether that person could fit into the fabric of society. 'I want you to consider', said the speaker, 'where these children would be if they were left uncared for, to fight for themselves in the world. Some would be in prison, not because of any real criminal tendency, but because of sheer inability to resist impulses to mischief and violence. Another class are those who cannot resist sexual impulses; in every colony there is a number who would be a menace to women and girls if they were allowed to be at large. Other older girls and women would be prostitutes, not because they are vicious, but simply because they are too weak to resist temptation and the lust of men. They are the women who, more than any others, spread the most terrible diseases. There are others who are a social menace, because they are unable to guard themselves from common danger, or observe even the most elementary rules of cleanliness and health. They fill our hospitals. Others become chronic unemployables, and encumber our workhouse machinery...' All these types, Mr Brock emphasised, needed segregation, not only for their own sake, but for the protection of society...*

The purpose and aim of a colony for mentally deficient people can be further deduced from rare observations in the literature by the Medical Superintendent of neighbouring Monyhull Colony, Dr AM McCutcheon. These aims were:

- To correct anti-social conduct,
- To develop self-respect and ensure happiness.
- To teach them various kinds of work for which they are best fitted by reason of their mental and physical condition, and to recover from

them some contribution, however small, towards the cost of their maintenance.

- To lead up to discharge if possible.
- To prevent the procreation of children, and so to stop the handing on of the blight to successive generations.

This, it was advocated was best achieved by 'segregation in institutions, preferably of the colony type' McCutcheon (1925).

General management

The following Great Barr Park Colony Institution Rules reflect a segregational ethos: Rule 97. The male and female patients shall be kept in separate homes, and as far as possible the younger patients shall be separated from the older. No member of the staff or patient shall be allowed to enter the premises of the opposite sex, except in discharge of some duty or with adequate authority. Any member of the staff transgressing this rule, unless a satisfactory explanation be given to the Medical Superintendent, shall be immediately dismissed. Rule 98. In visiting the female homes during the night the medical officers, unless they be women, shall always be accompanied by the head or some other female officer.

The following extract is taken from the rules of Leavesdon Hospital written in 1932 (Brown, 1995:9). It also reflects Leavesdon's segregational ethos.

The male and female patients shall be kept in separate wards, and no male nurse, servant or patient shall be allowed to enter any female wards, nor any female enter the male... During the day patients of both sexes shall be employed as much as practicable, especially out of doors; the men in gardening, husbandry and handicrafts, the women in occupations suited to their ability; and as a principle in treatment, endeavours shall be used to occupy the minds and bodies of the patients to induce them to take extended exercise in the open air, and to promote cheerfulness and happiness...

Before teatime no work other than hospital work is to be done by working patients, but after tea such patients may, if they so wish, do work for the nurses, provided such work is for the nurses' own use. No payment, either in money or kind is to be made for any work so done...

When the patients go to bed their clothes are to be folded up and placed on shelves provided or as otherwise directed...

Every patient is to be bathed once a week, unless exempted by medical order and not more than one patient is to be bathed in the same water...

The gate porter shall exercise a general observation to prevent the escape of patients and keep them from communicating improperly with person's outside,,,

The Medical Superintendent shall have paramount authority in the hospital...

Women were singled out as posing the greatest threat under the passing of the Mental Deficiency Act, largely because of the perception that illegitimacy and a rising birth rate among the lower classes were both attributable to feeble-minded women (Simmons, 1978; Barker, 1983). Walmsley (2000) suggests that young women and girls were taken into institutional care to protect them from abuse in the world outside, and that control was far more important than care.

Women were seen to be particularly vulnerable and those who conceived children 'out of wedlock' were often rejected and 'inevitably gave birth to crime-prone offspring' (Rafter, 1998: 35). Jordan (1976), the Medical Officer of nearby Monyhull Colony, advocated the value of segregation, believing it to be 'the main beneficial result to be obtained from the formation of colonies'.

Nurse C: *'They were pushed in because perhaps they'd had a baby at 13 or 15, or something like that. The parents couldn't cope with them and would push them out. Most of the girls were there for misbehaviour when they were younger, and of course vulnerable to men. When they were with us, I thought it was sad they had to stick to a routine, bed at a certain time, bath at a certain time, up at a certain time. In later years we were able to be more flexible.'*

Attendant T: *'The males and females were rigidly kept from each other. Except in Church on a Sunday morning, and even then they would be separated with staff between them. They only rarely went out into the community. I suppose that was it in those days. Something to be hidden away, that was the philosophy in those days, it wasn't due to the staff, medics or anybody at the hospital – it was law.'*

Nurse F: *'You only worked with females. The females and males were absolutely separated – they started to integrate around 1960/62.'*

Attendant A: *'There was an absolute ban on male staff being involved with female patients, you were in serious trouble if you were found on the female side.'*

Attendant S: *'Saturday they'd go round the lake, if they couldn't swim they could paddle, but fully clothed. No way could they undress, no contact between males and females at any time. Even at the cinema in the assembly hall, they were segregated. Also in the dance hall, males on one side, females the other. This also happened in Church.'*

'The way it was organised was not created by the people working in it. It was in fact part of the social policy which is law, and in Britain law is everything – there is no way you can put the person first and break the law.'

'Some sort of system had to be devised, the system that evolved in Britain in dealing with these people is trying to do something for them. It may have been up to its specification in the legalities, it may have been quite cruel in many ways. Most other industrial societies in the world have not got anything other near it. I think the system was as good as it could have been at the time, with the fact that it was there is something to be proud of more than critical of, because the people who were in the colony would never have been allowed to live a reasonable life outside at that time. They would today and that's the consequence of evolution.'

'The idea of selecting a piece of beautiful landscape, building these beautiful homes, you couldn't have selected a nicer place. An old estate that goes back several hundred years, beautiful green surroundings, woods, shopping areas, community outside, lakes inside, parks, gardens and greenhouses where patients worked.'

Attendant A: *'The term colony was used in those days as a more descriptive term than hospital. The colony system allowed them to live with people of the same ability or similar abilities – no one was better than anybody else, very rarely had trouble and they weren't looked down upon, not like today where they are looked down upon by society.'*

'The colony attitude I think it stems from the fact that there are people who live in a community with like needs and that the whole place was geared to the effective care and training of the mentally deficient person. Few people went out in those days, we never had a patient returned to us because they had failed in the community. When they went out, they were fit and able to take their part in society and they coped with society quite ably for many years afterwards. The name home was used rather than ward – it means so much more than a ward which is impersonal. A home is somewhere where people live, and so we didn't have wards in those days, they were homes.'

'Colony is a place where people with needs and like attributes are gathered together in surroundings of each one knowing what the other one needs and quite prepared to help them to achieve that need.'

Nurse F: *'It was a lovely place to be, and the grounds were kept so lovely and there used to be a male nurse to take about a dozen patients out with barrows and shovels.'*

Attendant T: *'It was self-contained and they were like people living in one of those stately homes, and everything was provided for you. Had there own gardens, grew there own fruit, own kitchens, all own cooking and there was a lot of the patients involved in this kind of thing, working, capable.'*

Attendant N: *'Then of course look at the grounds, they always had congenial surroundings and they were perfectly safe, they could wander around, didn't have to dodge traffic – and could set your mind at rest. Everyone was together, from a practical point of view, the doctors were there, the nurses, the chiropodists, hairdressers, dietician, recreational facilities on the spot, so there weren't any practical difficulties arranging that, because it was all sort of in one campus, and that was a great virtue in being in the colony, which I don't think people think about now.'*

Interviewee U: *'People admired Great Barr, you know, they came and saw the homes, saw that the patients were happy on the whole. There was a lot of criticism in the papers – sort of metaphors they would use, you know, 'Kept chained up'... sounded as if the patients were actually restrained, but they weren't. The only people restrained were those poor unfortunate people who were hydrocephalic, people with epilepsy, had to be given high doses so they wouldn't get harmed. You had got influences in politics where a certain amount of the 'politics of envy', I suppose the local politicians wanted to be in charge of it. I suppose the medico's seemed a bit lofty.'*

Attendant N: *'I suppose the most satisfying part, this applies more to the high grade patients, was seeing them go out, after a time, after they had been there several years, and it seemed that they had improved themselves of some way or another. To enable them to get out and a lot of them made good afterwards, and it sort of justified things.'*

Organised living

Great Barr Park Colony Institution Rule 100 states: During the day the patients shall be employed, as much as is practicable, in their special trades, and in suitable occupations in or out of doors. And endeavours shall be continually made to occupy the patients and to promote cheerfulness and happiness amongst them. (*Plate 5*)

Dr Jordan (Medical Officer at Monyhull) cited by Hutchings (1998) stated:

Carefully organised and directed work has been the most valuable agent in bringing about the improvement of the colonists... The true value of the work of the colonists is the educational effect it has on them as men and women. The constant aim of our training is to develop to the fullest extent every faculty of mind and body which can improve them in character and in capacity, and so make their lives more and more happy. Every one of the colonists is made the most of and it is astonishing how much that most is in the case of many of them.

Attendants and nurses give accounts of what a day for patients and staff was like where there was a structure of organised living

.

Attendant S: *'The first thing you would participate in was counting that everybody that was there, the night duty would go off then. Next was breakfast; all the patients would line up at the kitchen window, they were to take their food, our job was to see that they didn't spill it at the table.*
'Now the morning would be preoccupied with breakfast, possibly cleaning, bumping, tidying, clubs, actual good exercise. I never minded it, and the patients didn't either.'
'Maybe then go up to the central building, which was up the hill, to bring down the meals, the dinner, and you could take a dozen patients up with you and they'd help to push the wagon up and down. Dinner time, then a bit of relaxation, and football in the afternoon out in the fields, playing games and that was good. You would have a mixed team of patients and staff. As you moved into the evening things were more relaxed, tea-time, and a film show in the hall.'

Attendant B: *'The work was laid down. You had to get the breakfasts. The work people you would escort them to the workshops, farm people escorted to the farm and back again. In the home see that the beds were all made up and homes clean. The patients used to do a lot of work. Oh! We used to supervise woodcutting gangs, we used to get wood out of the woods, saw it up into little logs for the fires, and that was about it. It was about 99 percent supervision. You couldn't plan nothing for the day, only the basic things as I have said, just work gangs and all that. When things happened, you couldn't plan for nothing. The charge nurse would detail the work'.*
'We used to go out to the woods on woodcutting gangs. With their muscles, they could wield an axe better than an American woodsman. They could do everything.
'They used to scrap to get on the gangs, used to go for hard work. All the fields at the bottom of the hall, they used to weed that by hand, and they'd be kneeling down all day picking weeds – they used to love it didn't they... If you offered one of the chaps £10 to stop work – they'd prefer to go out and work for nothing. No problem finding work gangs. We didn't have to force

them to work – as a matter of fact we had to force them to get back in from the work gangs. The trouble was stopping them from work.'

Attendant D: *'The main thing about it was making mattresses and the hair in mattresses. They sewed the cover and filled them with mixed hair. There main job was mattresses and so we did that for quite a few years. They did a little bit of upholstery, but the main bits to upholstery was a bit too intricate.'*
'Everything was done by hand when I first went there. There was one lorry that's all. We had horses which were pulling the ploughs and ploughing the fields. There were no tractors at all. They fetched everything from the top hospital by barrows, to get a whole line of patients, using barrows to fetch from the homes, and that was part of their life, it was something for them to do. They got out of the homes you see, and that was the policy, Dr Mac's policy'

Attendant A: *'The patients that went out, they were trained to do things, trained to drive tractors, to manage horses on a farm, to plough fields, to sow, to reap and they could do it. They could take their part with a normal person at that particular job and be adequate in doing it.'*

Attendant S: *'I learnt something fundamental actually about people who probably had IQ's somewhere around 70/75 in the fact that they were quite obsessional, excellent workers in the particular job they had. But if you changed the routine in any way you blew the whole show. So what did I do, I sat on the bed without realising it, and one of the patients was 'bumping' under my feet. He didn't say, 'Clear off', and then settled down. Obviously, I got up and moved. Now whether I had a fag end or whatever, I put some ash on the floor. That started another one, and that resolved itself. Now the third one, I was looking out the window, and I suddenly heard this almighty crash. Three 'bumpers' went through the windows. So, obviously, I realised later I had exacerbated the boys to such an extent, they just couldn't take any more of me interfering with their work.'*

Nurse C: *'Of course you hadn't got television in those days so you've got to somehow keep them active – but mind you the patients had to work then. I mean there used to be two or three patients keeping the kitchens all nice and woe betide any other patient going in that kitchen to do anything. The patients used to do the bumping, patients used to do the dusting, keeping the place clean, which I think is good. The men worked out in the gardens.They used to have beautiful gardens and allotments, and men had to do physical exercise in the morning. Soon after breakfast they had to go out and exercise outside the homes, and the women of course had to work in the laundry and do the housework. You didn't get window cleaners coming in, the men used to come round, male patients had to come round with a male nurse and they'd do all the window cleaning – they were kept occupied.'*

'I had one of the girls to help me with my housework on a Saturday. The Committee – the Joint Board – allowed it and was the first trial that she was going out really, and then she'd go back. They had to be trusted. She'd come to me on a Saturday morning, she'd help me with my housework, and then she'd have to go, but I would have to pay Matron. I considered those trusted patients who shouldn't have been in, in the first place.'

Religion

Great Barr Park Colony Institution Rule 36 states: The Chaplains and the RC Religious Instructor shall be appointed by the Joint Board, and shall attend the Institution weekly to hold services and give religious instruction according to their respective churches to members of their own faith, under such arrangements as the Joint Board may make from time to time.

However, although the Joint Board arranged for such services, little account was made at a time of segregation of the impact personable and individual relationships and contact would have not only on the patient but also on the community of patients living in the home.

Attendant A: *'Mealtimes were taken as a family, they sat down at the table together. Grace was said before meals, prayers were said at night before going to bed, and the staff were expected to take part in prayers, not just for the patients, the staff also, it was a family living in a home.'*

Attendant B: *'For instance, the patients didn't like to be singled out. A Catholic Priest used to come on the home, and the first words he said to me were, "Point the Catholics out". That was the biggest mistake he ever made – to have them pointed out. He'd go to them individually and ignore the others, and that was the trouble. They used to hate outside visitors coming, and when they singled one out, that patient, for right or wrong was in trouble when they'd gone. It was disruptive things like that, they didn't think before they acted.'*

This practice of visiting patients and singling them out by religious denominational representatives was found to be of significance some 30 years later in 1974 at St. Margarets Hospital, when the following was reported (christiananswers.net).

Levi, I was to learn, had the mentality of a boy of nine years. Nevertheless I knew I should visit him, so as soon as I was back on my feet I found out where the hospital was and I went to see him. This was my first Jewish contact. Levi soon got to know me and showed his pleasure each time I visited him, in fact he became quite possessive when other patients tried to attract my attention....

Attendant N: *'In the Colony there were three religious services every Sunday. The RC Chaplain used to come in early in the morning, C of E Clergyman later in the morning, and Denominational service later on in the afternoon.*

Institution as a regulatory system

This can be summed up with the comment made by Attendant S: *'Stop treating the patients as if they were ordinary people.'*

A clique of staff at Great Barr were perceived as hardliners. They were staff who had come out of the war and who introduced elements of militarianism into their working relationships with patients and staff, and who ran the homes like barracks.

Nolan (1993:111) identifies those mental health nurses who had the ability to control, those who controlled through fear, and those who had an aptitude or skill for control, as opposed to the more aggressive posture adopted by 'bullies'. Those nurses who had had terrible experiences in the war directed their anger onto the patients, and some even felt that the patients were in a conspiracy against them so staff had therefore to assert their authority.

Attendant S: *'Now the first piece of instruction I ever had was that I had got to stop treating the patients as if they were ordinary people. This instruction came from the charge nurse... Implicit in this was the message, "You will never be any good at this job 'cos you know nothing about discipline and order"... This is what actually happened: "I believe you gave a patient a cigarette; I want you to watch this." Charge nurse to patient "The nurse has given you a cigarette hasn't he, well, which do you want, his cigarette or my butt end?" The patient threw away the cigarette and picked up the butt end and walked away. The charge nurse explained that we must be in control at all times – we could not allow feelings to interfere with the work.'*
'It was oppressive, repressive, inward looking, paranoid almost schizophrenic. All the labels you could put on individual people, the way these people behaved as a group of staff, it was there. Now the extent to which you suffered from any one of these situations depended on how you fitted in. So, you started off, they didn't want us there – the clique that were there.'

Attendant T: *'There was an element of staff, you know, who were hardliners, they didn't see the people as people, but some kind of object, it was just a job for them. I wasn't in the good books of some of the charge nurses, because I used to call these people by their name, as soon as I would know their Christian name, and so I'd say, "Oh! Hello, you are John, Michael or Bill", I used to call them by their name, and you had to be called Mister you see, which was like an infringement into an army rule. You know, you daren't drop the rank. But I bloody dropped the rank all the time. Patients would come and say, "Hello T," and the charge nurse would be glowing, and they couldn't stop them. The old brigade, they were really severe, you know. I don't know why it was. It was just like an acceptance of a way of life behaving around the job. You know, they weren't bad people at all, its just that, that was passed onto them, there had to be a shield between us and the patients. The ranks were the same, and you didn't speak to the ranks except on duty matters, and there was no social life with you and the charge nurse or people like that. To me the patients were people who needed special attention, support and help. I was quite pleased with the way I handled that side of training, I think we were like a breath of fresh air to the patients, people like me and J, and some of the young people who started coming in.'*

Attendant S: *'You started off as a Private, and you became a Corporal because you were behaving as Corporals wanted you to behave, and they were the first line of authority and then you became a Sargeant because you outgrew the Corporals and you behaved as a Sargeant wanted you. You could be qualified but that didn't get you into the commissioned rank, your behaviour got you into the commissioned rank, but you had to be qualified to even get into it. I was seen as officer material, but no sooner as I was seen as officer material, that I was also seen as I shouldn't be a Sargeant, because of my affinity of relationship with, or the way I handled a particular patient. There was no going back, you had to do it their way, and you had to be oblivious to the humiliation and the pain that was inflicted on the recipient.'*

Attendant T: *'A Bloke called Mr. T was there, he was a really hard character, quite a small man. He would come in, in the morning he said, "Upstairs, Mr ...," that was the directions. I had to go up and see what you were going to do yourself. He'd come up after about an hour and a half, walk around, "Pretty good," you know draw attention to something that you'd forgotten to deal with, it would be something silly, no conversation. He'd say, "Go down, and have your breakfast." The duties would be laid down by the charge nurse, that didn't apply entirely, but mainly it did.'*
'You daren't sit down with the charge nurse – this strictness and firmness, you didn't sit down with the charge nurse unless, you were invited, and you were never invited. That was it, it was unspoken.'

Attendant B: *'The charge nurse – what he said was law, but if the patients could see anybody was getting anything over a charge nurse, of course the whole place started. They all started having a little niggle and of course made things a hundred times more difficult. In later years we had the Friends of St. Margarets, they started it – outsiders. They used to visit the patients. If a patient had a grievance, at one time they used to come to us to sort it out. Instead of that they told these people, and you know what happens if they tell anybody else it magnifies... By the time you got to realise what was going on, a kind of gradual insidious complaint worked from little things that grew into a mountain, and when they got to the top of the mountain they didn't know what to do. I think that's when the rot started – having outside interference. Don't get me wrong, not only the staff were upset by these disruptions, the patients themselves were. They liked a nice orderly life.'*

Nurse C: *'There were one or two nurses who I didn't like at all, who I thought could be aggressive, which I didn't like at all. We had one nursing sister – she was a bitch. She picked fault with everything. She hit them with a towel, I don't know why she was like that, yet she'd only got to open her mouth and they'd be dead silence. She'd got them just like that in a nasty way really.'*

In contrast some nurses had the 'right' attitudes.

Nolan (1993:112) identifies that in the 1930s, 1940s and 1950s, respondents talked about mental health nurses who were positive role models, devoted to the patients, always calm and blessed with a sense of humour – the compassionate and caring. In much the same way, nurses in this study have identified what they consider crucial qualities of a good nurse.

Attendant S: *'Being introduced to this type of work reasonably early, about 20, 21. Meeting the right sort of official in charge was a key issue. Be introduced to the work by the right sort of people, I would still rate that probably. Mr C... got over to people like me, when I worked with him. I still think that was the way to introduce people to the world of caring, let them see people who have the right attitudes.'*

'Mr C was quiet and reserved, always ready to do you favours, and always treated the patients with dignity. Mr C had been a school teacher of some kind before the war, and he was injured during the war, and he had a completely different approach to the way we dealt with the patients on the homes. It was essentially something that I thought that if I'm going to get anywhere in this, or do anything in this, Mr C has got the right approach, the right sort of attitude, and the strange thing was all of us, and my kind of mates, all that was wrong with us was that we were completely lacking in

any kind of insight into any of the problems some patients could create.'

Attendant T: *'He was a really nice feller, he was austere, he had a rapport with you and especially if he saw you were interested in the children. I loved them, got on great with them, and I got on with him too. There wasn't too much formality, like. If I suggested something to him, he'd say, '"Go on, you carry on," he was very liberal.'*

Influences of the medical superintendent

Great Barr Park Colony Institution Rule 9 stated: The Medical Superintendent shall reside in the institution and have paramount authority in the institution, subject to that of the Joint Board; shall have control over all the officers, attendants, and servants, and shall superintend and direct their duties, as prescribed by the Institution Rules and Instructions. He shall be empowered to suspend any institutional officer, and shall report such suspension to the Joint Board at their next meeting.

Dr MacMillan was the first appointed Medical Superintendent for Great Barr Park Colony and so it seems fitting to have a perspective on his appointment from a member of his family, followed by observations of attendants and nurses on his role at the colony.

Interviewee U: *'This was a good appointment for him, it wasn't a very popular scope of work, people would be put off by thinking of handicapped people. He was appointed in 1929, and I think it was a matter that he had always taken up asylum work – he wanted to benefit their lives. We lived in a flat in a block next to the assembly hall... He was a good practical doctor, I don't know if he was a great one on modern psychology, I don't think he read a lot of it very well, analysis and that sort of thing. Freudianism and so on... But as a good practical man, he really boosted occupational therapy. It was one of the things that was coming along as a training idea for these people to keep them busy, so they were kept busy purposely.'*

Great Barr Park Colony Institution Rule 75 stated: The Clerk of Works shall work under the direction and control of the Medical Superintendent.

Interviewee U: *'He used to see the Clerk of Works every morning at 11.00 o'clock – that's when his day started, and then he'd visit the homes when necessary, and he was really keen on helping the patients and staff.'*

Great Barr Park Colony Institution Rule 20: In any case of difficulty or danger he [the Medical Superintendent] shall consult the visiting physician or call to his aid the specialist service of Hallam or Manor Hospitals, or in special circumstances, he may call to his aid in consultation any registered medical practitioner.

Interviewee U: *If some patient had some pain, he wouldn't have to fill in a form, he would ring up the Head of West Bromwich Hallam Hospital. Well, he'd ring up the Head, he knew these Heads by name, and they were all friends of the Walsall Manor Hospital and say, "So and so has appendicitis, can you get him in?" The patient would be whipped off that afternoon – that applied to all of the patients and staff.'*

'He was always a keen sportsman, he would be at every football and cricket match that was on. He would play golf and so on. He and his wife were always connected with social events in Walsall in various clubs. I mean he was in charge of all these people and particularly in organising their occupational therapy, and of course being a sportsman, he was keen on nurturing activities for them'

'I mean he mixed very much in Walsall where he was well known. He went to football matches and did medicals and spotting of injuries for the footballers, same with cricket, same with boxing... He did it voluntarily, he said it turned you into a more normal outgoing person, you understand people better, and you got vitality and energy.'

Great Barr Park Colony Institution Rule 15 stated: He [the Medical Superintendent] shall keep a journal, in which he shall make the following entries, *viz*: first, the name of every attendant and servant whom he shall have suspended, together with the date and cause of such suspension; and second, all escapes, accidents, deaths, and inquests since the last visit of the Joint Board…

Attendant A: *'In those days the ultimate boss who was the Medical Superintendent, he was God, and he dispensed his justice as one would do. Him and the Matron, if she wasn't God she was very near, if not on the same level.'*

Attendant T: *'Old MacMillan, he was lord and master of the whole place, and he could hire and fire any level of staff, just like that – no questions about it. He was a very good man, he was very interested in the residents that were there, you know the people that were there, and he would not tolerate any kind of misbehaviour by the staff towards them, and that was a good thing'*

'It was his rank, he was authority, like the army. MacMillan was like God – you wouldn't approach him without an appointment. The charge nurse would be frightened to death of him, terrified of him. Yet, I could never see any reason why they should have been. It was his rank to them, he was authority.

Some of them were ex-army so they were used to authority... MacMillan was a kind, good man. I think he had an interest in the patients, because he used to go to a lot of trouble to see them, and see them individually as well. He'd see them over a period of time and review them. He'd be actually reviewing them, and he'd review medication as well.'

Nurse C: *'They would have their yearly test – intelligence test. Well! It horrified me because of some of the questions they asked those patients. I couldn't have answered them myself. I was scared stiff sometimes if MacMillan turned to me and asked me the same question. I wouldn't have been able to answer it. I was disgusted with that, I really was, because some of those girls should never have been there.'*

Nurses' attitudes towards the medical staff

Although the Medical Superintendent and medical staff were in charge, the attendants and nurses were very much in control of the homes and what went on inside and controlled the information that went to the medical staff.

Attendant S: *'They saw the medical staff as people really who were trained in medical schools, and worked in general hospitals, not Colonies or subnormality hospitals. So, in actual fact they controlled the information they gave to doctors. Now, there's no way they would keep information from a doctor about someone having a high temperature. But they would certainly keep information about somebody who was standing in the toilet naked, or for throwing their porridge about, they wouldn't report that. In fact two of us reported this unfair treatment to the Medical Superintendent. He told us we had no authority to leave the home, and if we did it again we would be dismissed.'*

Points of change

As the NHS dawned and the colony was to come under a different kind of control, nurses at the colony were concerned about how these changes were going to impact on them personally, and on the patients.

Attendant B (p9): *'I'm not against the NHS, I think it's a good thing, but they tried to do too much, too suddenly. I mean you can't run a mental hospital like that, you have to talk to the patients, and gradually work them round to the idea. You couldn't say one day we'll do this and the next day we'll do the other, 'cause they couldn't take it in, they were regimented to that extent you know. The patients weren't encouraged to do things for themselves, they tried to put female cleaners on the homes to stop them cleaning windows or anything like that. Well the patients felt frustrated and for years they did these jobs. "That's my job," sort of thing, and once they did their job (the cleaners) there was trouble.'*

'If they had consulted the old hands, they had probably made a better job of it. There was no consultation at all, you do it or you don't. It was something like doing something for 20 to 30 years all your life and someone turning round and saying, "That's wrong, you just can't do it." Its like stopping a ship – it carries on a bit, doesn't it. They hadn't got a period like that – a transition, it was overnight.'

Nurse C: *'Today the patients have outsiders now, haven't they, doing this kind of thing, which is bad, 'cause I think they need to do something which would always equip them better for going out, be able to cope better and they used to take an interest in their work and it kept them occupied.'*

Attendant A: *'The role of the attendants changed quite considerably when the General Nursing Council became involved. They were more concerned about the nursing aspects than they were concerned about the recreational and occupational aspects, which again, in my humble opinion, were far more important to me than the medical aspects. It was a sad day really when the RMPA packed up. The direction that the GNC took was a bit detrimental to the actual people receiving the care. The GNC didn't, and as far as I know still with the new education bodies, do not understand the difference between disability, deficiency and the physically ill.'*

Interviewee U (p3): *'Now, of course, 1948, and you got the NHS. You got a different kind of councillor coming in. They wanted lay control not independent management, and of course he was always a very independent man, and he didn't always agree with them. You know he would stand for his corner, I think they found him a little intransigent. They tried to make him resign, and he did finally retire, but after a bit, they needed him back again. So he went back for another couple of years as Medical Superintendent, because they couldn't get anyone else who handled things, because he had the personal contact with every member of staff.'*

Striving towards ordinariness within a regulatory system

The core explanatory variable of the research results is *striving towards ordinariness within a regulatory system*. This process may appear almost paradoxical, as closed institutions such as the colony are not outwardly seen as positive environments in contemporary literature, and indeed in the context of contemporary person-centred philosophies within a citizenship model and human rights framework for legislation.

However, this provision for the mentally deficient was an example of a unique period in British social policy and history, where eugenics influenced the segregational model in the form of colonies for the mentally deficient.

The attendants and nurses within the research study, and identified within this chapter, have constantly referred to those qualities for striving towards ordinariness within a regulatory system. The colony system was not devised by attendants/nurses but through political legislation, and which, as a 'closed' institution, reflected society's solution to mental deficiency and was wholeheartedly embraced, therefore, by society

Attendants' and nurses' practices, through their accounts and throughout the themes identified, demonstrate qualities and enthusiasm for working and developing relationships with the patients. Discipline has been identified as a major form of control within the colony, and it was seen as necessary to establish a respectful and stable relationship. The numbers of patients, coupled with a broad spectrum of patient problems in the homes, and the small number of staff to sustain order meant that to establish a meaningful structure for patients and to keep them busy, a strategy was put into place so as to develop further potential for organised and conformed living.

Qualities to be found essential for nurses in developing an effective relationship with patients included having patience and a sense of humour, working, playing, and teaching, and almost living with the patients. In this way the nurse can help patients develop their potential. All these factors were identified and explored by nurses throughout this study.

Nurses saw patients as people, who were capable and who should be treated with dignity. These attitudes existed and prevailed amidst inappropriate views held, and abusive practices engaged in, by other staff who provided negative role models. These were the qualities needed to provide the motivational commitment to sustain, for most attendants/nurses, a lifetime of work within Great Barr Colony/St. Margarets Hospital.

References

Barker D (1983) How to curb the fertility of the unfit: The feeble-minded in Edwardian Britain. *Oxford Review of Education* **9**(3): 197–211

Brown K (1995) *The Leavesdon Hospital Story, 1870–1995*. Horizon NHS Trust

Charmaz K (2000) Grounded Theory: Objectivist and constructivist methods. In: Denzin NK, Lincoln YS (eds) *Handbook of Qualitative Research* (2nd edn) Sage, Thousand Oaks, CA: 509–36

Chester G, Dale P (2007) Institutional care for the mentally defective,

1914–1948: Diversity as a response to individual needs and an indication of lack of policy coherence. *Medical History* **51:** 59–78

Christian Answers (2004) Available at www.christiananswers.net/ evangelism/stories/judaism-tanner2.html. Accessed 13 December 2004

Dey I (1999) *Grounding Grounded Theory: Guidelines for Qualitative Inquiry.* Academic Press, San Diego, CA

Field P, Morse J (1985) *Nursing Research: The Application of Qualitative Approaches.* Aspen Systems, Rockville, MD

Frieze Stephens H (1933) Cheaper institutional care. *Mental Welfare* **13:** 8–13

Glaser BG, Strauss AL (1967) *The Discovery of Grounded Theory.* Aldine, Chicago

Glaser BG (1978) *Theoretical Sensitivity.* Sociology Press. Mill Valley, California

Hammersley D (1990) *Reading Ethnographic Research: A Critical Guide.* Longman, London

Hutchings D (1998) *Monyhull 1908–1998, A History of Caring.* Brewin Books, Studley,Warwickshire, UK

Jordan R (1976) My life story. *New Aspect Quarterley Magazine* for The National Society for Mentally Handicapped Children.West Midlands Region

McCutcheon A (1925) Institutional treatment of mental defectives with special reference to occupation. *Journal of Mental Science* **71:** 694–70

McDowell M (1930) *Simple Beginnings in the Training of Mentally Defective Children.* Law and Local Government Publications

Mitchell D, Smith P (2003) Learning from the past – Emotional labour and learning disability nursing. *Journal of Learning Disabilities* **7**(2): 109–17

Nolan P (1993) *A History of Mental Health Nursing.* Stanley Thornes, Cheltenham UK

O'Hara J (1967) *The Role of the Nurse in Subnormality. A Re-Appraisal.* Fred Esher Award Essay

Rafter NH (1998) Feebleminded women and the advent of Eugenic criminology.Chapter 2. In: Hahn N (ed.) *Creating Born Criminals.*1st edn. University of Illinois Press pp 35–54

RMPA (1931) *Manual for Mental Deficiency Nurses.* Bailliere,Tindall and Cox, London

Simmons HG (1978) Explaining social policy:The English Mental Deficiency Act of 1913. *Journal of Social History* **11**(3): 387–403

Stevens ARA (2000) Women superintendents: the contribution of Margaret MacDowall and other women managers of mental deficiency institutions in England. *British Journal of Learning Disabilities* **28:** 71–7

Strauss A, Corbin J (1990) *Basics of Qualitative Research: Grounded Theory Procedures and Techniques.* Sage, Newbury Park, California

Turner BA (1981) Some practical aspects of Qualitative Data Analysis: One way of organising the cognitive processes associated with the generation of Grounded Theory. *Quality and Quantity* **15**(3): 225–47

Walker D, Myrick F (2006) Grounded Theory: An Exploration of Process and Procedure. *Qualitative Health Research* **16**(4): 547–59

Walmsley J (2000) Women and the Mental Deficiency Act of 1913: Citizenship, sexuality and regulation. *British Journal of Learning Disabilities* **28:** 65–70

Walsall and West Bromwich (Barr Colony) Joint Board (1932) *Great Barr Park Colony.Institution Rules.* Walsall and West Bromwich (Barr Colony) Joint Board

Wiener CL, Wysmans WM (1990) *Grounded Theory in Medical Research.* Swets and Zeitlinger, Amsterdam

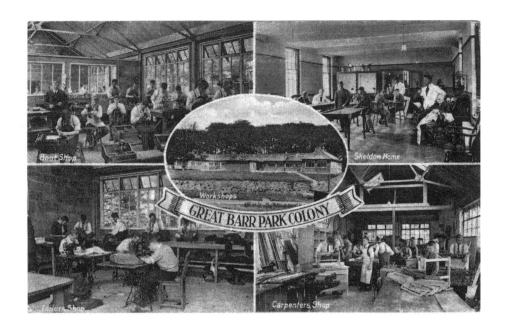

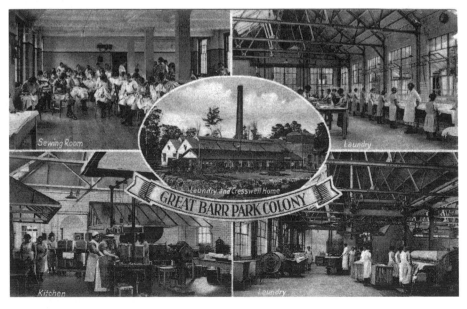

Plate 1. Great Barr Colony: Postcards depicting life and work.

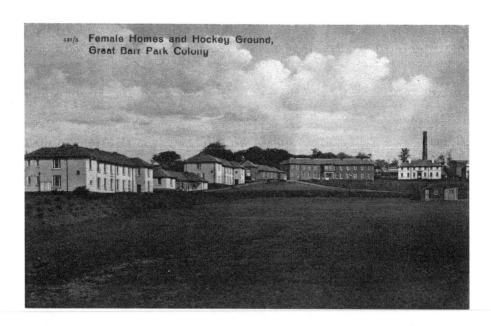

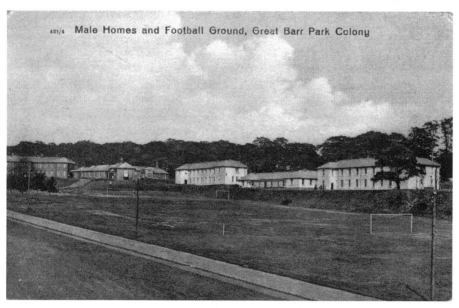

Plate 2. Great Barr Colony: Female homes and hockey ground (top), and Male homes and football ground (bottom).

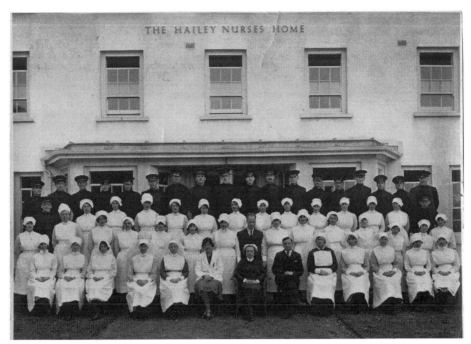

Plate 3. Great Barr Colony: Attendants and nurses c. 1928.

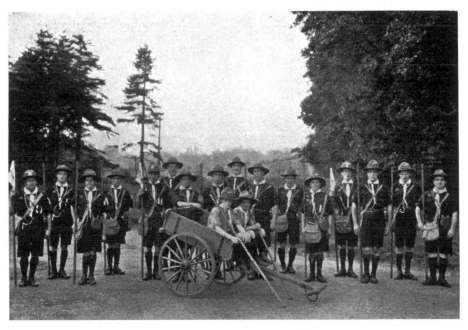

Plate 4. Great Barr Colony: Scouts.

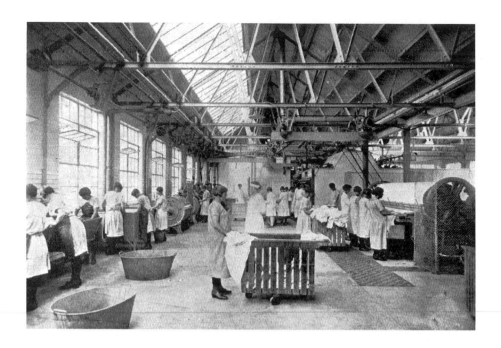

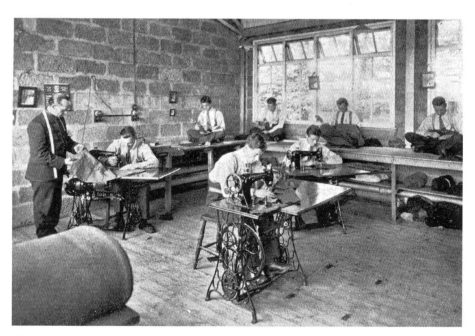

Plate 5. Great Barr Colony: Laundry (top) and tailors (bottom).

CHAPTER 3

Mental deficiency nursing and the GNC: A square peg in a round hole

Duncan Mitchell

Introduction

Learning disability nursing has an ambivalent relationship with its history. This is not surprising as the roots of the profession lie within the large institutions that dominated services for people with learning disabilities throughout much of the 20th century. Most of the learning disability nurses who completed their training before 1990 experienced life working in one of the institutions. Those who trained before the 1980s spent most of their training within various parts of a single institution.

With a small amount of prompting, such nurses will relate tales of the institutions that combine elements of humour, nostalgia, pride and shame for the conditions that many of the residents lived in. They will often describe people among the staff and residents who have remained in their memories as larger than life characters who had a profound effect on their careers and lives. Some recall a sense of camaraderie that existed in spite, or perhaps because of, the isolation and the poor working and living conditions within the institution. Many will also discuss the way in which the institutions declined and were replaced with community services that were often highly innovative and radical in their design and implementation. The ambivalence reflects an irony in that learning disability nurses were the main group of people who ran the institutions and who also played a significant part in their demise.

This chapter explores the origins of nursing for people with learning disabilities and the reasons why nurses became the main group of workers within learning disability institutions. The difficulties that the regulatory body for nursing had in incorporating learning disability nursing into its rules are discussed and reasons for its reluctance and eventual agreement to compromise are suggested.

In this chapter, the normal historical convention of using some of the language of the past when directly referring to historical events is used. This means that the term 'mental deficiency' nursing will be used as it was the language used throughout the 1920s (and indeed up until the 1950s in the UK). The chapter is mainly devoted to the work of the General Nursing Council (GNC) as it grappled with the question of whether work in mental deficiency could be described as nursing. Reference is also made to the Medico Psychological Association (MPA) that was granted a royal charter in 1926, becoming the RMPA. The RMPA was a significant player in both mental and mental deficiency nursing until the early 1950s and both influenced the GNC and organised its own training scheme. However, despite their influence, this chapter, as befits a volume about learning disability nursing, concentrates on the challenge that mental deficiency presented to the definition of nursing promoted by the GNC.

This story concerns a group of workers who, in the early decades of the 20th century, worked in a small number of institutions for people with learning disabilities. Variously known as institutions, asylums, or colonies their numbers were to grow for several decades until their decline that began in the 1960s and culminated in the closure of most of them by the 1990s. This part of the story is about definition and occupation position. In other words why did nursing become the main occupational group within the institutions?

Why nursing?

The reason that this group of workers became nurses was a mixture of assumption and coincidence: an accident of history. To explain this, consideration needs to be given to issues in the history of nursing generally as well as the development of care for people with learning disabilities.

The 1919 Nurses' Registration Act was the point at which in Abel Smith's words 'the profession had come of age', in that a campaign for state registration that had been going on for many years had borne fruit (Abel-Smith, 1960:99). The legislation for the first time introduced restrictions on the use of the term 'nurse' in that state registered would be added to those entered on what would become the GNC's register. Prior to this there was no exclusion to the term that was used, often, to describe women engaged in paid or unpaid care.

It would seem obvious to refer to women who worked with people with learning disabilities as nurses in the same way as women who worked in mental illness asylums were called nurses. Men, on the other hand, doing similar work were termed attendants. The term nurse was gender specific and encompassed all women involved in physical care. Prior to the 1919 Nurses Registration Act anyone could legitimately call themselves a nurse (Abel-Smith, 1960). Within institutions for people with learning disabilities this use of the terminology continued well beyond the 1919 Act when women workers continued to be referred to as nurses while men continued to be referred to as attendants, mirroring the practice in mental illness asylums. To some extent therefore it was an issue of semantics. The term nurse was used because it was the natural word for the job and for the women who did it.

The campaigns within nursing at the beginning of the 20th century however were aimed at restricting the use of the word nurse to trained nurses and in this they were partially successful. The inclusion of mental nurses and the virtual creation of mental deficiency nurses as a formal group was not in the minds of many of the campaigners. Nolan makes this clear when he describes the antipathy of one of the leading campaigners for nurse registration, Mrs Bedford Fenwick, to mental nurses and the general animosity directed towards them from the nursing establishment (Nolan, 1993).

Hospital and private nursing had claimed a proud history by reformers to separate it from the Sarah Gamp image portrayed by Charles Dickens in Martin Chuzzlewit (Dickens, 1844). Such reformers tended to emphasise the purity of the religious vocation and the discipline of the military as well as the new technical demands created by the science of medicine. Mental deficiency nursing was not able to construct such a history. The history of those working with people seen as being mentally defective was less clear because their history was unrecorded: this largely remains the case today. There is very little written about those who worked with people with learning disabilities and seemingly very little evidence upon which to build. Andrews, writing about the provisions for the mentally disabled in early modern London, claims that those who cared for the 'simple minded' were just as neglected as those who were cared for (Andrews, 1996). This emphasises the hidden history of this group of workers. Andrews explains that it was mainly women who cared for people with learning disabilities and these women were usually the parish nurses who looked after a variety of cases. Men did get involved but tended to only be concerned with the people who were considered to be more difficult to manage. Some parish nurses did tend to specialise and some, according to Andrews (1996), specialised in work with people with learning disabilities.

In the latter part of the 19th and early 20th century, workhouses that segregated people with learning disabilities employed people termed 'imbecile nurses' or 'epileptic nurses'. There is no evidence to suggest that these people were seen in any way as specialist but certainly had separate jobs to the work of other staff. A history of work with people with learning disabilities prior to the 20th century has yet to be constructed in a similar way to that of the history of nursing prior to formal institutional nursing. What is important is that those women who did the work were popularly called nurses and that their work with people with learning disabilities was seen as part and parcel of their duties as nurses.

This corresponds with other evidence suggesting that nurses, in this case the trained hospital nurses, were seen as a profession from which to draw people to work with people with learning disabilities, usually in an administrative function. In 1914, for example, the *Nursing Times* reported an 'interesting appointment' when the Matron of Paddington Infirmary was appointed to the post of provincial organising secretary for the Central Association for the Care of the Mentally Defective (*Nursing Times*, 1914a).

So it was not only the fact that female carers were popularly termed nurses that provides the past of learning disability nurses but the fact that hospital trained nurses were employed to work with people with learning disabilities as nurses. However, this was not necessarily nursing work but work carried out by nurses. Dingwall et al (1988) point out the importance of making this distinction clear when considering the history of nursing. They argue that it is difficult to draw a distinction between nursing and non-nursing work and in particular to define work that ought to be preserved for the nursing profession rather than that which could be carried out by a number of different occupational groups.

In two ways, therefore, we can trace a past in which nurses were involved in care for people with learning disabilities. Both ways, however, corresponded more to the notion of the work nurses carried out than they did to distinctively defined nursing work. Moreover, neither of these paths would have led naturally to a separate branch within the profession. If this is compared to similar cases of nurses working with other groups of people there were no corresponding supplementary registers set up. The early GNC introduced supplementary registers for mental, sick children's and fever nurses (the 'mental deficiency' branch was a part of the mental register). If the two ways in which a past can be traced for learning disability nurses are considered there are corresponding groups who would have had similar claims for a supplementary register or part of a supplementary register. People working with children outside of hospitals had often been termed nurses but this title did not continue into the 20th century: many adopted other titles such as 'house parent'. Nursery nurses retained a title of nurse but at no time became part of the nursing profession. Hospital-trained nurses working in epileptic colonies did not seek or gain a separate branch of nursing. Mental deficiency nurses did gain a separate branch yet from an examination of nurses' past there was no obvious reason for this. It would have been far easier to blend the mental deficiency nurses with mental nurses.

A new part of the profession

It may well be the case that if the Nurses Registration Act had been passed at the turn of the century rather than in 1919 there would have been no separate learning disability nursing. Although the MPA had briefly discussed a separate certificate before 1900 they were reluctant to develop such a scheme because of the lack of demand (RcPsych, 1895). They finally introduced a separate training during the First World War and the first MPA certificate for nursing in mental deficiency was awarded in 1919. The role of the GNC in the 1920s will be examined later but suffice to say at this point the GNC neither understood nor wanted the separate branch of mental deficiency nursing. The concern from nursing about the work was not new: the attempt to classify nursing into technical work that was highly valued and less sophisticated caring work had been a theme within nursing for some time. This is illustrated by a speaker at the International Congress of Nurses in 1902 who divided the insane into three classifications: mental exaltation (acute and chronic mania), mental depression (acute and chronic melancholia) and mental enfeeblement (dementia, paranoia, epileptic insanity, circular insanity, general paralysis, idiocy, imbecility) (Laird, 1902). The speaker then went on to talk about the first two classifications on the grounds that graduate nurses will be more likely to meet them than the third class. The latter apparently required less intelligent and scientific nursing and 'need but little more than custodial care or the attention given to any feeble patient'. The value given to perceptions of curing in contrast to caring is also demonstrated by the reluctance of hospital-trained nurses to work in anything other than managerial posts in mental deficiency institutions. This is illustrated by Margaret McDowell writing in 1924 of the lack of success that general hospital nurses found in mental deficiency work:

I think that the main reason is that cure is the main idea in nursing of sickness, whereas in the nursing of the underdeveloped what the world calls cure is rarely obtained, and people who aim for this get dissatisfied by their inability to achieve a definite end.

This reluctance to embrace work that did not fit into nursing's ideal of the new scientific work goes to the heart of the debate that repeats itself constantly about the role of learning disability nursing in the wider profession.

So if nursing did not want mental deficiency in the profession why was medicine, in the form of the MPA, so keen to introduce it? Here we need to look at the links with mental nursing which are such that one wonders why a separate branch of nursing needed to be formed. Carpenter (1985) argues that the medical profession wanted to organise the training of mental nurses because they wanted to prevent other groups from doing it. A trained nursing workforce certainly gave the medical superintendents a firmer control over the asylums. It also ensured dominance over one other group that had a legitimate claim on the control of training. The educational ethos of the early institutions had diminished but had never completely disappeared. Education remained important to the institutions but a distinction came to be drawn between the education of children and the training of adults. The training of adults within the institutions was vitally important: not necessarily to ensure their rehabilitation into employment and life outside the institution but to ensure the economic stability of the institution. The climate may have changed from education to containment but training was still necessary for effective control. The medical superintendents needed to control their workforce to control their asylums

Medical superintendents recognised this and by bringing all workers employed to work with people with learning disabilities into a nursing workforce trained by them, they would retain control of the institutions. Medical superintendents saw nursing as a vital element of the institutional regime as illustrated by one of their number, McCutcheon, writing in the *Journal of Mental Science* in 1925:

> *Considerable attention of late years has been paid everywhere to the raising of the standard of nurses in mental institutions, and I am strongly of the opinion that the work among defectives stands or falls very largely on the efforts of the nursing staff. If they are not properly trained, if they are not honest, and if they do not set the right tone with the patients, no amount of work done by the doctors or matrons can ever hope to succeed. From my own experience in mental hospitals and with defectives I consider that the defective is, if anything, the more difficult patient to deal with and on the whole I think he makes more demand on the nurses' patience and good temper, and that is why I consider that the nursing staff really determine the success or failure in an institution for mental defectives.*

This reflects an assumption that nurses were the natural occupational group to work in the mental deficiency institutions and also reflects an interest in the good quality and character of the workforce.

In addition to the interests of the medical superintendents there were also other significant pressures from trades unions and from the Board of Control which was the Government department responsible for mental and mental deficiency services. Unions were keen to add to their numbers by bringing another group of workers into their membership. In 1914 the medically controlled Asylum Workers Association carried a resolution that workers employed following the Mental Deficiency Act should be included with other asylum workers (*Nursing Times*, 1914b). The Association not only argued for the inclusion of mental deficiency nurses within its own ranks but was also active in campaigning for the inclusion of all mental nurses in nurse registration. The *Nursing Times* went so far as to claim that the Association was 'largely instrumental in getting recognition for mental nurses in the Nurses Registration Act' (*Nursing Times*, 1920).

Evidence for the extent to which pressure was applied to the GNC that was formed after the Registration Act is limited. What there is rather confirms the *Nursing Times'* view that it was medicine or at least medically controlled organisations that influenced the inclusion of mental deficiency nurses. To say that the pressure came entirely from the medical superintendents, however, would be to simplify the issue too far. The doctors themselves were continually being pushed into action by a Central Association set up by the Government to oversee local arrangements for the implementation of the Mental Deficiency Act (the initials CAMW – Central Association for Mental Welfare – will be used to describe this group). The Board of Control demonstrated the importance that they attached to training within the institutions in a circular to superintendents in 1916 (National Archives, MH51/239 28.2.1916):

The working of the Mental Deficiency Act is bringing a large and increasing number of young and trainable defectives into the institutions under the Board of Control. These defectives need lifelong support and care, and the urgent necessity of training them in industries so as to enable them to contribute to their own support and in manners and habits so that they will need the minimum amount of supervision, has become imperative.

The thrust of the circular was a plea for the improvement of training of staff who could in turn train the residents of the institutions. The Board reminded superintendents that they had already begun courses of training for teachers for the institutions.

However, instead of creating their own certificate for other workers, CAMW pressured the MPA to address the issue within existing structures. The MPA remained half-hearted about the separate certificate and although it lobbied hard for the inclusion of mental nurses into the Nurses Registration Act it was only after encouragement from the honorary secretary of CAMW that the MPA's education committee decided to act. They resolved that, in addition to the mental nurses, 'nurses who hold the certificate of the association for proficiency in nursing mental defectives should also be placed upon the supplementary register under clause 16(3) of the Nurses Registration Bill (RcPsych, 1919). Despite this reluctance it is clear that it was the MPA who were the main, if at times lukewarm, protagonists in the introduction of mental deficiency nurses into the regulations of the GNC.

That is not to say, however, that the GNC embraced mental deficiency nursing with enthusiasm, far from it. Mental deficiency nursing was almost totally ignored in the early part of the 1920s as the GNC became caught up in its own internal debates. The GNC acceded reluctantly to pressure to introduce and maintain mental deficiency nursing and tried to ensure that it followed the model of sick nursing. The model was totally unsuited for mental deficiency nursing but it was followed by the GNC in its quest for professional status. When this chosen model failed to turn mental deficiency nurses into sick nurses and the GNC failed to evolve a satisfactory alternative, mental deficiency nursing was marginalised within nursing.

The caretaker GNC and the inclusion of mental deficiency nursing

The caretaker GNC was set up by the Government following the Nurses Registration Act as a step towards an elected Council. Its early months were given over to making the rules for the operation of the Council and for the nursing registers. Dr. Bedford Pierce represented the MPA and was also, together with Tom Christian, the voice for mental nursing. The Caretaker Council was immediately involved in conflict as the various factions that had agreed an uneasy compromise to win support for the Registration Act began to break down (Rafferty, 1996). The crucial decision regarding mental deficiency nursing that was taken by the Caretaker Council was to include it within the rules; this both recognised its presence within nursing and marked its difference by making it a separate part of the mental supplementary register. The sequence of events is important because there seemed to be very little discussion until after its inclusion and although it is difficult to disentangle the decision making process within the Council it is possible to analyse and speculate upon the pressures that encouraged it to happen.

The first meeting of Council was held on the 11 May 1920 when a temporary committee was formed to write the rules. The formulation of the rules is important to this story because the Nurses Registration Act did not specify mental deficiency nursing as one of the supplementary registers. As far as the Act was concerned there was no need to include mental deficiency nurses at all. The Council was required only to create a general part and then supplementary registers for male nurses, for those trained in the nursing and care of persons suffering from mental diseases and for those trained in the nursing of sick children (Bendall and Raybould, 1969). At the second meeting of Council, Bedford Pierce moved that mental deficiency nurses be admitted to a separate division of the mental supplementary register and once this had been accepted, mental deficiency nursing remained as a separate element within nursing.

Following this initial decision there was a suggestion that Council should go further and create a completely separate supplementary register for mental deficiency nursing. On the 22 June 1920 Bedford Pierce wrote to the Chairman of the GNC that he had no objection to the suggestion that there should be a supplementary register for mental deficiency nurses. He felt, however, that it would be inconsistent with the Nurses Registration

Act. There was some discussion about the name of the new nurse but only of a perfunctory nature; in the same letter Bedford Pierce felt that the title 'mental defective's nurse' would be unsuitable because it was likely that the 's' be dropped and a 'reflection be cast on the nurse's intelligence'(National Archives, DT20/231, Bedford Pierce to Priestly, 22.6.1920). His suggestion of the term 'mental deficiency nurse' was the one that was eventually taken up, although when the GNC's mental committee reported to Council in August 1920 it was recommended that the formal title should be 'Registered Nurse for Mental Defectives' (National Archives, DT48/158, 16.7.1920)

Once a decision about the rules had been made by the GNC, ministerial approval was required: this was far from automatic and demonstrates the constraints that were placed on the GNC. The rules were sent by the Minister to the Board of Control for comment. They were particularly asked to give their opinion on whether they concurred with the proposal that the mental supplementary register contain a separate part for mental deficiency nurses (National Archives, MH55/475, Brock to Pell, 29.9.1920). In concurring with the Council's decision the Board explained that it saw mental deficiency nursing as being subsidiary to mental nursing (National Archives, MH55/475, Byrne to Pell, 15.10.1920):

> *Nurses adequately trained in the nursing of mental diseases have had in the course of their training sufficient experience of mental defectives to enable them to assume the responsibility of nursing and taking charge of mental defectives. The converse does not hold good: for there are many emergencies and propensities arising in mental disorders (from which mental defectives are largely exempt) how to meet and guard against which nurses can only be taught by additional experience.*

This indicates clearly that mental deficiency nursing was seen as a subsidiary category within a supplementary register and not suitable for equal status with the mental, children's and fever parts that were in turn only seen as additions to the general register.

Mental and mental deficiency nursing

The whole issue of supplementary registers had been controversial within nursing for some time and their existence had been a matter of compromise within the GNC (Rafferty, 1996). The *Nursing Times* summed up the mood in June 1921 when it commented:

> *The existence of supplementary registers at all is a necessary evil, and the ideal to be kept in view is not a number of little groups of nurses registered*

as specialists, but a great body of nurses who, in addition to their general training, have specialised in various departments of nursing.

This explains why the general part was pivotal to those who wished to have the title nurse and why other branches were marginalised as separate entities.

The whole issue of mental nursing was a particularly sensitive one. The GNC was dominated by general nurses as was its mental committee. The *Nursing Times* (1921) acknowledged this when, in October 1921, it concluded that mental nurses had a grievance in that they were represented only by a doctor and a male nurse and that expert advice would have to be sought before regulations or syllabuses were framed.

Mental and 'mental deficiency' nursing shared common ground in relation to the mainstream representatives on the GNC. Not only were there comparisons in terms of class and gender, there was also the issue of the nature of the work in similar institutions. Bedford Pierce argued that the subjects were similar and that the exams were identical for the first two years but that the place of training and the work was different (National Archives, DT20/231, Bedford Pierce to Priestly, 22.6.1920).

This shows an ambivalence of approach regarding integration and inclusion demonstrating both similarity and difference which was common in this period. It was the issue of sickness that was divisive between mental and mental deficiency nursing as it was uniting between mental and general. Although it was the case that there was a great deal within mental nursing that could not be described as sick nursing, according to the *Nursing Times* (1920), Bedford Pierce, for example, argued that 'it was difficult to distinguish between social service and what might strictly be called nursing', mental nursing could still be understood in terms of a general framework of cure as well as care. It was when 'sickness' was considered that mental deficiency was pushed well away from the mainstream in a way that mental was included in it. It is no surprise that in the very early months of the GNC mental deficiency was not an issue because it was subsumed under mental nursing. As soon as the regulations and the syllabus for the general and supplementary registers began to be discussed in detail it became clear that 'mental deficiency' was never likely to become a specialism of nursing whose practitioners could become general nurses with a shortened training. This was because they would not have the required experience of sick nursing. If they had been allowed through as a special case then the whole image of a general and supplementary register would collapse allowing in all manner of applications for supplementary registers to be created. This had been the fear of many of those who had campaigned for state registration for nurses because it would dilute the professional development of nursing (Rafferty, 1996).

Mental deficiency nursing becomes an issue for the GNC

The issue of mental deficiency nursing appears to have lain dormant from October 1920 until April 1922. The rules, which included a general register and four supplementaries, with a separate division for mental deficiency nursing in the mental supplementary, had been signed by the Minister of Health in July 1921. In April 1922 it was proposed by the Mental Nurses Committee that a small conference be held to discuss the syllabus for 'training for mental defectives' (National Archives, DT48/158, 5.4.1922). The proposed syllabus was that for mental nurses with an additional section for mental deficiency. The mental nurses' syllabus was the one developed by the MPA.

The conference was held on 3 May 1922. The morning was spent considering the issue of mental nursing and the afternoon considering 'mental deficiency'. Medical superintendents from the Royal Albert, Darenth Park and the Royal Eastern institutions attended; the need for such expertise was justified by the chairman because 'no one on the council had any experience of their special work and their advice would be most valuable' (National Archives, DT48/158, 3.5.1922).

Unlike the morning session, when the mental nurses were represented by a matron and a chief male nurse, there were no 'mental deficiency' nurses present. The total lack of involvement within the GNC and MPA of 'mental deficiency' nurses until well after the Second World War reveals their marginal status in comparison to other branches of nursing.

The conference was the first to consider the complex issues of the syllabus and the recognition of institutions. All county asylums were recognised for the training of mental nurses but the Mental Nurses Committee would not recognise any 'mental deficiency' institutions until the Board of Control provided a list of institutions recognised for training (National Archives, DT48/158, 3.5.1922).

This approach, which seems to have been one of wait and see, was maintained until December 1922 when the Mental Nurses Committee was forced to consider the issue by the application of Monyhull Colony for recognition as a training school for mental deficiency nursing. The shorthand minutes of an exchange between three members of the mental nurses committee demonstrate the committee's confusion about the issue (National Archives, DT6/97, 6.12.1922):

> *Bedford Pierce: I do not know anything about the mental deficiency institutions.*
> *Christian: They are very obscure.*
> *Herringham: Who can tell us anything about them?*

> *Bedford Pierce: I think nobody but the Board of Control.*
> *Herringham: If you cannot help us what are we to do? We have to go to*
> *somebody else.*
> *Bedford Pierce: I thought of replying that we shall send them one of the*
> *syllabuses and say we have not yet gone over institutions for recognition*
> *for mental defectives and will let them know when we have.*

The Committee was clearly floundering, the members had no knowledge about mental deficiency and did not know what to do about it. Between 1923 and 1927 there was a flurry of discussion about the issue of syllabuses and recognition of institutions for the training of mental deficiency nurses. These were initially being held within the context of the wider debate affecting mental nurses. 'Mental deficiency' nursing was sometimes part of and sometimes sidelined by these discussions. What followed was a catalogue of deferred discussions by the GNC and MPA. It is quite clear that there was an issue but that no-one knew enough about the subject and there was not the will to drive discussions and a decision through. Another period of incompetent management of mental deficiency nursing arises reflecting a confusion of thinking and approach to the issue similar to the whole history of learning disability nursing.

The Mental Nurses Committee of the GNC had before it in its meeting of October 1923 an agenda item considering the 'the position of nurses for mental defectives as regards training, examination and admission to the register' (National Archives, DT48/158, 13.10.1923). This item was deferred although items after it were discussed. It was again deferred at the meeting of 5 December 1923 and the shorthand notes are again illuminating in the way they show how members of the mental committee were thinking (National Archives, DT6/97, 5.12.1923):

> *Bedford Pierce: None of us has any knowledge of this.*
> *Donaldson: The MPA have a special certificate of their own.*
> *Bedford Pierce: We are too.*
> *Yapp: I think we should find out about the MPA and see if we can improve*
> *upon it.*
> *Bedford Pierce: There are three ways. One, to apply to the Board of*
> *Control. I don't want to do that. Two, apply to MPA and ask what they*
> *do. A confession of weakness. Three, we could call another conference*
> *of institutions.*

It was agreed to discuss the issue at a conference to be held a week later on 13 December (National Archives, DT48/158, 5.12.1923). The committee's lack of knowledge about 'mental deficiency' was such that two members, Dr Smedley and Miss Yapp, were asked to obtain information about institutions involved in the training for 'mental defectives' before the next meeting (National Archies, DT48/158, 5.12.1923). The Committee's ignorance of the subject is compounded by the fact that they felt they could gain an understanding within a week.

If the conference on 13 December 1923 between the GNC and MPA discussed the issue of mental deficiency nursing then it was not recorded in the minutes. When the full GNC met on 29 December 1923 the Mental Nurses Committee reported that it was not in any position to make any recommendations regarding training for mental deficiency because it was awaiting further information (*Nursing Times*, 1923). The matter continued in a similar way in 1924 when it became clear not only that the Mental Nurses Committee was unable or unwilling to discuss 'mental deficiency nursing' but that it was increasingly looking to the MPA for help. Dr Smedley reported back in February 1924 that he had visited Darenth Training Colony but was not able to report back to the Committee. He had not gained much information and was still 'in doubt as to exactly what are the nursing duties of mental deficiency work' (National Archives, PRO, DT6/97, 6.2.1924). Dr Smedley was asked by one of the nurses on the Committee whether he would rather not call them nurses and this suggests that the crux of the problem was that although the Committee members knew very little about mental deficiency work, what they did know was very difficult to reconcile with their understanding of nursing. The matter was deferred again until after the next conference with the MPA and was also deferred in March 1924 (DT48/158, 6.2.1924 and 5.3.1924).

The full extent of the difficulty can be seen in the minutes of the joint meeting between the Mental Committee and the MPA: the two groups that were responsible for developing and maintaining training for mental nurses deferred the discussion. This was because the Board of Control had set up a small committee to consider the issue (National Archives, DT48/158, 2.4.1924). There is little evidence to indicate why the various groups behaved in the way they did. My assumption is that the Board had become anxious that despite asking for action from the MPA it was not forthcoming and it had therefore set up a group to move the matter forward.

In May 1924 the GNC Mental Nurses Committee recommended the first seven hospitals as suitable for training 'mental deficiency' nurses (National Archives, DT 48/158, 6.5.1924). By the end of the year the GNC agreed that the syllabus for mental nurses be issued, although an expected report had still not been received from the MPA or the Board of Control whom the GNC believed were meeting in joint committee (National Archives, DT 5/3, 19.12.1924). The Council clearly could not wait any longer but was still unable to devise a syllabus for mental deficiency. The Council felt totally reliant on outside bodies.

GNC's reluctant action

The impression gained from reading the minutes of the Mental Nurses Committee is that it would have continued to remain in ignorance of the situation and in a state of inaction until encouraged to act. The effect of the inaction was to push mental deficiency nursing to the margins by ignoring it. It was forced to the attention of the Committee by information that all too clearly spelt out the flaw in the assumption that underlined the rules of the Council. The GNC intended that the preliminary examination should be the same for all nurses, it had an important function in not only setting the same standard between the general and the supplementary registers, but also defined nursing as sickness or bedside nursing. Mental deficiency nursing had been accepted under the GNC but did not conform to its most central criteria for nursing. This had been apparent before 1925 but began to be taken seriously after the letters concerning individual institutions were received. The first of these was received by Stratton, who was the male nurses' representative on the GNC, complaining that there was no sick nursing at the Manor, Epsom which had been recognised for training in mental deficiency nursing (National Archives, DT 6/98, 4.3.1925). The second was from a male nurse at the same institution who complained that he was unable to take the examinations because there was no opportunity for him to practise bedside nursing (National Archives, DT 6/98, 1.4.1925). Later in the year the emphasis moved to Farmfield Colony whose nurses could not be examined because 'they did not know what the training was' (National Archives, DT 6/98, 6.5.1925). When Farmfield was discussed at the July meeting members seemed frustrated by a lack of knowledge on mental deficiency and Bedford Pierce repeated his, by now familiar, refrain of 'nobody knows anything about these mental defectives' (National Archives, DT 6/98, 1.7.1925).

A series of discussions and visits were then held to try to gain information on mental deficiency nursing. Farmfield Colony and Darenth Training Colony were visited by members of the Mental Nursing Committee who were shocked at both the lack of bedside nursing and the conditions within the institutions. In October 1925, for example, two Committee members, Miss Wiese and Miss Du Sautoy, visited Darenth Training Colony and found that they were not only unwelcome but were not allowed to visit the male side at all. They found that the wards, that contained up to 100 children, were unclean and crowded and there were no activities for the children. They reported that the nurses looked as if they were 'a very inferior type' and recommended that the colony should not be recognised for training and that other visits should take place to improve on the Committee's total lack of knowledge (National Archives, DT 6/98, 2.12.1925).

The summaries of the reports which are available within the Mental

Nurses Committee minutes indicate a total preoccupation with the issue of sickness nursing (National Archives, DT 48/158). Miss Weise pointed out that when patients at Darenth were sick they were nursed in their own wards and trainee nurses would not be able to get the required experience of bedside nursing unless sick patients were transferred to an infirmary ward. Another member of the GNC got to the heart of the issue when he stated that the only solution was to establish a separate specific examination instead of a general preliminary examination for mental deficiency nurses. The consequence would be that mental deficiency nurses would not therefore be eligible for reduced training in general hospitals. This was the GNC's main dilemma. Mental deficiency nurses could not, unlike mental nurses, be shoehorned into the existing arrangements for preliminary examinations because they could not practise the required amount of bedside nursing. To set up a separate preliminary examination would destroy the principle of one register with supplementaries rather than several registers. The idea put forward by Miss Weise that sick patients be taken from their own wards to special sick wards so that nurses could do their training was one of the most bizarre suggestions to come out of the GNC. This demonstrates the problem that the GNC had in trying to use a general nurse training to improve standards in mental deficiency work.

In addition to the complaints about the lack of bedside nursing from within nursing itself the GNC was encouraged to act by external influences. The minutes of the Mental Nurses Committee indicate this when they record two letters sent to them, one from the RMPA and one from the Board of Control. Reading summaries of the correspondence it becomes clear that everyone was expecting someone else to do something, the result being that little was done at all. Mrs Pinsett, a Commissioner of the Board of Control, had written to the GNC asking why nothing had been done. The GNC had expected the RMPA to take a lead on something about which they themselves felt that they had no expertise and the RMPA was waiting for guidance from the Board of Control. Despite the fact that individual commissioners such as Pinsett were taking an interest, the Board of Control generally was lukewarm about the whole issue of mental deficiency which it had shelved in the second half of the 1920s as it concentrated on mental illness policy (Thomson, 1998). The confusion was not helped by the fact that some of the leading figures in mental deficiency were members of both the RMPA and the Board of Control and did not always seem clear about the capacity in which they were acting.

The Mental Nurses Committee decided to recommend to Council that a conference be called early in 1926 for representatives of leading institutions and for others interested to discuss the training and examination of mental deficiency nurses (National Archives, DT48/158, 2.12.1925). Apart from this recommendation the Mental Nurses Committee remained hopelessly confused and divided. They could not agree on a proposal to abandon the preliminary examination for mental deficiency nurses because that would mean abandoning the principle of one portal of entry. They could not agree to the desirability of bedside nursing experience with some members suggesting that it was not that important and others, like Pierce, arguing that 'if we call them nurse they ought to know something of nursing' (National Archives, DT 6/98, 12.1.1926). There was even a suggestion made several times by different people that the Council leave mental deficiency alone altogether. The response to the last suggestion made by Herringham was that 'it is too late to object': the Council was legally bound to register mental deficiency nurses because of the 1919 Nurses Registration Act (National Archives, DT 6/98, 2.3.1926). This was quite erroneous because the Act did not require the registration of mental deficiency nurses. There was a similar response, again by Pierce, to the attempt by Herringham to question the validity of mental deficiency nursing in the Council meeting of December 1925. Herringham suggested that (National Archives, DT 6/3 18.12.1925):

The point for us to consider is whether such persons enter into the definition of a sick nurse at all. It requires to be very carefully considered before the Council comes to a decision on the proposal of the Mental Nurses Committee to call a conference. The care to be exercised by a nurse for mental defectives is nothing more than a sort of companion or children's nurse. It is not sick nursing and I don't know whether there is enough of it to enable us to register such cases.

There was no careful consideration recorded in the minutes because Pierce merely defended the position of mental deficiency nurses by saying that the question was determined by the Act.

The discussions were designed to culminate in a conference between the GNC, RMPA and Board of Control to consider the whole issue of mental deficiency nursing. The conference exposed the differences within the GNC, particularly between the nurses, who argued for single portal entry and Pierce and Herringham who argued for a training based on the work that was needed rather than for bedside nursing (National Archives, DT 6/98, 2.3.1926).

According to the *Nursing Times* the conference was adjourned but only after some form of compromise in principle was agreed upon. The majority present felt that mental deficiency nurses filled an important role and that there ought to be some arrangements whereby they receive bedside training to meet the criteria of the GNC and then spend time on the 'educative and psychological side of the work, co-operating with the teachers' (*Nursing Times*, 1926a).

The conference was far from conclusive and perhaps this was the reason for it not being publicised. It did, however, change the direction of the discussions for the future. It appears that the day was dominated by a draft syllabus put forward by the Board of Control. This suggested that the second and third year of the training be spent in special training, with the first year concentrating on bedside nursing and passing the preliminary examination (National Archives, DT 48/158, 2.3.1926).

The Board of Control continued to exert pressure on the GNC: the chairman of the Mental Nurses Committee reported that together with the chairman of Council he had met with Dr Rotheram of the RMPA, Mrs Pinsent of the Board of Control and others (National Archives DT 48/158, 3.4.1926). After the meeting it was decided to organise the first final examination specifically for mental deficiency nurses and to hold it in October of 1927.

The *Nursing Times,* although excluded from the conference, gave an account of the activities and the 'important' proposals of the Board of Control. The Board, they reported, believed that a distinct syllabus was necessary because there were differences between the mental and mental deficiency nurses that needed separate examination. The differences noted were 'the nature of mental disorder, objects of treatment and reasons for special care' (*Nursing Times*, 1926b). But in addition to these differences the issue of sick nursing was again the crucial element.

It is suggested that all nurses of mental defectives should be required to produce evidence that they have attended, in the two years after their preliminary examination, 24 lectures or demonstrations on sick nursing, and to have received certain practical instruction. In view of the difficulty experienced by these nurses in securing sufficient bedside instruction for passing the preliminary examination, the GNC, it is stated, was considering modification of that examination (*Nursing Times*, 1926b).

The 1926 conference was supposed to clear up the issue that the presence of mental deficiency nursing created for the GNC. Like other events in this period it only served to emphasise the difficulties of trying to fit the square peg of mental deficiency work into the round hole of the GNC's understanding of nursing.

An anomoly within nursing

Following the conferences in the early part of 1926 there seems to have been a continuation of confused activity. In June of 1926 the Education Committee of the RMPA felt that the issue of the syllabus for those nursing the mentally defective was not urgent and should be postponed until a paper on the subject appeared in the next *Journal of Mental Sciences* and the matter had been discussed at the conference of the National Asylum Workers Union (RcPsych, 1926). The article, written by the medical superintendent of the Manor, Epsom, appeared in the July 1926 issue of the journal. The author was very clear that the mental deficiency nurse was concerned with the 'healthy as well as the sick defective' but was also needed to work with a wide range of people. In short he was arguing that mental deficiency nurses ought to be able to work in all sections and with all types of people in the larger colonies. He placed the mental deficiency nurse very firmly in nursing (Frieze Stephens, 1926):

> *But though much of the work is not among the actively ill, it should not be forgotten that first and last and all the time she is a nurse. She represents the type of modern nurse, whose activities are concerned chiefly in the maintenance and improvement of bodily health, the hygienic educator, whose duties lie largely in the prevention of disease, in the detection of the early signs and symptoms of illness, rather than in the treatment of established disorders; nevertheless, she should know what to do, and how to do it, in the event of sickness, for she may not always enjoy the facilities of a colony hospital or clinic.*

He argued for a complete separation of mental and mental deficiency nursing. His syllabus led to further discussions within the Mental Nurses Committee of the GNC. The nurses on the Committee were clearly unhappy with the idea of diluting the preliminary examination to enable mental deficiency nurses to take part but were also unwilling to jettison the one portal of entry into nursing and develop a separate training as Stephens suggested. The discussion prompted an examination of the meaning of the word 'nurse', with one member stating that mental deficiency work was not nursing but educational. The emphasis was again on sickness nursing: Dr Pierce, for example, explained that if nursing meant 'a knowledge of sick nursing and nothing else' then the preliminary examination must not be compromised. Miss Cowlin compared mental deficiency with sick nursing (National Archives, DT6/98, 6.7.1926):

> *It is helping to restore the damaged mind. You can't restore mental defectives. It is not like mental. It is an educational problem only.*

With such a definition of nursing it is not surprising that the issue of mental deficiency nursing frustrated the Mental Nurses Committee and the rest of the GNC who were trying to promote nursing as a technically competent professional body defined by its ability to work with sick people. There were some defenders of a definition of nursing that would incorporate mental deficiency work, but this was only on the basis of widening the definition of sickness (National Archives, DT6/98, 7.9.1926):

> *Weise: lots of these people are helpless, a helpless person is a sick person.*
> *Pierce: The feeling is that the word nursing really means caring for the bodily wants.*
> *Cox Davies: It is not confined to that. There is more to that whether nursing the brain or the body.*

This debate gets to the heart of the nature of mental deficiency nursing. It was perceived as an anomaly within nursing because of its lack of a role in sickness nursing. Mental deficiency work, by its very presence within nursing, challenged a strict definition of the latter. If mental deficiency nursing was not defined by sick nursing, however, how could it be defined? An examination of the syllabus gives us some indication of the work from the point of view of the RMPA and the Board of Control.

The main requirement of a mental deficiency nurse was the ability to manage a group of people living in a defined area within a mental deficiency institution. This involved total care and control in which a nurse was needed to ensure that the part of the institution for which they were responsible ran smoothly and efficiently (RcPsych, 1932).

The wide range of skills demanded of a mental deficiency nurse reflected the requirement for nurses to manage units within the mental deficiency institutions with as little outside help as possible. A section on the principles of mental deficiency nursing went on to outline the importance of the nurses' personality and character to the management of mental deficiency. The intriguing part of the syllabus was not the basic requirements but the additional or special part of the final examination. Having completed the written examination, candidates were required to specialise in one of four parts, A, B, C and D. In the RMPA's syllabus these four parts are described as bedside nursing, special methods of teaching mentally defective children, the teaching of mentally defective adults, and, finally, physical training, drill, dancing, indoor and outdoor amusements (RcPsych, 1932). This reflects the varied work of mental deficiency nurses as well as the continued emphasis on education and training. However there was no commonality of approach and managers of institutions used the training and qualification of mental deficiency nurses to meet their own needs. Some institutions may have used all four parts of the scheme, others may have been more restrictive. It is also possible that some nurses qualified with experience in only one part of the syllabus. The latter was the GNC's suspicion when negotiating integration of the RMPA nurses in the 1940s (National Archives, DT16/241). If this was the case the

GNC's antipathy to mental deficiency nursing can be explained by its need to establish a national standard for nursing rather than to allow local flexibility. The problem for mental deficiency nursing within the GNC, however, was not based on the principle of a common standard but on the nature of its definition which, for the GNC, was through the preliminary examination.

There was some flexibility within the GNC among those who felt that the preliminary examination was essential in raising standards within general nursing. Herringham, for example, felt that it would be better to have a separate examination for mental deficiency nurses if they could not reach the general standard. This would have caused problems for the advocates of the principle of a single general register followed by post-registration supplementaries and also caused problems for representatives of the RMPA. Sensitive to suggestions of inferiority of mental nurse training the RMPA argued that the GNC should keep the preliminary examination for all nurses (National Archives, DT48/158, 6.7.1926). There was, however, no suggestion about how mental deficiency nurses could gain the necessary experience in bedside nursing to pass the examination. The problem was for mental deficiency rather than mental nurses and it appears that the RMPA was ensuring a similar place of power in the mental deficiency institutions that it had in the mental. One way of doing this was by at least influencing, if not controlling, the training of workers within the institutions. This is illustrated by the rescinding of the RMPA's regulation that mental deficiency institutions without a resident medical officer could train nurses under the RMPA's scheme (RcPsych, 1926).

The minutes of the GNC meeting of July 1926 summed up the difficulty facing the Mental Nurses Committee that had still to come up with a report on the syllabus and examinations. The first issue was whether mental deficiency nurses were required to have experience in bedside nursing and the second was whether the present syllabus was adequate for the needs of the nurses. Yet again there was no report. The *Nursing Times* summed up the issue when decrying the fact that after all there was only one candidate for the examination when it reported Pierce as defending the position, pointing out that (*Nursing Times,* 1926c):

> ...*wide questions of principle affecting the policy of the Council are involved and he predicted that with the growth of institutions up and down the country this branch of nursing is destined to become a very important service.*

This links the discussions firmly back to the social policy context; institutions were being planned and built and there was soon to be a further Mental Deficiency Act. It becomes clear that the RMPA, although late in its enthusiasm for a separate branch of nursing, had taken steps to ensure that it was to control the institutions and the workers within them. It seems that at this point, it was the RMPA who was as insistent on a common preliminary examination as the GNC.

In September 1926 the Mental Nurses Committee of the GNC recognised that it was unlikely to get any help from other bodies and would have to take action itself to move the matter forward. At this stage it still felt ignorant of the nature of mental deficiency nursing and decided to invite representatives of the work to discuss the issue. For the first time this involved not only medical superintendents but mental deficiency nurses themselves. The committee invited Dr Frieze Stephens, Miss Rose, Matron of Tooting Bec Institution, Miss Cullwick, Matron of Monyhull Colony, and Mr Galley of the Manor, Epsom (National Archives, DT 48/158, 7.9.1926). The two matrons were unable to attend so the Committee met only with Dr Stephens and Mr Galley on 28 September. The record shows that both men supported the Council's policy of insisting on a common preliminary examination, arguing that it ensured a higher standard of nurses and that this was better 'even if it meant a smaller number of nurses coming onto the register' (National Archives, DT 48/158, 28.9.1926). Meanwhile the RMPA was waiting for the GNC to take a lead before it continued its own deliberations and adjourned its special committee regarding mental deficiency until the GNC declared its view on the syllabus of the Board of Control (RcPsych, 1926).

The GNC finally took a decision when it confirmed the report of the Mental Nurses Committee in October 1926. The preliminary examination was to remain the same for all branches of nursing and the final examination for mental nurses should 'continue to cover an all round training in this department of nursing' (National Archives, DT5/3, 15.10.26). The *Nursing Times* warned that the problem had not been solved and that the difficulty was still that of bedside nursing. It felt that the policy of the GNC was that 'we know it is difficult but please do it' (*Nursing Times*, 1926d). The ultimate aim of the GNC was still, according to the *Nursing Times,* to establish the principle that a nurse in a special branch should be fully trained in general nursing before specialising. The matter of the syllabus had still not been settled and while the RMPA was waiting for the GNC, the minutes of the Mental Nurse Committee of the GNC reveal that the GNC was waiting for the RMPA to submit a report (National Archives, DT 48/158, 2.11.1926).

The GNC's policy falls at the first hurdle

Prior to the decision regarding the preliminary examinations the GNC had tended to put off some of the decisions about recognition of institutions for training. Some of the larger institutions had been recognised on the principle that they were very similar to the asylums recognised for mental nurse training. It had been an individual application that had provoked much of the controversy in the first place and now that a decision had been made there would be applications that would have to be examined under the agreed regulations. It was not long before the policy was put to the test. All applications from mental or mental deficiency institutions had first to go to the Mental Nurses Committee that made recommendations to Council.

The first application that was to come before the Committee was that of the Starcross Institution. The secretary of Starcross asked for a relaxation of the rules because six months bedside nursing was not practical. The problem seemed particular to male nurses and the Committee was not prepared to approve Starcross for training until provision had been made for male nurses to nurse the sick (National Archives, DT 48/158, 29.3.1927). By September 1927 the Mental Nurses Committee was satisfied that such provision had been made but was concerned that there was no resident medical officer at Starcross. The October meeting of the Mental Nurses Committee had the benefit of a report of a visit to Starcross, the results of which opened up the whole issue again. Dr Smedley had looked up the list of special schools approved by the Board of Education and found that Starcross was registered as a special school for mentally deficient children and also as an institute for ineducable children. 'He considered that there could be little, if any training for nurses working in the special school' (National Archives, DT 48/158, 4.10.27). The Committee felt that they could not approve Starcross for the following reasons: there was no training in sick nursing, no registered nurses to give instruction, no sister tutor, no lectures from a medical officer, and no experience in nursing the more severe type of cases. The Committee would have realised that at least some if not all of these problems would have been apparent in most of the mental deficiency institutions at the time. Yet again the Committee agreed to look at the issue and the October meeting decided to open up the whole matter by resolving (National Archives, DT 48/158, 4.10.27):

...that the question of the training of nurses for mental defectives should be brought up again with a view to revising the rules on the system of making this a special class of nursing and given a special training.

The logic of the situation is inescapable. Most of the mental deficiency institutions could not possibly meet the GNC's criteria for sick nursing in terms of numbers of beds, variety of cases and medical direction. The GNC was not prepared to alter its criteria and there was no group prepared to force them. The policy was supported by the RMPA which was trying to establish control of the institutions and their role in training as a way of doing this.

The Board of Control wanted a trained workforce to ensure segregated colonies and institutions that were self-sufficient and they saw an element of sick nursing as being important in ensuring such self-sufficiency. It seems that they were preoccupied with a trained workforce of some description and were prepared to go along with the GNC's rules to achieve this. In the middle of all this were the institutions, particularly the smaller ones who could not meet the regulations. The circle could not be squared. A clear comparison can be drawn here with the position of fever nurses. Some of the small fever institutions were affected by similar policies and could not meet the criteria. The Minster of Health forced the GNC to back down and to recognise training schools despite their inability to meet the criteria; in effect the GNC had to alter the criteria (Bendall and Raybould, 1969). Altering the criteria for mental deficiency nursing would have separated the mental deficiency branch from that of mental and essentially set up a separate supplementary register. That would have brought into question the one issue that no group wanted to face, this was whether work in mental deficiency institutions was true nursing. The October meeting of the Mental Nurses Committee deferred the issue until the election of a new General Nursing Council and the indecision continued while the idea that workers in mental deficiency institutions were nurses became more entrenched.

Conclusion

This chapter has examined debates within the GNC to throw light on why work with people with learning disabilities became part of the nursing profession. It has been argued that rather than some grand design it was a mixture of coincidence and organisational self-interest. The coincidence was the timing of the Nurses Registration Act that coincided with the implementation of the Mental Deficiency Act. Workers within institutions that were created under the Act were thought to require regulation and the infant General Nursing Council reluctantly and eventually provided the means. The importance for contemporary learning disability nursing is that their anomalous status within the nursing profession is far from new and that arguments about whether this work really is nursing have been active since the profession of nursing established its regulatory framework in the 1920s.

References

Abel Smith B (1960) *A History of the Nursing Profession*. Heinemann, London

Andrews J (1996) Identifying and providing for the mentally disabled in early modern London. In: Wright D, Digby A (eds) *From Idiocy to*

Mental Deficiency: Historical Perspectives on People with Learning Disabilities. Routledge, London

Bendall R, Raybould E (1969) *A History of the General Nursing Council for England and Wales 1919—1969*. HK Lewis and Co Ltd, London

Carpenter M (1985) *They Still Go Marching On, a Celebration of COHSE's First 75 Years*. COHSE

Dickens C (1844) *Martin Chuzzlewit*. London, Ballantyne Press

Dingwall R, Rafferty AM, Webster C (1988) *An Introduction to the Social History of Nursing*. Routledge, London

Frieze Stephens H (1926) The training of mental deficiency nurses. *Journal of Mental Science* **July:** 444–5

Laird S (1902) The International Congress of Nurses, Nursing the Insane. *Nursing Record and Hospital World* **1**(3): 166–8

McCutcheon M (1925) Institutional treatment of mental defectives, with special reference to occupation. *Journal of Mental Science* **71:** 694–703

McDowell M (1924) Letter to the editor. *Studies in Mental Inefficiency* **5**(2): 42–3

Nolan P (1993) *A History of Mental Health Nursing*. Chapman and Hall, London:

Nursing Times (1914a) An interesting appointment. *Nursing Times* **8**(8): 1001

Nursing Times (1914 b) Asylum Workers Association. *Nursing Times* **30**(5): 713

Nursing Times (1920) General Nursing Council. *Nursing Times* 20(11): 1360

Nursing Times (1921) Comment. *Nursing Times* **11**(6): 1921

Nursing Times (1923) General Nursing Council. *Nursing Times* **29**(12): 1248

Nursing Times (1926a) Nurses for mental defectives. *Nursing Times* **3**(3): 223

Nursing Times (1926b) Nurses for mental defectives. *Nursing Times* **22**(3): 458

Nursing Times (1926c) The nurse for mental defectives. *Nursing Times* **24**(7): 650

Nursing Times (1926d) Nurses for mental defectives. *Nursing Times* **23**(10): 939

Rafferty AM (1996) *The Politics of Nursing Knowledge*. Routledge, London

RcPsych (1895) *Education Committee Minutes.* 26.6. 1895

RcPsych (1926) *Education Committee Minutes*, 12.6.1926 / 12.7.1926 /Sherlock to Daniel, 8.12.1926

RcPsych (1919) *Education Committee Minutes*, 20.2.1919

RcPsych (1932) *Syllabus for the Examinations for the Certificate of Proficiency in the Nursing of Mental Defectives*, RMPA, 1932. This is the earliest syllabus available in the archives of the Royal College of Psychiatrists and is a revised version of earlier ones

Thomson M (1998) *The Problem of Mental Deficiency: Eugenics, Democracy and Social Policy in Britain c 1870–1959*. Clarenden Press, Oxford

Section Two:

Perspectives

CHAPTER 4

From the workhouse to citizenship: Four ages of learning disability

Tony Gilbert

Introduction

This chapter considers shifts in the way social policy has approached the question of learning disability from the 1970s onwards by focusing on the ideas or discourses that underpin policy development. However, to identify and fully appreciate these shifts we need to consider a longer trajectory enabling the tracing of continuity and change across the period rather than change alone (Emerson, 2005). Therefore, while the balance of the chapter is weighted towards the post-1970s, the journey begins in the mid-1800s; roughly the time specialisation within the Poor Law started to separate lunatics from the mass of the poor and destitute (Digby, 1996) laying the foundations for modern learning disability services (Neugebauer, 1996; Gladstone, 1996). Tracing continuity and change has particular advantages. It circumvents the assumption that this period is one of inevitable progress: a shift from darkness and ignorance towards enlightenment. Conversely, it also avoids the search for a 'lost or romantic age' of community and mutual support crushed under the relentless process of industrialisation (Rushton, 1996).

Taking a lead from contemporary academic shifts in the analysis of social policy (Lewis, 2000; Fink, 2004) this chapter aims to render explicit the discourses embedded in social policy during particular periods that underpin outcomes for all concerned, rather than becoming lost in the detail of particular policy interventions. In the process, four 'ages of learning disability' are described, which provide metaphors for the overarching strategy (Dreyfus and Rabinow, 1982) (*Table 4.1*) towards people with learning disability in that period: age of the workhouse; age of the colony; age of normalisation; and age of citizenship. As with any typology, these metaphors work as 'ideal types', that is, simplified models emphasising the main policy and service configurations at the time.

A second essential component to this analysis is the recognition that implementation of policy tends to proceed in fragmented ways producing

Table 4.1: The four ages of learning disability: Timeline

1850–1910	1910–1970	1970–1995	1995–present
Age of the workhouse	Age of the colony	Age of normalisation	Age of citizenship

wide variations both across and within regions and between specific localities, producing what is discussed here as the micro-politics of caring; the specific possibilities produced for those involved in particular localised configurations of services. One advantage of using metaphor is that it enables us to identify how particular discourses 'spill over' into subsequent ages. Mental deficiency colonies, for example, provided the dominant service model in the early 20th century. Nevertheless, the legacy of the colony model continues. Contemporary policy in the shape of *Valuing People* (Department of Health, 2001a) wrestles with the final closure of the colonies albeit in their later guise as learning disability hospitals, thus ensuring that traces of the discourses that produced the Mental Deficiency Acts (1913, 1927) live on. At the same time, the redevelopment of these buildings preserves part of their legacy for future generations.

Historical perspectives of learning disability also require us to consider the extent to which the population of people with learning disability has retained similar characteristics over time. Presently, the population of the UK is ageing, as is the age profile of people with learning disability, with life expectancy extending from 30 years in the 1930s to 66 plus years today (Bigby, 2004). This, in part, contributes to an anticipated increase of 1% in the total population of people with learning disability (Department of Health, 2001a). People with Down syndrome are living longer but apparently experiencing Alzheimer type changes leading to early onset dementia (Evenhuis et al, 2001). In the early part of the 20th century, many detainees of colonies were young able-bodied people detained under mental deficiency legislation as 'moral defectives'. In addition, a brief look at a purpose built colony in the early 20th century with its two storey villas and extensive farmlands quickly indicates that people with multiple disabilities formed a lesser proportion of the population.

The chapter concludes by considering potential developments in this relationship between social policy, people with learning disability and the range of workers involved in supporting this policy as the age of citizenship extends. The reader should note the terminology used often takes nomenclature from the period as a means of maintaining consistency between the discourses used and the subject positions established. While it is recognised that many people find these terms offensive, these terms are part of the social construction of learning disability. They encompass the legal, lay and medical descriptions of the people targeted by policy at that time and are therefore critical to understanding the histories of learning disability (Rushton, 1996).

Social policy and social construction: Discourse and the 'micro-politics' of learning disability

In itself, social policy is a somewhat ambiguous idea and as such attracts a range of attempts at definition. Usually definitions include a view on the role of the State in redistributing wealth from the most to the least well off in society, alongside establishing mechanisms protecting vulnerable sections of the community from the full effects of market forces, or from abuse and exploitation by unscrupulous characters (Lewis, 2000). The exact role of the State in this process changes over time. In the Victorian and Edwardian periods, the *laissez-faire* approach characterising early 19th century politics gradually gave way as the State increasingly intervened in the management of private concerns. This produced the great public programmes that established clean water and asylums, as well as a wide range of interventions concerned with things as far apart as school meals and early forms of pension.

Following the Second World War the post-war settlement in the UK produced a commitment between political parties to a new form of citizenship, a social citizenship (Marshall, 1996), based on the idea of a 'Welfare State' organised and managed on behalf of the population. Since the 1980s the respective roles of the State, the market and individuals/families, have progressively reconfigured to the point where, in contemporary terms, the role of the State is one of organising or co-ordinating the activity of a myriad of organisations across the statutory and independent sectors rather than the direct provision of services (Clarke and Newman, 1997); a shift paralleled by rhetoric, placing an increasing emphasis on individual responsibility, market-based (welfare) choices and self-management with people supported by rather than reliant on the State.

Adding further complications to these shifts is the reality that social policy progresses in fragmented and uneven ways (Lewis, 2000). In some cases, policy outlined at national level lacks the levers and drivers necessary to make things happen. For example, the Royal Commission in 1957 recognised the need to develop community-based services (Digby, 1996), a position later reinforced by the 1971 White Paper *Better Services for the Mentally Handicapped*. However, it was only in the 1990s with the passing of NHS and Community Care Act (1990) that a real shift towards community-based services began to take place. Historical and contemporary relationships between key agencies provide important insights into the micro-politics of specific localities and analysis of the relative importance given to developing services supporting people with learning disability. This also relates to priorities given to initiatives within specific services and critically it provides evidence of power relations and the localised exercise of power (Thomson, 1996; Gilbert, 2003). Existing relationships between local NHS and Local Authorities influence the role afforded to each in the development of community services. Moreover, such local configurations often determine the role constructed for the independent sector.

Other important considerations concern policy initiatives, which cross cut learning disability policy with unintended consequences. Policy developed in areas, for example childcare or adult social care, had the impact of causing revisions of policy either nationally or more locally resulting in policy making by default. Thomson (1996) identifies this effect in the way the expansion of welfare in the early 20th century affected practice concerning the mentally defective. Recently, the British Government published a Green Paper entitled *Independence, Well-being and Choice* (Department of Health, 2005) addressing social care for adults, including adults with learning disability; policy triggered partly because of the restructuring of Social Services, Health, and Education Departments, following the implementation of *Every Child Matters* (Department of Health, 2003). Further revisions to learning disability services will no doubt arise because of the White Paper *Our Health, Our Care, Our Say* (Department of Health, 2006), which seeks further mergers between what is left of Social Services departments (adult services) with the Primary Care Trusts.

A social constructivist approach to the question of learning disability enables exploration of the relationship between policy and discourse, highlighting ideas and meanings underpinning practices and interventions alongside the range of roles and identities produced. Essentially, the myriad of interactions occurring between individuals across multiple social institutions produce knowledge and experience of the social world. Such institutions are defined as sets of administrative processes, procedures and norms that bind a particular set of activities rather than necessarily being bounded by a physical setting, delimiting practice within each age (Mackintosh, 2000). Institutions include families, schools, workplaces, leisure centres, health and social services, churches, clubs, etc. This creates a space for social interactions which bring people into contact with a range of discourses or specific forms of knowledge underpinning social (language-based) practices maintained by these institutions (Potter, 1996), condensing emotions, attitudes and values within practices and so institutionalising meaning and experience. Together these activities inform opinions about particular sections of the community and produce the relationship between power and knowledge underpinning the micro-politics of any social milieu. In this context, power, rather than a coercive force, is productive, circulating the innumerable interactions between individuals creating particular possibilities for action (Foucault, 1980, 1984a).

Social construction gives primacy to the role of ideas over the role of the individuals concerned. Other accounts credit great men and women as the authors of particular ideas, for example, Francis Galton (1822–1911) as the creator or 'founding father' of eugenics. In contrast, social construction assumes discourses, a priority to great men and women, have an important role as conduits for particular configurations of discourse rather than as 'authors of the text' (Fairclough, 1992), developing the meanings associated with specific discourses and practices in an iterative process with other less prominent individuals and groups. Evidence of activity gathered through evaluation and research, disseminated in a range of professional and academic journals, further strengthens discourse. Outcomes are scrutinised from a range of sources and recorded, observed and reported on in a variety of ways, e.g. clinical records, management audits, and professional notes, which are collated, analysed, commented on and disseminated through a variety of media to provide evidence that further informs the very discourses on which social policy is developed.

Social constructivists use the concept of discourse to include all forms of communication: text, verbal, pictures, images, music, film, etc. along with the language and language-based practices supporting activity. These discursive formations are dynamic and therefore historically and culturally specific. Processes of interdiscursivity and intertextuality transform discourses as they have contact and merge with other discourses over time. In addition, 'orders of discourse' reconfigure from period to period with particular discourses losing credence or being displaced by emerging discourses. Indeed, we see this process across the history of learning disability with the dominance and then decline of moral, eugenic and medical discourses in the early to mid-20th century while the 1970s saw the advent of normalisation as hegemonic discourse (Brown and Smith, 1992). Latterly, citizenship is providing fresh discursive configurations (Walmsley, 1993; Kings Fund, 1999; Duffy, 2003; Fripp, 2005; Gilbert et al, 2005). It is of course entirely possible for a dominant discourse to decline only to re-emerge later in more refined forms as happened with the psychiatry of learning disability.

Such discourses inform and, informed by social policy, underpin the design of services and related processes and procedures. Once established as practice, e.g. supported living and person-centred planning, power/knowledge creates particular possibilities for clients, carers and workers while closing other possibilities. Recognising the relational nature of this process in creating possibilities and options for individuals, families and communities through the multiple interactions of users, workers and others is critical. Through interaction, mutual interpretations of meaning and events are generated which then fix people in particular social positions, shaping the very identities of those involved producing what is referred to as subject position, i.e. carer, nurse, social worker, person with learning disability, or person with challenging needs. It is of course possible to have multiple subject positions. In addition, acceptance of multiple perspectives and an assumption that there is no fixed truth(s) to discover is core to a social constructionist approach as all are products of human activity.

Viewing social policy as relational and the critical importance of subject position is central to this discussion (Lewis, 2000; Fink, 2004). The process of identifying people as having a learning disability is part of the process of defining those without learning disability. Constructed in comparison with non-learning disabled people, people with learning disability are identified as 'other' (Digby, 1996; Hall, 2001) and subjected to processes and procedures that separate, categorise and classify to what extent they differ from biological, psychological and social norms (Gilbert, 1995, 2003). At the same time, these differences become the concern of specialised workers who manage individuals through specific forms of practice relevant to each historically specific turn, thus reproducing their own identities as an outcome of interactions with the target group and related individuals, such as parents, carers, administrators, managers and policy makers. Identities of workers therefore develop in a way that is mutually dependent on the development of the 'other'.

Thus the formation of the identities of 'imbeciles' within mental deficiency colonies was inextricably linked with the identities of the attendants and mental welfare workers embedded within the institution. Later, in similar ways, the identities of the mentally handicapped persons in group homes and day centres are inextricably linked with the identities of day service officers, residential care workers, mental handicap nurses and social workers involved in managing community care services. Integral to this process is the social construction of space. Social policy defines social and institutional spaces. Space is critical to understanding the micro-politics of services and relates to both physical and social space, and who has rights of ownership. We can identify professionally dominated spaces such as workhouses, colonies, hospitals and a variety of group homes and day centres. Some spaces are private such as the homes of parent/carers although even here policy and regulation penetrate. Other spaces such as the homes of people with learning disability bounded by legal tenancy agreements produce new dynamics of space linked to citizenship (Gilbert et al, 2005).

What emerges from this brief overview is that understanding the emergence and development of social policy in relation to people with learning disability requires a multi-dimensional matrix. This matrix has to take account of policy, discourse, service developments and the subject positions produced. It also has to be sensitive to historical or temporal shifts and the importance of the spaces within which practices take place.

Age of the workhouse: Harmless idiots and dangerous lunatics?

The age of the workhouse (*Table 4.2*) is possibly the most ambiguous of the four ages put forward. The workhouse, offered here as the metaphor for the dominant service model, did not have as its central remit the management of people now considered as having a learning disability. Workhouses managed the poor and, as the 19th century progressed, not only provided relief to the destitute but also distinguished the deserving from the undeserving poor establishing the principle of 'less eligibility' (McClimens, 2005), evident in welfare policy today. For people with learning disability a number of other options (or spaces) existed; family-based relief, boarding out, and private and public 'idiot asylums'. Critically, people with learning disability retained a presence within communities for, as a group, policy had not yet set out to identify and manage their lives in specialised and segregated spaces. Provision also differed within the countries of the UK; special provisions such as the idiot asylums founded in the second half of the 19th century were not universally available. In the absence of other options, the workhouse was the backstop, the common denominator. One feature of the period is evident; community-based support was of central importance (Rushton, 1996) despite opinion being divided on its benevolence (Digby, 1996).

We begin the discussion around the mid point of the 19th century as the provisions of a plethora of legislation including the 1834 Poor Law (amendment) Act, the Lunacy Acts (1845, 1862), the Asylums Acts (1806, 1853) and the Idiots Act (1886) settled into place. Legislative output mirrored growing social and political concerns over 'national efficiency' focusing on the 'fitness' of the population and ability of the working class to defend the declining military and economic status of the British Empire (Mort, 1987). Nevertheless, both idiocy and lunacy had been legally proscribed conditions since the end of the 15th century. Central to concerns of this period was the need to separate idiots from lunatics as the King had greater responsibilities for the care of the latter than the former (Neugebauer, 1996). Lunatics and their families were entitled to the King's protection for their person and property without charge, whereas the King could charge idiots for their protection making them a more lucrative prospect. Moreover, idiots often contributed to their keep undertaking tasks in workhouse kitchens or similar (Rushton, 1996).

Legal and moral discourses distinguished the concepts of lunacy and idiocy. Characterised by a temporary loss of powers of thought and reason with the anticipation of recovery, lunacy was afforded a different status to idiocy which was considered permanent. No such recovery of rationality and thought was expected (Digby, 1996; Goodey, 1996). The social status of each shifted according to their fiscal worth, with idiots privileged in early modern

Table 4.2 The Age of the Workhouse 1850–1910

Discourses	Policy	Subject positions	Service developments	Spatial	Temporal
• Idiocy ≠ lunacy • Idiocy a condition apparent since birth • Idiots harmless • Idiocy a sub-human condition • Growing concerns over national efficiency • Benefits of education and training • Managerialism	• Poor law: less eligibility • Specialisation of poor law with Lunacy Acts • Origins of policy separation between idiots and lunatics • Separation of harmless idiots from dangerous persons • Community-based support key	• Idiots – thieves and vagabonds • Harmless idiots • Deserving poor • Sub-human • Workers • Ambiguous	• Workhouse • Boarding out • Private and public idiot asylums	• No specialised or segregated spaces specifically for idiots • Idiot asylums few and far between with progressive ethos • Schools for idiots – again a progressive ethos	• Population of idiots largely able-bodied many capable of simple work • Industrialisation continued movements from the countryside to the towns

times for the potential discussed above whereas in the mid to late 19th century this reversed due to the potential for recovery (Neugebauer, 1996). Definitions of idiocy and lunacy developed in opposition to one another: a dichotomy establishing idiots as 'other', supported by philosophical discourses promoting idiocy as a sub-human condition (Goodey, 1996), thus creating separate trajectories in social policy and practice that remain today.

Both Neugebauer and Rushton note that administration of relief to idiots had been organised and documented in Poor Law records for some time with Rushton commenting on the style of the records, which reflected the exercise of local power (micro-politics) rather than reflecting recognition of specific need. Managerialist discourse dominated the recording of transactions reflecting criticisms of welfare provision in later periods (Clarke and Newman, 1997; Gilbert, 2005a). In contrast, Andrews (1996) remarks on the invisibility of what he refers to as the mentally disabled noting that the majority of poor law parish records in London fail to refer to idiots or similar persons. Digby (1996) observes that at this point idiots only had walk-on parts on the social stage, usually as thieves and vagabonds.

This period has also been marked for the origins of medical domination of learning disability. However, Wright (1996) notes that medical practitioners had only a peripheral role at the time signing the 'Reception Orders' required by law to certify idiots prior to admission to an asylum. Moreover, this involved negotiating the grounds for certification with parents and family members, particularly fathers, who usually countersigned on behalf of the family (Wright, 1996). Thus, definitions of idiocy grew out of discourse fusing lay perspectives largely concerned with the ability to learn, protect oneself and competently engage in self-care with an administrative discourse concerned with the requirements of Reception Orders. Critical to certification was establishing the fact that the condition had persisted since birth.

Indeed, rather than a medical concern idiocy was an educational issue. A body of work, such as that of Edward Seguin (1866), provided a discourse of specific educational and training techniques as the means to improve the general habits of selected idiots. Potential to learn and train in aspects of work and self-care determined admission to the voluntary idiot asylums founded in the latter half of the 19th century which also operated with the expressed goal to return the person to his or her family following a period of training, often anticipated as five years. Certified idiots considered un-trainable were refused admission (Gladstone, 1996). Reflecting the growing prominence of this optimistic discourse of education and training for idiots the late 19th century saw the establishment of the first special schools. Gladstone (1996:155) notes that by 1903 there were special schools in London and 50 other authorities. However, Emerson (2005) notes this optimism soon slipped away as the expected gains failed to emerge, an interesting observation as an optimistic educational discourse re-emerged in the 1970s in the guise of behaviour modification (Scheerenberger, 1987) dominated by clinical psychologists (Race, 1999).

Therefore, the key discourses at the time were educational in relation to the training of idiots and managerial in terms of the identification of idiots, the administration of relief and the issuing of Reception Orders. Subject positions for people certified as idiots identified persons in need of protection, lacking capacity for rational thought or potential for recovery, a condition persisting since birth but not necessitating confinement to specialised managed spaces. Control over the individual's life and property rested with the family, with the medical profession's role limited to confirming idiocy. Worker's identities are ambiguous. Outside of the medical practitioners, there are earlier references to keepers and nurses in the context of boarding out. Lunatic asylums and workhouses had attendants but medical control of idiocy is somewhat overstated as many of the idiot asylums lacked a resident medical superintendent well into the 20th century (Gladstone, 1996; Jackson, 1996). Andrews (1996) concludes that research on the identities of these workers is as neglected as the identities of idiots themselves.

Age of the colony: Eugenics, heredity, pauperism and the parasitic feeble-minded

The decline of optimism in the potential of idiots to learn coincides with the rise of probably the darkest period in the history of learning disability. Heralding the dawn of the age of the colony (*Table 4.3*) are the conclusions of the Royal Commission on the Care and Control of the Feeble Minded (1908) and passing of the 1913 Mental Deficiency Act, leading to the establishment of a large-scale service that aimed to segregate the 'mentally defective'. This 'age' includes the later transition to 'mental subnormality' and the advent of the hospital system under the British National Health Service. Combining the colonies and the hospitals under one 'age' highlights the continuity in discursive structure, which maintained a service model based on the use of highly specialised and segregated spaces. Mental deficiency colonies had similarities with the asylum model implemented in the latter half of the 19th century for the management of lunatics. A number of colonies were purpose built with a familiar two-storey 'villa' type arrangement of buildings with some single storey buildings set around an administration block. However, a large number of buildings and sites commissioned as colonies had previously functioned as workhouses, lunatic asylums, epileptic colonies and homes for inebriates, private and voluntary idiot asylums, and special schools.

Mental deficiency colonies materialised as a consequence of the emergence in the late 19th century and early 20th century of a new discursive

Table 4.3: The Age of the Colony 1910–1970

Discourse	Policy	Subject positions	Service developments	Spatial	Temporal
• Mental deficiency and eugenics • Extended to include anti-social behaviour • Sexuality – hereditary pauperism and moral deficiency • Different from the normal population • Medicalisation • Education discourse challenging discourse of mental deficiency	• Mental Deficiency Acts • Identification and compulsory detention • Segregation and no reproduction	• Mentally defective as dangerous, predatory parasitic and deceitful – different from the normal population • Feeble-minded women the most dangerous • Workers as wise to the ways of the defective exerting control to render them useful	• Large-scale development of the mental deficiency colony • Special contraception • Guardianship order • Reinvented as hospitals post-1945 • Emergence of psychiatry as manager of mental deficiency	• Development of specialised segregated spaces in colonies • Shifting of those identified as mentally defective from the general population to the colonies • Gender segregation to prevent reproduction	• Mental deficiency not harmless • Military and economic tensions in the developed world • Decline of eugenics as scientifically valid • Establishment of the Welfare State • Population of mentally defective showing changes with increasing dependency

structure that was to dominate in one form or another for the next 80 years. 'Harmless idiots', once separated from dangerous persons and lunatics, and ejected from the asylums (Richardson, 2005) are now 'a problem'. Redefined under the Mental Deficiency Act (1913) as idiots, feeble-minded, imbeciles and the morally defective, this section of the population is targeted with a wholly unsympathetic discourse aimed at identifying and segregating the 'dangerous' feeble-minded and other defectives from the rest of the population. Underpinning this discourse are the key concerns of Victorian Britain: sex, sexual practices and reproduction, echoing Foucault's (1984b) observation that the Victorian period saw an unparalleled expansion in discourses concerning sexuality and sexual practices. Four key concerns dominated debates: the Malthusian couple, the masturbating child, the hysterical woman and the perverse adult (Weeks, 1985), all of which have consequences for people with learning disabilities (Gilbert, 1998).

Provisions of the Act also extended beyond the colony walls placing under guardianship orders large numbers of people designated mentally defective who remained living with their families. Not only were parent guardians paid but, as Thomson (1996) observes, it would be wrong to place family-based and statutory care in opposition. Both affected each other in negotiations over the local implementation of the Act. Moreover, the category of moral defective provides an interesting development as it extended the social construction of learning disability to include a new social group, and technologies of social control to a new range of behaviours (Gladstone, 1996). Apparently immoral behaviour, usually sexual promiscuity in women and a lack of employability in males, constructed as a deficiency in the capacity to reason morally, established for politicians, scientists and a range of professionals a scientific link between antisocial behaviour and a congenital underdevelopment of the brain. This occurs despite no evidence of a general inability to reason.

This new discourse of mental deficiency grew to dominate political and social debate in the 20 years or so preceding the Mental Deficiency Act. Articulated by enthusiasts of the time, including Francis Galton, Winston Churchill, Mary Dendy and Alfred Tredgold, this discourse claimed a 'scientific morality'. Concepts from the emerging sciences of genetics and psychology, in particular work establishing the 'Intelligence Quotient' as the scientific measurement of intelligence, are articulated with concerns over the physical and moral 'fitness' of the British working class. These concepts merged with racist ideas about the supremacy of the British Race and the Empire (Digby, 1996), thus establishing eugenics as a credible and scientific means of managing the population (Jackson, 1996; Richardson, 2005). Eugenicists postulated that pauperism was hereditary thus constructing poverty as a question of reproduction rather than the distribution of wealth.

Eugenics, paralleled in the USA, under the Mental Hygiene Movement (Digby, 1996), and in Europe, saw the mentally defective or, more accurately, the 'feeble minded' as predatory, parasitic and dangerous to the 'quality' of the race. Most dangerous was the feeble-minded woman who provided a threat to both the family and the nation (Jackson, 1996; Cox, 1996).

Eugenicists' zeal focused on the potential for 'unfit' persons to reproduce. Across the Western world, this led to debates and policies aimed at preventing procreation with the wholescale segregation of the mentally defective, first from the community and second a gender-based segregation from one another. Most countries debated and implemented either explicitly or implicitly sterilisation of the mentally defective, medical abortion and the possibility of programmes of euthanasia, but few went this far. The UK adopted segregation, Sweden and the USA added sterilisation and infamously Nazi Germany implemented a programme of euthanasia (Atkinson et al, 1997; Emerson, 2005). Elements of this sterilisation policy remain today (Keywood, 1995; Brammer, 2005). However, it would be wrong to credit eugenicists with inventing a discourse that supported genocide since philosophical and religious discourses proposing extermination of defectives had persisted for centuries (Goodey, 1996). What the eugenicists achieved was credibility for earlier discourses by adding objective scientific rationale for separating human beings from a sub-human strata and a way of establishing membership of either group by objectively and scientifically measuring intelligence. Therefore, discursively, eugenics achieved the status of science and truth.

Segregation was the primary objective of eugenicist's policy. Education and training of mental defectives provided important distractions as they aided the running of the institution and relieved some of the financial burden (Jackson, 1996). However, there was to be no notion of a return to the community. As such, eugenicists were scathing of the voluntary idiot asylums for their policy of rehabilitation to the community and the special schools for their discourse supporting a continuum of mental ability rather than a sharp divide between the fit and the unfit (Jackson, 1996). Eugenicists were committed to the idea of compulsory life-long segregation, a spatial contraception, ensuring that every defective died without passing on his or her 'horrible tradition'. Convinced by the hereditary basis of mental deficiency they placed considerable effort in tracing the defective relatives and ancestors of people identified as feeble-minded disseminating their scientific searches and conclusions in a range of medical and other respected scientific journals. This provided a self-fulfilling process reinforcing the truth and power of the discourse. Jackson notes increasing interest in the topic in the last decade of the 19th century from medical practitioners who up to now had shown little interest outside of the few that had a personal interest in the area, such as Langdon-Down, Little and Tredgold.

Mental deficiency colonies established the first large-scale service model for people with learning disabilities, producing a specialisation within medicine that would become a distinct branch of psychiatry (Atkinson et al, 1997). Supported by disciplines of medicine and psychology the Royal Medico-Psychological Association (RMPA) developed the first qualifications in working with the mentally defective, establishing the idea that specialist knowledge was required to manage them (Mitchell, 2002; Gilbert, 1995). Alongside, a variety of texts emerged, including academic journals, which explored the identification, definition and management of the mentally defective. Subject positions for the mentally defective held a deviant identity and unbridled sexuality in need of segregation and management. In contrast, staff trained and wise to the ways of the defective, skilled in surveillance and management rendered defectives docile and productive, ensuring the effective running of institutions. The eugenics' response to mental deficiency was not without its discontents. Older discourses persisted as research continued to emerge, which challenged notions of a clear dividing line between the normal population and the mentally defective (Pearson and Jaederholm, 1914; Jackson, 1996).

The period following the Second World War brought the advent of the Welfare State and a new conception of citizenship (Marshall, 1996). Eugenics lost credence, partly because of the horrors of the concentration camps in Europe where the Nazis killed some 70000 disabled people in euthanasia programmes (Richardson, 2005) and partly due to the advent of the National Health Service in the UK. The transition to the NHS reinvented mental deficiency colonies as mental deficiency hospitals and converted the workers from attendants to nurses. Medical discourses subordinated the excesses of eugenics. Focusing on genetics and the causation of mental deficiency, the moral tone of eugenics was subdued and the idea of hereditary pauperism largely discredited. The qualification for workers moved under the auspices of the General Nursing Council (GNC). The transition from colonies to hospitals, and attendants to workers produced new subject positions for both 'patients' and 'workers' making a significant contribution to the conversion of the mentally defective from dangerous and deviant to sick and in need of care. The GNC qualification as a nurse for the mentally defective (RNMD) cemented workers within medical discourses alongside notions of sickness and cure, and their associated practices.

However, the physical and spatial presence of the service changed little. Sexual discourse focused on hygiene and venereal disease, particularly syphilis, as the hospitals retained the policy of spatial contraception. Changes in the structure of the population of people with learning disability, in particular those living in the hospitals saw a greater proportion with high support needs due to high levels of physical, sensory and mental disability. Numbers of severely disabled children and adults began causing accommodation problems in facilities that were already overcrowded and designed for a largely ambulant population. The large two- and three-storey blocks that made up the bulk of the accommodation in mental deficiency hospitals was unsuitable. In addition, the conditions in many of the hospitals were very poor, particularly those with buildings inherited from previous centuries, problems well known to the British Cabinet at the time of the inception of the NHS but which, due to institutionalised medical power in the wider NHS, remained largely unchallenged up to the late 1960s (Klein, 1989). Possibly the first major change in the discursive structure of the service was the passing in 1959 of a new Mental Health Act which removed many of the features of the older structure. Out went the terminology of mental deficiency to be replaced by 'mental subnormality'. Also removed was the idea of compulsory detention for life. The Act established the rights of individuals, unless subjected to specific detention orders, to leave the hospital should they wish. At the same time the Act promoted the idea of community-based services managed by local authorities.

Age of normalisation: From patients to clients and consumers

At the start of age of normalisation (*Table 4.4*), over 50 000 people of all ages were resident in long-stay mental subnormality hospitals (Mittler, 1978). Klein (1989) identifies the role of Richard Crossman, then Secretary of State for Health and Social Security, in breaking the medical stranglehold on the allocation of NHS resources that prevented shifts to the long-stay sector comprising mental subnormality, psychiatric and geriatric hospitals. In 1969, Crossman opportunistically sanctioned the first of a series of public inquiries into practices in mental subnormality hospitals. Initiated following complaints of ill treatment and mismanagement (Department of Health and Social Security, 1969, 1971, 1974, 1978) these inquiries discredited the role of mental subnormality hospitals along with medicine's ability to manage mental subnormality itself, thus opening the discursive space around people with learning disabilities in ways not seen for over a century. Public outrage over the management of the population of people with learning disability was not limited to the UK; similar inquiries were occurring in the USA (Scheerenberger, 1987; Emerson, 2005). Government responses in both cases produced rhetoric of a new deal for people with learning disability through either policy declarations (Department of Health and Social Security, 1971) or presidential announcements such as John F Kennedy's revitalised humanitarianism (Scheerenberger, 1987).

Opening this discursive space marked the start of a period of major change

Table 4.4 The Age of Normalisation 1970–1995

Discourse	Policy	Subject positions	Service developments	Spatial	Temporal
• Revitalised humanism • Normalisation • Sexuality • Education • Medicine discredited to re-emerge later • Consumerism • Managerialism	• Better services for the mentally handicapped • NHS and Community Care Act • Case management • Division of health and social care • An ordinary life • Uneven developments • Micro-politics	• Vulnerable members of society • Nursing identity contradicts normalisation • Life history work – alternative identity for people with learning disability • Welfare consumer • Community nurses/workers	• Deinstitutionalisation • Locally based hospital units • Ordinary housing • Day centres central to community-based services • User involvement • Advocacy	• Segregated spaces in isolated hospitals reduced • Specialised spaces emerging across local communities • Dispersal of welfare across independent sector • Increased emphasis on role of the family in providing support • Children no longer admitted to hospitals	• Inquiries discredit hospitals • Margaret Thatcher – New Right see the end of the welfare consensus • Reduced role for the State • Welfare a problem • Recession and high unemployment • Increasing dependency of population

in the management of people with learning disabilities across the developed world (Scheerenberger, 1987; Emerson, 2005). Deinstitutionalisation of people with learning disabilities began, linked to rhetoric of community care: an idea that was to provide the basis for policy development to the present despite a number of reincarnations. The hegemony of the medical model fractured allowing not only a new configuration of discourse but also the emergence of new power relations, albeit only among the different professionals involved (Race, 1999). People with learning disabilities had to wait some time before their participation became essential (Department of Health, 2001b). Multi-disciplinary team working and multi-agency approaches developed as much as a bastion against the excess of medical power as they were attempts to co-ordinate activity across a range of interests. Discursively, a configuration of three core discourses: normalisation, sexuality and education dominate the strategy of community care for people with mental handicaps. Sexuality and education had clear continuities with earlier discourses while normalisation, an influence in Scandinavian countries for some time (Emerson, 2005), was a relatively new entrant to the UK. Nevertheless, we should remind ourselves that community-based options for people with learning disability existed in the 19th century.

Normalisation provided an optimistic discourse and a basis for coherent change although it would take some time before services felt its full impact. Hegemonic in its influence, normalisation provided the organising discourse for learning disability services subsuming discourses of sexuality and education in a new discursive structure promoting community presence, and participation in everyday lives, personal relationships and socially appropriate behaviours. A dynamic discourse, normalisation has undergone a number of different interpretations and configurations following periods of application, evaluation and revision (cf. Bank-Mikkelson, 1969, 1980; Nirje, 1972; Wolfensberger, 1972, 1983a; O'Brien and Tyne, 1981). Influenced by mid-range sociological theories focusing on deviance and labelling (Barnes, 1996) and more latterly devaluation (Race et al, 2005), power relations produced by discourses of normalisation opened up a range of new possibilities for the design of services and relationships between people with mental handicaps, carers, professionals and the communities where they lived. Reversing the principle of segregation and block treatment established in the age of the colony normalisation, later social role valorisation (Wolfensberger, 1983a; Race, 1999; Race et al, 2005), promoted individuality, choice and presence within the community. Commitments that ensured the management of personal lives of people with learning disabilities were going to take a new turn establishing techniques dedicated to the micro-management of every individual by a range of 'experts'. Central to this has been a succession of technologies designed to enable this micro-management such as 'Individual Programme Planning' (Blunden et al, 1987), 'Life Planning' (Jenkins et al, 1988), 'Shared Action Planning' (Brechin and Swain, 1987), through to case (care) management and brokerage models (Brandon, 1991).

Early concerns in the age of normalisation focused on the search for a new residential model to accommodate people presently in hospital, which would have three key functions. First, it would provide humane living arrangements ending the great dormitories and gender segregation of the subnormality hospitals; second, it would provide a physical presence in the local community; and third, it would fracture the power block represented by the institutionalised interests cemented in the workings of the subnormality hospitals (Ryan and Thomas, 1980). A number of 'experiments' in providing community-based housing options for people with mental handicaps emerged, such as the 'Locally Based Hospital Units' (Felce et al, 1980) established in the then Wessex Health Region. Accommodation centred on a 25-bedded hostel type residential building within local communities providing accommodation on a mixed gender and mixed ability basis.

Within a short period, opinion shifted, accepting the maximum size for accommodation as eight places. *An Ordinary Life* (Kings Fund, 1980) promoted further reductions in maximum size to four places. Opinion remained divided to the relative effectiveness of each model (Felce et al, 1980; Felce, 1989; Emerson and Hatton, 1994; Hatton and Emerson, 1996). However, each, in its own way, supported the advance of normalisation principles.

Nevertheless, some 'ordinary life' projects were compromised by joining two or more four-bedroom houses together, or four-bedroom bungalows built on campuses of similar bungalows. Early Scandinavian influence waned replaced by American discourse emerging from community living projects such as ENCORE (East Nebraska Community Office of Mental Retardation). Ironically, while US models of de-institutionalisation were prominent this represented something of a triumph of rhetoric over reality for, as Digby (1996) points out, the overall numbers of people in US institutions changed little once the expansion of the private sector institutions is taken into account.

Education, largely concerned with the management of behaviour and vocational training, and the management of sexuality provided the pillars on which programmes of normalisation and deinstitutionalisation rested. Major programmes developed aimed at promoting socially appropriate behaviours among the mentally handicapped, who were now conceived as residents or clients rather than patients, while also increasing competencies in these areas in the supporting professionals and carers. Educational discourse, while providing a rationale for vocational activities in day services, was nevertheless dominated by psychological techniques informed by operant conditioning. Focusing on both adaptive and maladaptive behaviour it produced a range of approaches designed to develop individual skills as well as techniques for the modification and change of undesirable behaviours. Emerson (2005) highlights the utility of these techniques, harnessed to support community presence. As noted earlier, this provided discursive continuity with the optimism surrounding the training programmes for idiots in the late 19th century. Emerson also notes Tizard's earlier (1954) assertion that the young feeble-minded who formed the majority of the population in mental subnormality hospitals could, after a period of training and education, return to the community, demonstrating further discursive continuity with earlier times.

Educational discourse made two major contributions. First, it promoted the development of day centres as core provision in learning disability services in contrast to options for paid work (Powell and Flynn, 2005). Second, it produced the social construction of challenging behaviour and its management by non-medical approaches (Blunden and Allen, 1987; Emerson, 2001). Behavioural approaches mounted a challenge to the use of poly-pharmacological approaches to managing behaviour that developed during the later stages of the age of the colony. The significance of this challenge concerned the prescription of medications when doubts existed over the efficacy and ethics of using powerful poisons to subdue learned behaviours (Tyler, 1997). As the prescription of anti-psychotics provided much of the basis for psychiatry's continuing foothold in learning disability these doubts further undermined its role.

New discourses of sexuality accompanied the shift to community-based services. Ideas of a deviant sexuality central to discourses of mental deficiency, configured in the spatial contraception of the colony and hospital models, gave way. Community houses followed a normal gender mix while many hospitals attempted to provide a mixed gender environment in wards. Consequentially a new approach was required. Yet, we would be mistaken to see this development as a new freedom for people with learning disability. It certainly opened up new possibilities. However, it remained that the sexuality of people with learning disabilities, considered as incomplete, therefore required management by an array of specialists and support workers (Gilbert, 1998). Discursively, we can identify two major themes within sexuality at this point: first, a focus on promoting and supporting the development of living arrangements and personal relationships with appropriate behaviours and a degree of safety; second, a concern over sexual abuse linked with broader concerns about abuse and its consequences on behaviour (O'Callaghan et al, 2003). It had soon become clear that the movement from hospitals to small community housing had not removed the threat of sexual exploitation or other forms of abuse. At the same time, concerns around consent questioned the nature of many of the relationships formed between mentally handicapped people and between mentally handicapped and non-mentally handicapped people (ARC/NAPSAC, 1993; Craft, 1994; Brown and Thompson, 1997; Department of Health/Home Office, 2000).

Discrediting the mental subnormality hospitals brought changing political imperatives and different roles for professionals concerned (Johnson, 2001). The emergence of discourses of normalisation and the decline of medicine in mental handicap seriously challenged the appropriateness of the nursing qualification in mental subnormality. Initially raised by the Briggs Committee report (Department of Health and Social Security, 1972) into the structure of nurse education and later reinforced by the majority report of the Jay Committee (1979), which called for the end of the nursing qualification and the establishment of a new caring profession for what it referred to as the mentally handicapped. Proponents of the majority report of the Jay Committee were highly influenced by the discourses which underpinned the Seebohm Report (1968) that established the ground for the emergence of a new generic social work profession in the early 1970s while the dissenting minority held to the preservation of the nursing qualification (Williams, 1979a, b).

However, the political tide was changing with the election of a 'New Right' Government under Margaret Thatcher in 1979, strongly opposed to public sector professions in any guise and antagonistic toward social work in particular (Langan, 1993). Drawing on discourses from the user movement (Clarke and Newman, 1997) and anti-professional stances of academics such as Illich (1979), the new administration's agenda did not include establishing any 'new caring professions'. It had a very different programme. Consequently, leaving the question of the role of 'nurses for the mentally handicapped' to be determined by changing events rather than policy, such events periodically revived the debate (Chief Nursing Officer, 1985; Cullen, 1991; Sines, 1993; Kay et al, 1995). Nevertheless, a new syllabus (English National Board for Nursing, Midwifery and Health Visiting, 1985) saw the discourse of normalisation refashion somewhat the focus and identity of these workers. Subject positions shifted, orientating away from associations with medical nursing and illness towards education and behaviour management alongside community presence. Ideas of supporting moves towards independence in definitions of nursing (Henderson, 1991) rearticulated with discourses of enablement and empowerment begin to provide a bridge between discourses of nursing and normalisation, a feat of discursive gymnastics as normalisation was fundamentally opposed to associations that promoted images of the mentally handicapped as sick (Wolfensberger, 1983b).

This discursive space also opened up possibilities for new configurations of qualifications as institutions looked to resolve continuing uncertainty provoked initially by the Jay Committee's conclusions now compounded by ongoing changes in the relationship between health and social services, as community-based services were established. In this space, a number of courses leading to joint qualifications with social work were established (Brown, 1994). However, social work had its own problems, least of all was learning disability, as childcare failures continued to haunt the profession and the political environment became increasingly hostile to its role and function (Langan, 1993). This period also saw a significant development in the management of people with mental handicaps away from institutional settings such as hospitals with the gradual establishment in most areas of community mental handicap teams (Hall and Russell, 1985). Locked within the normalisation discourse, community teams extended support to people with learning disabilities living in the home with 'family carers' or people with learning disabilities living independently. This established new technologies for the micro-management of people with mental handicaps while extending the capacity for surveillance far beyond anything achieved in the age of the colony. Alongside this, new roles emerged for workers in the community. Critically, these new roles provided the foundations that would support the shift in provision that was to take place with the implementation of the National Health Service and Community Care Act (1990).

Exploring the micro-politics of the closure of hospitals and the development of community-based services is of central importance to understanding why developments took diverse shapes and proceeded at different paces in different areas. Analysis of micro-politics identifies localised configurations of power and the specific way the discursive structure provided by normalisation and its associated discourses is organised. Cautioning against seeing deinstitutionalisation as a smooth and uncontested movement of hospital closure alongside the development of community-based services, Emerson and Hatton (1994) note the different pace of change across the four countries of the UK, between the English regions, and within specific localities. Moreover, they note the wide variation in the type of services established, influenced by local policy, service infrastructure and culture. Micro-politics determine the key organisations providing particular services in a locality, which in turn produced a number of innovative and imaginary approaches to maximising opportunities to develop responsive services. In some areas health services retreated to providing only specialist peripatetic services, in other areas social services took a lead role while in others independent sector organisations were invited or created to take developments forward. Particular examples of innovation and new possibilities emerged in the local implementation of joint management, joint financing and joint commissioning arrangements (Rose, 1993; Gilbert and Rose, 1998).

The early 1990s brought a decisive shift in the configuration of the discourse of normalisation through exposure to new political commitments seeking to establish market-based approaches to welfare. The passing of the NHS and Community Care Act (1990) brought new impetus to deinstitutionalisation as the then Conservative Government sought to reconfigure expectations of the State in relation to welfare. A revised discourse of community care emerged, shifting responsibility for continuing care away from the statutory sector to the private and voluntary sector and/or the family (Clarke and Newman, 1997). Normalisation and its associated discourses of education and sexuality were now configured in a discursive structure dominated by discourses of consumerism and managerialism; ideas concerning user involvement became refashioned through the emergence of a 'new' subject position where service users became welfare consumers (Clarke and Newman, 1997). Subsumed in the process was a longer standing discourse of participation or advocacy committed to political involvement and change. In addition, the Act promoted user involvement and managerialism as further challenges to professional dominance of service development and delivery. Consumerism aimed to promote choice through market-based options rather than professional definitions of need while managerialist discourse subjugated professional priorities to management imperatives using technologies such as target setting, budgeting, standard setting, audit, and quality. Processes such as participation and advocacy became institutionalised in organisational procedures linked to managerial priorities, leading to criticisms that managerialism bureaucratised involvement to meet priorities of organisations not the needs of service users (Beresford et al, 1997).

Case management and brokerage, often deployed through community mental handicap teams, extended managerialist discourse to individualised care planning. Moreover, this enabled managerialism to penetrate the discrete corridors of individual communities and the myriad of interactions enclosed in personal lives. Furthermore, competitive tendering introduced new disciplinary processes to bear on organisations developing community-based services, sometimes with painful consequences (Gilbert, 2005b). At the same time, financial constraints saw social service departments redrawing eligibility criteria in line with Government interpretations where 'needs only existed where resources were available' (Langan, 1998). Learning disability in itself was no longer a sufficient condition to receive a service while attempts to define and separate out healthcare from social care undermined many of the joint working and joint financing arrangements established in the period prior to the Act. In addition, this separation reinforced the principle that healthcare, free at the point of need, was quantitatively and qualitatively different from social care, which became increasingly means-tested providing echoes of the Poor Law and its discourse of the deserving and undeserving.

Moreover, this reordering of 'healthcare' in learning disability provided an anchor for the re-emergence of medicine, or more accurately psychiatry, as a powerful discourse laying claim to primacy over a range of behaviours through a newly configured discourse of mental illness in learning disability (Moss and Patel, 1993; Moss et al, 2000). This notion was rejected by psychiatry itself based on the assumption that people with learning disability lacked the maturity of intellect required to experience mental illnesses (Borthwick-Duffy, 1994). This newly configured discourse extended the social construction of learning disability to another range of behaviours and social contexts, including criminal justice (Holland et al, 2002), thus cementing further the position of psychiatry in the management of certain sections of the population with learning disability. The discourse of mental illness in learning disability also re-established the legitimacy of the use of anti-psychotic medications on behaviours. However, the involvement of medicine in learning disability through either psychiatry or general practice has continually failed to resolve many of the problems experienced by people with learning disability seeking to access 'ordinary' healthcare (Kerr et al, 1996; Mencap, 1998; Department of Health, 1999, 2001a; Scottish Executive, 2002).

In a parallel development given impetus by the discourses of user-involvement and consumerism underpinning the NHS and Community Care Act a range of methods for 'giving voice' to the concerns and experiences of people with learning disabilities developed (Walmsley, 2001; Boote et al, 2002). Choice and participation were also integral to the discourse of normalisation (O'Brien, 1987) although often limited in practice to consumerist rather than political applications (Gilbert, 2005a). Advocacy for people with learning disability began in the 1970s (Wolfensberger, 1977) and a number of advocacy groups emerged at a local level throughout the UK in the 1980s along with a national movement under the umbrella of 'People First' (Goodley and Ramcharan, 2005). Learning disability also began to interest oral historians who produced accounts of the life experiences of people with learning disability (Atkinson et al, 1997), opening up space for what Foucault (1984a) described as subjugated knowledges. These once discredited voices of people such as learning disability service users provide the embers of resistance, which establish the basis for the emergence of alternative subject positions for people with learning disability; subject positions they themselves had a hand in designing (Digby, 1996; Atkinson et al, 1997).

As we look back from the mid 1990s, the age of normalisation has brought profound changes in the social position of people with learning disability. Subject positions have shifted from that of a dependent with little choice and no meaningful opinion to one of an active consumer of welfare services consulted about service development and change. However, people with learning disabilities remain largely dependent on these services for their access to social life with, in many instances, a single service providing the range of support. More recently, the role of day centres attracted scrutiny (Dowson, 1998). Once the bedrock of community-based services, day centres, ironically, now replaced hospitals as the symbol of segregated and institutional approaches supporting people with learning disability. In particular the 'Changing Days' project offered alternative models for work, leisure and education (Wertheimer, 1996).

People with learning disability are present in an ever-increasing range of social spaces albeit located in the expanding independent and voluntary sectors, a direct response to the statutory sectors' reconfigured role as a co-ordinator of services rather than direct provider. Technologies of care management, brokerage and individual care planning extend both the range and complexity of methods managing the lives of people accompanied by an ever-increasing array of professionals and support workers. Growth of the independent and voluntary sector is also having a profound impact on the organisations operating there with many now resembling the statutory sector organisations they replaced in terms of size and complexity, management structures, qualifications of staff, etc. Indeed, many organisations now reconfigured as independent organisations, were once part of statutory sector organisations. Equally, the sector remains almost exclusively funded by public money, therefore, from a fiscal perspective, maintaining the significance of the Welfare State despite the managerial discourse promoting competitive tendering and contract monitoring.

Age of citizenship: Learning disability in the 21st century: Rights and responsibilities, obligations and risk

The shift to the age of citizenship (*Table 4.5*) is more subtle than shifts between other ages. Emerging in the mid to late 1990s we are still in the very early days of the age of citizenship and its promise is yet to be revealed. Nevertheless, enough time has passed to identify the re-configuration of discourses around intellectual disability as well as emerging consequences. Possibly the most significant discursive shifts in intellectual disability emerge from its ambiguous and contested relationship with the Disability Movement which, while not focusing on intellectual disability as such, has had profound effects on the way disability in general is conceived (Wistow, 2005). Challenging conceptions of disability through the articulation of 'the

Table 4.5: The Age of Citizenship 1995–present

Discourse	Policy	Subject positions	Service developments	Spatial	Temporal
• Social model of disability • Citizenship and human rights • Responsibility and obligation • Social exclusion • Social capital • Decline of normalisation • Sexuality • Education • Communitarianism • Managerialism • Risk	• Disability Discrimination Act • Direct payments • *Valuing People* • *Our Health, Our Care, Our Say* • Merging of adult social services and PCTs • Tactics of social inclusion • Three trajectories produced: self-managing; empowered; risky • Six keys to citizenship	• Three trajectories – self-managing: citizens, tenants, workers, parents, employers – empowered: damaged subjects – risky: dangerous • Workers: subject position and identity linked with role in managing risk	• Support for ordinary lives/ supported living • Personal care plans • Re-invented case management • Decline of the day centre • Work opportunities • Parenting support • Personal assistants employed directly by individuals	• Myriad of spaces across social fabric • Own space created via tenancies and other forms of home ownership • Specialised workers enter space controlled by individuals • Increased role for the market • Welfare services increasingly dispersed across independent and voluntary sector	• End of State as a direct provider for adult community care services • Intellectual disability in itself no longer sufficient condition for welfare • Anticipated rise of 1% in population of people with intellectual disability

social model of disability', this movement rejected ideas of impairment, normalisation and 'quota' approaches to promoting social roles for disabled people, substituting a theoretical and political model emphasising the social nature of the barriers excluding disabled people from work and other aspects of political and social life (Finklestein, 1980; Oliver, 1990).

Defining itself as a 'new social movement' pursuing a 'civil liberties' approach in line with other identity movements such as those based on gender, sexuality and race (Hughes and Paterson, 1997), the Disability Movement reversed the subjugation of discourses of participation by consumerism, and linked with a broader debate concerning citizenship and human rights. This culminated in claims of major political successes with the passing of the Disability Discrimination Act (1995) and the Community Care [Direct Payments] Act (1996) (Beresford et al, 1997; Morris, 1997). Direct Payments, although not extended to people with learning disabilities in the first instance, laid the groundwork offering 'real' power to users, as they become 'real' consumers with the potential to employ their own support staff. The Disability Movement also provided further challenges to the domination of services and service delivery by the institutionalised interests of welfare professions as well as inertia from the legislature in enforcing laws against discrimination. Hegemony of normalisation waned for, while it was sympathetic to the idea of citizenship, its underlying theoretical structure of devaluation, deviance, labelling and stigma struggles with the concept, especially when compared to the social model of disability. However, Race et al (2005) make a sterling attempt to reconcile the gap by drawing out the connections between the frustration of citizenship and the experience of being devalued. Nevertheless, normalisation's simplistic conceptualisation of social integration marked by 'community participation' meant this remained an elusive goal with little evidence of achievement. A theoretical oversight, which is largely the consequence of differences in the conception of citizenship between the USA, where Wolfensberger developed the concept, and the UK, where there is a stronger tradition of social citizenship. A critical limitation is now policy demanded social inclusion as a central aim provoking a search for more sophisticated approaches, mainly by looking to sociological discourses; in particular, those already associated with citizenship, such as social capital, community development, communitarian theory and neighbourhood studies.

Nevertheless, normalisation had gone a long way, establishing physical presence in communities although, as Bigby et al (2002) note, this was often in anonymous public spaces. Choice had become an essential criterion in social policy. However, normalisation and deinstitutionalisation had a growing band of discontents. Among others, Chappell (1992) criticised normalisation as a professionally dominated discourse focused on service delivery incapable of promoting the political and social advancement of people with intellectual disability. Operationally, divisions materialised over how to interpret normalisation. In particular, disagreements related to the extent to which people's lives should be organised and managed in community homes, e.g. choice versus structured support. Alongside this emerged documented failures of community homes to promote good practice and quality of life (Emerson and Hatton, 1994). Others (Kinsella, 1993; Kinsella and Ward, 1993a, b) argued that deinstitutionalisation guided by normalisation principles had not gone far enough. Critical of the way people with intellectual disabilities remained dependent on professionals and other workers for access to community facilities through the residential home model, they called for the establishment of 'supported living' where people with learning disabilities lived in their own homes supported by workers. Significantly, the pivotal role afforded by Day Centres in the lives of people with intellectual disability had seen normalisation principles applied in a contradictory way contributing to the maintenance of large-scale segregated institutions (Wertheimer, 1996; Whittaker and McIntosh, 2000). Moreover, Skull (1984), in a damning analysis, argued with justification that deinstitutionalisation has been successful insofar as it has established another form of institutional model or trans-institutionalisation. In contrast, there were a range of views that deinstitutionalisation has gone too far. Cox and Pearson (1995) provide echoes of the original discourse of 'asylum' in making the case for village or campus communities where people with learning disabilities can live in safety with support.

The election of New Labour in 1997 provided a significant policy shift in the strategy of community care. The consumerist and managerial discourse that provided impetus for the shifts of the 1990s now articulated with a communitarian discourse (Sachs, 1997) promoting social inclusion, citizenship and civic responsibility, producing a reciprocal relationship between rights, responsibilities and obligations. The publication of *Valuing People* (Department of Health, 2001c) encapsulated New Labour's philosophy of social inclusion and citizenship establishing, in policy terms, the shift from the age of normalisation to the age of citizenship. *Valuing People* waters down the rhetoric of other policy documents that focus on individual obligations to manage themselves as a prerequisite for welfare entitlements encapsulated in statements such as: 'Government's role is to help people to help themselves'. Nevertheless, the discourse of citizenship promoted in *Valuing People* remains conditional. Citizenship as the new organising discourse for discourses about learning disability (normalisation, sexuality and education), is partnered by a powerful discourse of risk and associated technologies of risk management.

Promoting citizenship for people with intellectual disability brings two related challenges. First, citizenship is a complex and contested concept, therefore it is uncertain when it is achieved and then, to what extent. Second, in the context of UK policy, access to citizenship is largely dependent on participating in paid work (Lister, 1998; Department of Social Security, 1999; Scott, 2000) while access to work remains problematic for people with intellectual disability. Exploring the contested nature of citizenship, Riley (1992) describes it as a cluster concept bringing together a range of contradictory positions with no single fixed or agreed meaning. Lewis (1998) suggests that debates over citizenship involve three elements: ways of conceptualising the relationship between the State and individuals; questions of inclusion and exclusion; and a particular social status and entitlements. Further complications arise when the dynamic nature of citizenship is taken into account as the form citizenship takes is historically and culturally specific, varying systematically between societies (Turner, 1990) and within the same society (Lewis, 1998). In Western society, notions of citizenship underpinned by discourses of capitalism, nationalism and patriarchy (Humphries, 1996; Riley, 1992) promote particular relations of power to produce an instrumental equality between citizens while inequalities and exclusions persist (Taylor, 1996).

Van Steenbergen (1994) points out that citizenship is primarily about social participation and to this end possibly the most important integrating factor is work, a relationship lost in normalisation theory. However, barriers to accessing paid employment continue to frustrate people with intellectual disability with consequences for their sense of adulthood and self-esteem (Jenkins, 1989; Fripp, 2005; Powell and Flynn, 2005). Croft and Beresford (1996) observe that a confused language of rights and responsibilities surrounds citizenship as employment is an obligation from which many disabled people feel excluded. Interestingly, Powell and Flynn (2005) locate the failure to establish paid work as a viable option for people with intellectual disability with the Government White Paper *Better Services for the Mentally Handicapped* (1971). In many ways this was a landmark policy statement. However, it produced a contradictory position towards paid employment with profound implications for the development of services. Articulating a discourse of normalisation, vocational education, employment and training, Better Services, rather than establishing a vision promoting appropriate work opportunities for people with intellectual disability such as those provided by social firms, focused its aims of community care by expanding the role of Day Centres. Thus, the expectation was established that the majority of people with learning disability would not participate in paid employment (Powell and Flynn, 2005).

An associated hazard in discourses of citizenship for people with intellectual disability is the persistence of an underlying moral discourse of rights and duties producing a second-class position as 'welfare subject' for people reliant upon welfare for day-to-day support (Lewis, 1998). This position is compounded by the notion of 'active citizenship' promoted in social policy, which maintains an obligation to contribute through taxation, charitable giving and active volunteering. It also requires a supply of welfare subjects as beneficiaries of charitable giving and volunteering (Walmsley, 1993), thus creating circumstances where the socially disadvantaged provide a kind of conscience fodder for the self-esteem of respectable citizens (Barton, 1993). This echoes the objectives of the Poor Law where individuals were considered unable to be both beneficiaries of Government and to exercise control over it (Spiker, 1990).

At an operational or service level the contradictory nature of discourses of citizenship are apparent promoting different outcomes for people with intellectual disability depending on the way these discourses configure. In a study involving managers in a range of statutory and independent sector services in one English county, tensions were identified between residential care and supported living models regarding the model of citizenship promoted (Gilbert et al, 2003, 2005). Four core discourses related to citizenship were identified: work, consumption, participation, and community. All services tended to value work but enabled access in a range of ways. Many examples of work involved volunteering or work experience divorcing labour from reward (wages). However, the role and potential of social firms (CETEC, 1997) was highly valued. In contrast to the majority of disadvantaged groups levels of consumption were high although this is largely due to costs of support, i.e. staff wages, etc. Participation was interpreted in consumerist terms, i.e. using shops and local facilities, rather than as a vehicle for political and social enhancement, leaving advocacy as a care-plan activity. Consequently, there was little evidence of people with intellectual disability participating in the management of the services. Where this did occur it was linked with organisational imperatives such as quality monitoring (Gilbert et al, 2005).

The final area, 'community', provided a complex picture. Residential care models tended towards paternalistic but communitarian approaches to citizenship. People with intellectual disabilities remained dependent on the services that supported them to mediate access to work and community. This often involved voluntary work for either the community or another disadvantaged group, e.g. older people, producing a hierarchy of groups whose citizenship is compromised (Walmsley, 1993). Conversely, supported living models provided a different status: the citizen-tenant, constructing a legally defined space by the use of legal tenancy agreements. In addition the use of housing, unemployment and supplementary benefits produced an 'instrumental equality' with other members of society by using the same benefit platform relied on by other members of the community unemployed and in need of housing. Participation occurred only in consumerist terms as the model did not contain commitments to community-based activity such as work or leisure activity, drawing criticism from some quarters and reflecting Emerson and Hatton's (1994) observations that some services make use of normalisation to justify a lack of structure in people's lives with reservations over the 'quality of life' achieved (Gilbert, 2001).

Duffy (2003) provides a way for service users and providers to avoid philosophical and theoretical tensions and contradictions surrounding citizenship for people with intellectual disability. Offering an approach to support reflecting the familiarity of the 'framework of service accomplishments' (O'Brien and Lyle, 1987) used successfully to promote normalisation, Duffy's 'Six Keys' approach provides a framework for citizenship comprising: self-determination; direction; money; home; support and community life; unifying significant areas of social and economic life 'person-centred planning' and 'service brokerage'. Person-centred approaches (Department of Health, 2001c), the most recent manifestation of technologies for micro-managing individuals' lives, are used to negotiate individual and/or cultural differences in expectations of citizenship. However, while managerially expedient, avoiding the tensions and contradictions underpinning discourses of citizenship also ignores the power inequalities cementing the social and political position of people with intellectual disability. Shifts in policy from consumerist ideas of 'choice and independence' to political notions of 'control and interdependence' are about power relations, as are the continuing inequalities in social care experienced on the basis of gender, age, race and ethnicity (Wistow, 2003, 2005). Moreover, advancing these issues relies on a dynamic concept of citizenship, warts and all.

Central to analysing the relationship between citizenship and social policy is recognition of the role of discourses of risk in contemporary strategies of government. In particular, questions concerning how technologies of risk management operate to divide the population of people with intellectual disabilities on their ability or willingness to conform to expectations concerning citizenship obligations. Linking with the discourse of social inclusion, risk and citizenship provide a discursive structure more capable of supporting what Rose (1996) describes as 'management through the community'. Risk, alongside the idea of 'self-managing' individuals, provides central pillars in contemporary approaches to managing populations. Division of the population based on risk represents new, subtler forms of social control, assigning different destinies to individuals based on their potential to respond to the requirements of a market philosophy (Petersen, 1997). Correspondingly, Taylor Gooby (1993) concludes that welfare citizenship may develop simultaneously in different directions for different groups producing very different experiences.

In the context of intellectual disability, we can identify three broad trajectories. The first trajectory concerns people who manage their own lives with little intervention outside of the normal range of support and are willing and able to conform to the general norms and obligations of society. This group tends to use ordinary community facilities and services, e.g. primary care, schools, work, etc., involving the professionals based therein. A second trajectory includes a group of 'damaged subjects' who require help and support to meet these commitments and become self-managing, although many never fully achieve this status. Such individuals are often targeted by discourses of empowerment (Rose, 1996) and supported in ordinary community facilities by a range of professional and support workers based in specialist services for people with intellectual disabilities, e.g. community development workers, case managers, resource (day) centre officers, social workers, speech and language therapists, etc. People in this trajectory inhabit specialised spaces and have a presence in the community but often in the anonymous spaces noted by Bigby et al (2002). The final trajectory, reserved for a group of people who fail to meet this commitment to self-manage due to risky behaviours, are often subject to legal restrictions over their movements. Services are highly specialised and frequently use segregated and secure facilities reproducing a social context reminiscent of the age of the colony. These include private hospitals and secure NHS facilities, court diversion schemes, etc., and involve professionals such as psychiatrists, psychologists, nurses and social workers. Links with local communities are minimal and conditional.

Furthermore, discourses of risk have restructured professional activity to mirror political imperatives (Johnson, 2001), with trends towards client group-based rather than discipline-based identities (Hughes, 2003). Managing populations increasingly concerns professionals managing complex and unpredictable situations and is therefore almost exclusively located with predicting and developing strategies to minimise risk (Rose, 1996, 1999; Petersen, 1997; Kemshall, 2002). Situations that are more predictable have increasingly been managed at arms length through protocols and similar technologies devolving a range of activities, once the preserve of professional workers such as learning disability nurses, to an array of support workers and family carers across the independent and voluntary sectors. In certain instances this involves contracting with workers in the broader 'health industry' such as personal trainers and exercise specialists. This consists of constructing the relative status of health and social care professionals in the context of their role in managing risk and their ability to interpret and apply a growing range of specific 'risk-based' discourses while at the same time having to manage the expectations of users and carers underpinned by discourses of participation and partnership (Gilbert, 2005b). Consequently, leaving these professions to manoeuvre and compete for prominence by laying claim to competence in the management of certain forms of risk, e.g. challenging behaviour (Emerson, 2001), mental health (Moss et al, 2000; Morley, 2006; Alison, 2006), parenting (Booth and Booth, 1994), sexuality (Parkes and Hodges, 2006), and physical health (Gulliford et al, 2001; Alborz et al, 2003).

These discourses of citizenship and risk continue to make use of the discourses of sexuality and education that supported normalisation. The discourse of sexuality has seen further specialisation articulated with citizenship and human rights discourse to produce a complex discourse concerning homosexuality (Cambridge, 1996; Parkes and Hodges, 2006), erotic behaviour (Williams et al, 2000) and parenting (Booth and Booth, 1994; Feldman, 2004; Llewellyn and McConnell, 2005). Parenting and intellectual disability provide a particularly contentious area. At one and the same time promoted as a right and contested by a risk discourse concerned with child protection, this discourse leaves parents with intellectual disabilities vulnerable to concerns over reproduction echoing the eugenicists and the age of the colony drawing draconian forms of professional intervention rather than support (McGraw and Sturmey, 1993; Booth and Booth, 1994; Booth et al, 2005).

Physical health is also associated with a discourse of risk, highlighting failures of health services to manage people with intellectual disability while also noting the range of risky lifestyle behaviours in which they engage (Kerr et al, 2003; Mencap, 1998; Rogers et al, 1999; Broughton and Thomson, 2000; Northfield and Turnbull, 2001; Department of Health, 2001a, d; Gulliford et al, 2001; Smiley et al, 2002; Scottish Executive 2002). Educational discourse has started to target people with learning disabilities with health promotion and health education strategies (Kerr, 1998; Department of Health, 2001a) although links with public health are limited as yet (Alborz et al, 2003). In addition, discourses of gender (Walsh et al, 2000), age (Bigby, 2004; Hogg et al, 2000; World Health Organization, 2000; Factor, 2004; Cox et al, 2005; Wertheimer, 2005), race and ethnicity (Sham, 1996; Emerson and Hatton, 1999; McGrath et al, 2002), have extended discourses of risk to articulate the experience of people with intellectual disabilities with experiences of people from these social groups in the general population. This creates new areas of concern, extending the social construction of intellectual disability to groups previously invisible, and in addition rendering these sections of the population visible to a more general surveillance of the population.

The final area of risk concerns what are described as 'transitions', a special case of the construction of space where the space is actually a void causing individuals to fall between services, sometimes with catastrophic consequences. Transitions can relate to movements between one point in the life cycle, such as adolescence to adulthood (Hudson, 2006; Department of Health, 2001a, 2003; Williams and Hoadley, 2005) or adulthood to older person (Bigby, 2004; Thompson and Wright ,2001). Alternatively, these spaces may occur between services in multi-disciplinary and multi-agency working as evidenced in a number of inquiries concerning issues such as child abuse, domestic violence and deaths of older people (Department of Health, 2003, 2005; Amiel and Heath, 2003).

So what might we expect of future developments? For one, recent social policy has firmly divided children and family services from services for adults although the discourses of social inclusion, well being, choice, participation and improving health, are evident in policy for both adults and children (Department of Health, 2003, 2005, 2006). Probably the clearest theme separating the two service areas is the intention to shift the majority of all adult services to the independent sector leaving the reorganised partnerships between Primary Care Trusts and adult social services as commissioners rather than providers of community services. These moves, underpinned by a consumerist/choice discourse, position the independent and voluntary sectors as flexible, innovative and more user-friendly when compared with the statutory sector. The rhetoric of partnerships camouflages the power relationships within the commissioner/provider relationships retaining a dominant position for the State operated via contracts and quality monitoring mechanisms. Children services, in comparison, retain greater statutory duties and consequently retain a position in statutory services.

Second, mirroring Hughes' (2003) observation that client group rather than professional group will be the key factor identifying occupational groups in the future, these shifts in policy around adult and children services are likely to further the division between qualification and profession for individual workers. This is something that intellectual (learning) disability nurses and social workers have experienced for some time, where role requirements and titles bear little resemblance to initial professional education programmes. However, paradoxically, the increasing surveillance of the health and social care workforce through registration and periodic re-registration may retain some form of collective identity. Nevertheless, this poses challenges for bodies representing professions as the rhetoric around modernising health and social care professions takes hold (Department of Health, 1998, 1999). In particular, the focus on client groups undermines the ethos of social work as a generic qualification with specialisation through further training and higher qualification taking place post-qualification. In contrast, intellectual disability nursing, which is essentially a client-based qualification, may further suffer from the narrow vision of NHS workforce planning that has tended to focus only on NHS requirements ignoring the wider involvement of this organisational group across the social care sector.

To consider the possible implications of these changes for the subject positions of workers, in particular intellectual disability nurses, we need to return to the three trajectories referred to earlier and explore these in the context of discourse of citizenship for people with intellectual disability. The centrality of person-centred planning (PCP) to the way policy is unfolding, albeit in a variety of guises, is discursively located with ideas of individuals as citizens and participants and as such is contrasted with older individual planning technologies that objectify people in a profession/worker dominated process (Jukes, 2006). Dissemination is presently taking place of an emerging body of evidence on the efficacy of PCP as an approach to managing the lives of people with learning disability (Duffy, 2002; Cole and Lloyd, 2005; Emerson et al, 2005; Adams et al, 2006; Jenkins and Parry, 2006; McIntosh and Sanderson, 2006; Sanderson et al, 2006a, b).

This process, which exemplifies the relationship between power and knowledge central to the study of discourse and social policy (Gilbert, 2003), involves experiences of PCP converted into various forms of text. A range of audiences consume these texts, e.g. personal records, reports of service developments, research reports, articles in journals, chapters in books and official policy documents at various levels. The circulation of these texts further reinforces the original practice, i.e. PCP, to the point that its role is beyond challenge and it functions as truth. Early evaluations of PCP are that it has mixed benefits. There is an increase in activities for a number of groups in a range of contexts but less effect observed for other groups, such as people with autism, mental health problems, emotional difficulties and behavioural problems. Yet the impact of PCP on social inclusion and therefore citizenship is minimal. Researchers (Emerson et al, 2005) conclude that PCP is an evolutionary rather than radical development. It is a cost neutral approach that builds on existing service capacity, which possibly benefits poorer quality services rather than high quality services where capacity is limited. Despite this, researchers call for increased investment in research, staff training, service targets for PCP and monitoring systems to ensure that all services adopt PCP, thus establishing a general tactic for furthering the practice of PCP, ensuring its status as truth within the lives of people with intellectual disability.

Nevertheless, this research further reinforces evidence of a range of issues concerning people with learning disability, such as work (paid, work placements or voluntary work), advocacy, leisure and day-time opportunities, health, housing, direct payments and relationships. Technologies of PCP connect these concerns with the discourse of citizenship and associated discourses of managerialism and risk. The reinvention of case management in line with the citizen discourse of PCP provides the overarching mechanism to co-ordinate activity. Possible future roles for workers will be located with the three trajectories discussed previously alongside the central aim of social inclusion while incorporating the range of specific issues noted here, creating a myriad of spaces limited by only imagination and ingenuity. Rhetoric within policy and research calls for leadership and commitment to advance the possibilities opened up by the configuration of the discourse, which effectively shifts responsibility from the State to individual workers within local services.

In the context of the first trajectory, this includes people who manage their own lives and generally conform to the general norms and obligations of society. Workers are likely to emerge as mediators working on the general themes of social inclusion and health inequalities enabling access by introducing ideas and/or translating these into understandable formats through information and support. These workers are most likely to operate outside of statutory learning disability services promoting the notion of the 'self-managing individual' central to contemporary discourse of citizenship, although some may operate from bases within PCTs in the context of public health, health promotion and relationship-based activity, especially parenting. In such instances, workers may employ more specific person-focused approaches, such as those described by Jukes and Aldridge (2006). Employment and employment-based activity will provide a range of challenges for workers while political activity (advocacy) has the potential for important developments, e.g. people's councils, etc.

We can also predict an increase in the range of existing commercial or independent sector services targeting people with intellectual disabilities as they gain confidence in using earnings or monies from direct payments or individual budgets. For example, the range of self-reflexive activities engaged in by the general population has increased significantly (Gilleard and Higgs, 2000), e.g. yoga, exercise, beauty and health treatments, cosmetic surgery, etc. Health clubs may offer tailored services attracting people with intellectual disability either directly or via their general practitioner. The leisure industry might look to attract people with intellectual disability to particular activities, while home and kitchen design firms may develop specific lines. Banks, insurance brokers and building societies could also have interests, especially if dowries, trusts and mortgages become commonplace among people with intellectual disabilities. In each case, knowledge and skills in communication with people with intellectual disability are required for successful transactions. However, it is less likely that any of these workers would be responsible for developing and implementing either PCP or engaged in case management.

The second trajectory involves 'damaged subjects' who require support to move towards self-management. This provides a different set of opportunities for workers, where, again, the core themes of social inclusion and health inequalities apply. Workers would be involved in developing and implementing PCP and case management from bases within the independent and voluntary sectors, heavily influenced by managerial discourse and ideas of partnerships and multi-agency working. Alternatively, they may be direct employees of people with learning disability themselves, reflecting a new role and subject position for people with learning disability as employers and managers of staff. Key areas for workers remain those noted above: work (paid, work placements or voluntary work), advocacy, leisure and day-time opportunities, health, housing, direct payments and relationships. Although it is likely that the majority of workers will have a general knowledge of all the key areas they may have a specific interest in one or two areas in a traditional skills mix model and may employ a number of the person-centred approaches (Jukes and Aldridge, 2006). Managerialism in this sector requires skills in competitive tendering and project management as the sector is characterised by short-term funding opportunities, many of which are located with notions of innovation and flexibility. For workers who remain in the statutory sector, managerialist discourse will drive most activity, i.e. case management, service commissioning and contract monitoring. Workers are likely to have general rather than profession-specific titles and occupational role descriptions, e.g. service manager, development worker, and support worker with subject positions that reflect their general role within social care.

The final trajectory, those that fail to self-manage, will continue to draw on a range of professionals including intellectual disability nurses and social workers to anticipate and manage risks associated with a range of antisocial or self-harming behaviours. Medical and psychiatric discourse is likely to dominate alongside technologies of risk management. In this area, workers are most likely to retain occupational roles and titles and associated subject positions. Alternatively, they may adopt titles and subject positions linked to specific therapies, i.e. behavioural therapist or cognitive behavioural therapist, engaging a number of specific person-centred approaches (Jukes and Aldridge, 2006). Other roles/titles and subject positions may be linked to specific activities such as court diversion, vulnerable adults or epilepsy nurse specialist. The statutory sector is most likely to retain some provision here, especially in relation to children, although the independent sector is also active in parts of this provision, e.g. secure facilities and services for people with intellectual disability with emotional, behavioural or mental health issues. Community intellectual disability teams are also likely to remain within the statutory sector working with people with learning disabilities across both of the areas previously discussed on a case referral basis. Case management approaches involving specific risk management strategies are likely to be the tasks for workers operating from this third trajectory with PCP subjugated by and to risk management. Citizenship and social inclusion remain only long-term possibilities for people with intellectual disability sited in a trajectory characterised by segregation and social exclusion.

Summary and conclusion

The age of citizenship should represent the endpoint of the journey for people with intellectual disability from disavowed to inclusion as citizens in their own right. However, as described earlier, a significant trend in contemporary social policy is the production of different trajectories for different sub-groups of a population. The once apparently homogenous population of people with learning disability that existed in the 'ages' of the colony and later normalisation now subdivides on the basis of willingness or ability to comply with the obligations of citizenship with corresponding social spaces for the able, those to be empowered and the risky, along with consequent subject positions. Within this, for some, the spectre of the colony remains. Moreover, as we can see from the shifts occurring since the mid-19th century the social context is never static. Contested areas such as citizenship will be subject to future challenges and revisions while the vulnerability of people with learning disability means that such revisions maintain a constant threat to their position and status.

Social inclusion remains the objective but it requires accepting and cohesive communities into which people can integrate. This is further complicated in contemporary social policy by the way work remains the central route to citizenship and inclusion providing an elusive goal for many people with learning disabilities. Eugenics-type discourses continue to question the viability of the less-than-perfect foetus, devaluing disabled people in general, while competition for scarce resources brings threats of marginalisation. Nevertheless, significant achievements in material and social gains are evident, and probably the most effective safeguards are property rights and political participation. Property rights can bestow a legally constituted 'space' from which individuals can resist certain interference in their lives while also providing the basis for financial security and creditworthiness. Political participation in a vibrant democracy makes available a forum where those in danger of marginalisation have public recourse to resist powerful forces in society. For many marginalised groups these forces include both the market and the activity of the professionals. Relationships with professionals preserve for people with intellectual disability the status of 'other' while maintaining surveillance of everyday activity under the guise of support. Partnership working offers the opportunity for professionals to manage expectations of users and carers while anticipating risk and retaining capacity to deploy technologies of social control.

Work, social inclusion, participation, financial security, legal protection and appropriate support provide the basis for advancing citizenship. However, while it is beyond the capacity of services that support people with intellectual disability to resolve the contested and ambiguous nature of citizenship, one of the biggest threats to advancement is a lack of understanding among many people involved in the lives of people with intellectual disability over what citizenship entails. Formulaic representations may meet managerial agendas but for real progress, a more sophisticated understanding is necessary. The multi-dimensional matrix referred to earlier provides a basis for such an understanding, taking account of numerous factors including policy, discourse, service developments, and the relative subject positions produced while remaining sensitive to historical or temporal shifts, and the importance of the spaces within which practices take place. Central to this process is identifying discourses embedded in social policy and practice while an awareness of the threads of continuity and change occurring over time enable the identification in the present the once discredited moral and scientific positions from an earlier age.

References

Adams L, Mansell J, Beadle-Brown J (2006) Individual planning: An exploration of the link between quality of plan and quality of life. *British Journal of Learning Disabilities* **34**(2): 68–76

Alborz A, McNally R, Swallow A, Glendinning C (2003) *From Cradle to Grave: A literature review of access to healthcare for people with learning disability across the lifespan.* National Co-ordinating Centre for NHS Service Delivery and Organisation Research and Development. NCCSDO, London

Alison M (2006) Cognitive behaviour therapy. In: Jukes M, Aldridge J (eds) *Person-Centred Practices: A Therapeutic Perspective.* Quay Books, London

Amiel S, Heath I (2003) *Family Violence in Primary Care.* Oxford University Press, Oxford

Andrews J (1996) Identifying and providing for the mentally disabled in early modern London: In: Wright D, Digby A (eds) *From Idiocy to Mental Deficiency: Historical perspectives on people with learning disabilities.* Routledge, London

ARC/NAPSAC (1993) *'It Could Never Happen Here': The Prevention and Treatment of Sexual Abuse of Adults with Learning Disabilities in Residential Settings.* Association of Residential Care, Derby

Atkinson D, Jackson M, Walmsley J (1997) *Forgotten Lives: Exploring the History of Learning Disability.* BILD, Kidderminster

Bank-Mikkelson NE (1969) A metropolitan area in Denmark: Copenhagen. In: Kugel R, Wolfensberger W (eds) *Changing Patterns in Residential Services for the Mentally Handicapped.* President's Committee on Mental Retardation, Washington DC

Bank-Mikkelson NE (1980) Denmark. In: Flynn RJ, Nitsch KE (eds) *Normalisation, Social Integration and Community Services.* pro-Ed, Austin TX

Barnes C (1996) Theories of disability and the origins of the oppression of disabled people in western society. In: Barton L (ed) *Disability and Society: Emerging Issues and Insights.* Longman, Harlow

Barnes M, Prior D (1995) Spoilt for choice? How consumerism can disempower public service users. *Public Money Management* **15**(3): 53–8

Barton L (1993) The struggle for citizenship: The case of disabled people. *Disability, Handicap and Society* **8**(3): 235–48

Beresford P, Croft S, Evans C, Harding T (1997) Quality in personal social services: The developing role of user involvement in the UK. In: Evers A, Haverinen R, Leichsenring K, Wistow G (eds) *Developing Quality in Personal Social Services: A European Perspective.* Ashgate, Aldershot

Bigby C (2004) *Ageing with a Lifelong Disability: A guide to Practice, Program and Policy Issues for Human Services Professionals.* Jessica Kingsley Publications, London

Bigby C, Frederico M, Cooper B (2002) *Not Just a Residential Move but Creating a Better Lifestyle for People with Intellectual Disabilities: Report of the Evaluation of Kew Residential Services Community Relocation Project 1999–2001.* Department of Human Services, Melbourne

Blunden R, Allen D (1987) *Facing the Challenge: An Ordinary Life for People with Learning Difficulties and Challenging Behaviour.* Kings Fund, London

Blunden R, Evans G, Humphreys S (1987) *Planning with Individuals: An Outline Guide.* Mental Handicap in Wales Applied Research Unit, Cardiff

Boote J, Telford R, Cooper C (2002) Consumer involvement in health research: A review and research agenda. *Health Policy* **61:** 213–61

Booth T, Booth W (1994) *Parenting Under Pressure: Mothers and Fathers with Learning Difficulties.* Open University Press, Buckingham

Booth T, Booth W, McConnell D (2005) The prevalence and outcomes of care proceedings for involving parents with learning difficulties in the family courts. *Child and Family Social Work* **10**(4): 353–60

Borthwick-Duffy SA (1994) Epidemiology and prevalence of psychopathology in people with mental retardation. *Journal of Consulting and Clinical Psychology* **62**(1): 17–27

Brammer A (2005) Learning disability and the law. In: Grant G, Goward P, Richardson M, Ramcharan P (eds) *Learning Disability: A Life Cycle Approach.* Open University Press, Buckingham

Brandon D (1991) *Direct Power: A Handbook on Service Brokerage.* Tao, Preston

Brechin A, Swain J (1987) *Changing Relationships: Shared Action Planning with People with Mental Handicap.* Harper and Row, London

Broughton S, Thomson K (2000) Women with learning disabilities: Risk behaviours and experiences of the cervical smear test. *Journal of Advanced Nursing* **32**(4): 905–12

Brown H, Smith H (eds) (1992) *Normalisation: A Reader for the Nineties.* Routledge, London

Brown H, Thompson D (1997) Service responses to men with intellectual disabilities who have sexually abusive or unacceptable behaviours: The case against inaction. *Journal of Applied Research in Intellectual Disability* **10**(2): 176–97

Brown J (1994) *The Hybrid Worker.* University of York, Department of Social Policy and Social Work, York

Cambridge, P. (1996) Men with learning disabilities who have sex with men in public places: Mapping the needs of services and users in south east London. *Journal of Intellectual Disability Research*, **40**, 241–51.

CETEC (1997) *Definition of Social Firms agreed. European Confederation of Co-operatives and Social Business.* CETEC Conference, Linz: Austria

Chappell AL (1992) Towards a sociological critique of the normalisation principle. *Disability, Handicap and Society* **7**(1): 35–51

Chief Nursing Officer (1985) *The Role of the Nurse in Caring for People with Mental Handicap.* Chief Nursing Officer CNO/(85)5, London

Clarke J, Newman J (1997) *The Managerial State.* London: Sage.

Cole A, Lloyd A (2005) *Shaping the Future: Together.* Foundation for People with Learning Disabilities, London

Cox C, Pearson M (1995) *Made to Care: The Case for Residential and Village Communities for People With a Mental Handicap*. The Rannoch Trust, London

Cox D, Weze C, Lewi C (2005) *Cerebral Palsy and Ageing: A Systematic Review*. Scope, London

Cox P (1996) Girls, deficiency and delinquency. In: Wright D, Digby A (eds) *From Idiocy to Mental Deficiency: Historical Perspectives on People With Learning Disabilities*. Routledge, London

Craft A (ed) (1994) *Practice Issues in Sexuality and Learning Disabilities*. Routledge, London

Croft S, Beresford P (1996) The politics of participation. In: Taylor D (ed) *Critical Social Policy – A Reader, Social Policy and Social Relations*. Sage, London

Cullen C (1991) *Caring for People: Community Care in the Next Decade and Beyond: Mental Handicap Nursing*. Department of Health and Social Security, London

Department of Health (1998) *Modernising Social Services, CM4169*. The Stationery Office, London

Department of Health (1999) *Making a Difference- Strengthening the Nursing, Midwifery and Health Visiting Dontribution to Health and Healthcare*. The Stationery Office, London

Department of Health (2001a) *Valuing People: A new Strategy for Learning Disability for the 21st Century. CM 5086*. The Stationery Office, London

Department of Health (2001b) *Nothing About Us Without Us: The Service Users Advisory Group Report*. The Stationery Office, London

Department of Health (2001c) *Valuing People: A New Strategy for Learning Disability for the 21st Century Towards Person Centred Approaches. Planning with People: Guidance for Partnership Boards*. The Stationery Office, London

Department of Health (2001d) *Seeking Consent: Working with People with Learning Disabilities*. The Stationery Office, London

Department of Health (2003) *Every Child Matters. CM 5860*. The Stationery Office, London

Department of Health (2005) *Independence, Well-being and Choice. CM 6499*. The Stationery Office, London

Department of Health (2006) *Our Health, Our Care, Our Say: A new direction for community services. CM 6737*. The Stationery Office, London

Department of Health/Home Office (2000) *No Secrets: Guidance on Developing and Implementing Multi-Agency Policies and Procedures to Protect Vulnerable Adults from Abuse*. Department of Health, London

Department of Health and Social Security (1969) *Report of the Committee of Inquiry into Allegations of Ill Treatment of Patients and Other Irregularities at Ely Hospital, Cardiff*. Cmnd 3975. HMSO, London

Department of Health and Social Security (1971) *Report of the Farleigh Hospital Committee of Inquiry*. Cmnd 4557. HMSO, London

Department of Health and Social Security (1972) *Report of the Committee on Nursing. Cmnd 5115*. HMSO, London

Department of Health and Social Security (1974) *Report of the South Ockendon Hospital Committee of Inquiry*. Paper 124, HMSO, London

Department of Health and Social Security (1978) *Report of the Committee of Inquiry into Normansfield Hospital*. Cmnd 7357, HMSO, London

Department of Health and Social Security/Welsh Office (1971) *Better Services for the Mentally Handicapped*. HMSO, London

Department of Social Security (1999) *Opportunity for All: Ending Poverty and Social Exclusion*. The Stationery Office, London

Digby A (1996) Contexts and perspectives. In: Wright D, Digby A (eds) *From Idiocy to Mental Deficiency: Historical Perspectives on People with Learning Disabilities*. Routledge, London

Dowson S (1998) *Certainties Without Centres? A Discussion Paper on Day Services for People who have Learning Difficulties*. London: Values Into Action

Dreyfus HL, Rabinow P (1982) *Michel Foucault: Beyond Structuralism and Hermeneutics*. Harvester, Brighton

Duffy S (2002) *Care Management and PCP*. Valuing People Support Team, London

Duffy S (2003) *Keys to Citizenship: A Guide to Getting Good Support for People with Learning Difficulties*. Paradigm, Birkenhead

Emerson E (2001) *Challenging Behaviour: Analysis and Intervention in People with Learning Difficulties* 2nd edn. Cambridge University Press, Cambridge

Emerson E (2005) Models of service delivery. In: Grant G, Goward P, Richardson M, Ramcharan P (eds) *Learning Disability: A Life Cycle Approach*. Open University Press, Buckingham

Emerson E, Hatton C (1994) *Moving Out: The impact of re-location from Hospital to Community on the Quality of life of People with Learning*

Disabilities. HMSO, London

Emerson E, Hatton C (1999) Future trends in the ethnic composition of British Society and among British citizens with learning disabilities. *Tizard Learning disability Review* **14:** 28–31

Emerson E, Routledge M, Robertson J, Sanderson H, McIntosh B, Swift P, Joyce T, Oakes P, Towers C, Hatton C, Romeo R, Knapp M (2005) *The Impact of Person Centred Planning*. Foundation for People with Learning Disability, London

English National Board for Nursing, Midwifery and Health Visiting (1985) *Caring for People with Mental Handicaps*. English National Board for Nursing, Midwifery and Health Visiting, London

Evenhuis H, Henderson C, Beange H, Lennox N, Chicoine B (2001) Healthy ageing – adults with intellectual disabilities: physical health issues. *Journal of Applied Research in Intellectual Disabilities* **14**(3): 175–94

Factor A (2004) *Ageing with a Developmental Disability. Presentation to the White House Conference on Aging*. Rehabilitation Research and Training Centre on Aging with a Developmental Disability. University of Illinois, Chicago

Fairclough N (1992) *Discourse and Social Change*. Polity Press, Cambridge

Felce D (1989) *The Andover Project: Staffed Housing for Adults with Severe or Profound Mental Handicaps*. British Institute for Mental Handicap, Kidderminster

Felce D, Kushlick A, Mansell J (1980) Evaluation of alternative residential facilities for the severely mentally handicapped in Wessex: Client engagement. *Advances in Behaviour Research and Therapy* **3:** 13–8

Feldman MA (2004) Self-directed learning of childcare skills by parents with intellectual disabilities. *Infants and Young Children* **17:** 17–31

Fink J (2004) Questions of care. In: Fink J (ed) *Care*. Sage/Open University, London: 1–42

Finkelstein V (1980) *Attitudes and Disabled People: Issues for discussion*. World Development Fund, New York

Foucault M (1980) Two Lectures. In: Gordon C (ed) *Power/Knowledge, Selected Interviews and Other Writings 1972–1977*. Harvester Press, London

Foucault M (1984a) *Space, Knowledge, Power*. In: Rabinow P (ed) *The Foucault Reader*. Penguin, Harmondsworth

Foucault M (1984b) The history of sexuality. Volume 1. Right of death and power over life. In: Rabinow P (ed) *The Foucault Reader*. Penguin, Harmondsworth

Fripp N (2005) Work, learning and leisure: The journey towards fulfilling lives. In: Grant G, Goward P, Richardson M, Ramcharan P (eds) *Learning Disability: A Life Cycle Approach*. Open University Press, Buckingham

Gilbert T (1995) Nursing: Empowerment and the problem of power. *Journal of Advanced Nursing* **21:** 865–71

Gilbert T (1998) Sexual health and people with learning disabilities. In: Morrissey M (ed) *Sexual Health: A Human Dilemma*. Mark Allen, Wiltshire

Gilbert T (2001) *Social Welfare, Care-Planning and the Politics of Trust. PhD Thesis*. The Open University, Milton Keynes

Gilbert T (2003) Exploring the dynamics of power: A Foucauldian analysis of care planning in learning disability services. *Nursing Inquiry* **10**(1): 37–46

Gilbert T (2005a) Managerialism and trust: Exploring discourses of care. *Journal of Advanced Nursing* **52**(4): 1–10

Gilbert T (2005b) Impersonal trust and professional authority: Exploring the dynamics. *Journal of Advanced Nursing* **49**(6): 568–77

Gilbert T, Cochrane A, Greenwell S (2003) Professional discourse and service cultures: An organisational typology developed from health and welfare services for people with learning disabilities. *International Journal of Nursing Studies* **40**(7): 781–93

Gilbert T, Cochrane A, Greenwell S (2005) Citizenship: Locating people with learning disabilities. *International Journal of Social Welfare* **14:** 287–96

Gilbert T, Lockyer T (1995) Levels of intervention. Gilbert T, Todd M (eds) *Learning Disabilities: Practice Issues in Health Settings*. Routledge, London

Gilbert T, Rose SJ (1998) Commissioning and providing services. In: Thompson T, Mathias P (eds) *Standards and Learning Disability*. 2nd edn. Baillière Tindall, London

Gilleard C, Higgs P (2000) *Cultures of Ageing: Self, Citizen and the Body*. Prentice Hall, London

Gladstone D (1996) The changing dynamic of institutional care. In: Wright D, Digby A (eds) *From Idiocy to Mental Deficiency: Historical Perspectives on People with Learning Disabilities*. Routledge, London

Goodey CF (1996) The psychopolitics of learning and disability in seventeenth century thought. In: Wright D, Digby A (eds) *From Idiocy to Mental Deficiency: Historical Perspectives on People with Learning Disabilities*. Routledge, London

Goodley D, Ramcharan P (2005) Advocacy, campaigning and people with learning difficulties. In: Grant G, Goward P, Richardson M, Ramcharan P (eds) *Learning Disability: A Life Cycle Approach*. Open University Press, Buckingham

Grant G (2005) Healthy and successful ageing. In: Grant G, Goward P, Richardson M, Ramcharan P (eds) *Learning Disability: A Life Cycle Approach*. Open University Press, Buckingham

Gulliford M, Morgan M, Hughes D, Beech R, Figeroa-Muñoz J, Gibson B et al (2001) *Access to Healthcare: Report of a Scoping Exercise for the National Co- ordination Centre for NHS Service Delivery and Organisation Research and Development*. NCCSDO, London

Hall S (2001) The spectacle of the other. In: Wetherell M, Taylor S, Yates SJ (eds) *Discourse Theory and Practice: A Reader*. London, Sage

Hall V, Russell O (1985) Community mental handicap nursing – the birth, growth and development of the idea. In: Sines D, Bicknell J (eds) *Caring for Mentally Handicapped People in the Community*. Harper and Row, London

Hatton C, Emerson E (1996) *Residential Provision for People with Learning Disabilities: A Research Review*. Hester Adrian Research Centre, University of Manchester, Manchester

Henderson V (1991) *Nature of Nursing: A definition and its implications for practice, research, and education: reflections after 25 years*. National League for Nursing Press, NY, NY

Hogg J, Lucchoino R, Wang K, Janicki MP (2000) *Healthy Ageing – Adults with Intellectual Disabilities: Ageing and Social Policy*. World Health Organization, Geneva

Holland T, Clare ICH, Mukhopadhyay T (2002) The prevalence of 'criminal offending' by men and women with intellectual disability and the characteristics of 'offenders': Implications for research and service development. *Journal of Intellectual Disability Research* **46**(Suppl 1): 6–20

Hudson B (2006) Making and missing connections: Learning disability services at the transition form adolescence to adulthood. *Disability and Society* **21**(1): 47–60

Hughes B, Paterson K (1997) The social model of disability and the disappearing body: Towards sociology of impairment. *Disability and Society* 12(3): 325–40

Hughes L (2003) The workforce for social work and social care. In: Kendall I, Harker L (eds) *From Welfare to Wellbeing: The Future of Social Care*. Institute of Public Policy Research, London

Humphries B (1996) Preface. In: Humphries B (ed) *Critical Perspectives on Empowerment*. Venture Press, Birmingham

Illich I (1979) *Disabling Professions*. Marion Boyars, London

Jackson M (1996) Institutional provision for the feeble-minded in Edwardian England: Sandlebridge and the scientific morality of permanent care. In: Grant G, Goward P, Richardson M, Ramcharan P (eds) *Learning Disability: A Life Cycle Approach*. Open University Press, Buckingham

Jay P (1979) *The Report of the Committee of Enquiry into Mental Handicap Nursing and Care*. Department of Health, London

Jenkins J, Felce D, Toogood S, Mansell J, De Kock U (1988) *Individual Programme Planning*. BIMH, Kidderminster

Jenkins R (1989) Barriers to adulthood: Long-term unemployment and mental handicap compared. In: Brechin A, Walmsley J (eds) *Making Connections: Reflecting on the Lives and Experiences of People With Learning Difficulties*. Hodder and Stoughton, London

Jenkins R, Parry R (2006) Working with the support network: Applying systemic practice in learning disability services. *British Journal of Learning Disabilities* **34**(2): 77–81

Johnson T (2001) Governmentality and the institutionalization of expertise. In: Purdy M, Banks D (eds) *The Sociology and Politics of Health: A Reader*. Routledge London: 135–43

Jukes M (2006) Person-centredness. In: Jukes M, Aldridge J (eds) *Person-Centred Practices: A Therapeutic Perspective*. Quay Books, London

Jukes M, Aldridge J (eds) (2006) *Person-Centred Practices: A Therapeutic Perspective*. Quay Books, London

Kay B, Rose S, Turnbull J (1995) *Continuing the Commitment: The Report of the Learning Disability Nursing Project*. Department of Health, London

Kemshall H (2002) *Risk, Social Policy and Welfare*. Open University Press, Buckingham

Kerr M (1998) Primary healthcare and health gain for people with learning disability. *Tizard Learning Disability Review* **3**(4): 6–14

Kerr M, Dunstan F, Thapar A (1996) Attitudes of general practitioners to caring for people with learning disability. *British Journal of General Practice* **46**: 92–4

Kerr M, McCulluck D, Oliver K, Mclean B, Coleman E, Law T et al (2003) Medical needs of people with intellectual disability require regular reassessment, and the provision of client and care held reports. *Journal of Intellectual Disability Research* **47**: 134–45

Keywood K (1995) Sterilizing the woman with learning difficulties. In: Bridgman S, Mills S (eds) *Law and Body Politics: Regulating the Female Body*. Dartmouth Publishing Co, Aldershot

Kings Fund (1980) *An Ordinary Life: Comprehensive Locally-based Residential Accommodation for Mentally Handicapped People*. Kings Fund Centre, London

Kings Fund (1999) *From Care to Citizenship: A Kings Fund Position Paper*. Kings Fund, London

Kinsella P (1993) *Supported Living: A New Paradigm*. National Development Team, Manchester

Kinsella P, Ward L (1993a) Supporting Roles. *Community Care* **976**: 25–25

Kinsclla P, Ward L (1993b) Home Rules. *Health Service Journal* **103**(5365): 20–2

Klein R (1989) *The Politics of the NHS*. 2nd edn. Longman, London

Langan M (1993) The rise and fall of social work. In: Clarke J (ed) *A Crisis in Care: Challenges to Social Work*. Sage/Open University, London

Langan M (1998) The personal social services. In: Ellison N, Pierson C (eds) *Developments in British Social Policy*. Macmillan, Basingstoke

Lewis G (1998) Citizenship. In: Hughes G (ed) *Imagining Welfare Futures*. Routledge/Open University Press, London

Lewis G (2000) Introduction: Expanding the social policy imaginary. In: Lewis G, Gewirtz S, Clarke J (eds) *Rethinking Social Policy*. Open University/Sage Publications, London

Lister R (1998) From equality to social inclusion: New Labour and the welfare state. *Critical Social Policy* **18**(2): 215–25

Llewellyn G, McConnell D (2005) You have to prove yourself all the time: People with learning disabilities as parents. In: Grant G, Goward P, Richardson M, Ramcharan P (eds) *Learning Disability: A Life Cycle Approach*. Open University Press, Buckingham

Mackintosh M (2000) Exchange and the metaphor of exchange: Economic cultures in social care. In: Lewis G, Gewirtz S, Clarke J (eds) *Rethinking Social Policy*. Open University/Sage Publications, London

Marshall TH (1996) Citizen and social class. In: Marshall TH, Bottomore

T (eds) *Citizenship and Social Class*. Pluto, London

McClimens A (2005) From vagabonds to Victorian values. The social construction of a disability identity. In: Grant G, Goward P, Richardson M, Ramcharan P (eds) *Learning Disability: A Life Cycle Approach*. Open University Press, Buckingham

McGrath CW, Bhaumik S, Thorpe CF, Watson JM, Taub NA (2002) Prevalence, morbidity and service need among South Asian and white adults with intellectual disability in Leicestershire, UK. *Journal of Intellectual Disability research* **46:** 299–309

McGraw S, Sturmey P (1993) Identifying the needs of parents with learning disabilities: A review. *Child Abuse Review* **2:** 101–17

McIntosh B, Sanderson H (2006) Value Added. *Community Care* **20/4:** 30–1

Mencap (1998) *The NHS – Health for All?* Mencap, London

Mitchell D (2002) A contribution to the history of learning disability nursing. *Nursing Times Research* **7**(3): 201–10

Mittler P (1978) *Helping Mentally Handicapped People in Hospitals: A Report to the Secretary of State for Social Services*. Department of Health and Social Security, London

Morley P (2006) Solution-focused practice. In: Jukes M, Aldridge J (eds) *Person-centred Practices: A Therapeutic Perspective*. Quay Books, London

Morris J (1997) Care or empowerment: A disability rights perspective. *Social Policy and Administration* **31**(1): 54–60

Mort F (1987) *Dangerous Sexualities: Medico-Moral Politics in England Since 1830*. 2nd edn. Routledge, London

Moss S, Emerson E, Kiernan C, Turner S, Hatton C, Alboraz A (2000) Psychiatric symptoms in adults with learning disability and challenging behaviour. *British Journal of Psychiatry* **177:** 452–6

Moss S, Patel P (1993) The prevalence of mental illness in people with intellectual disability over 50 years of age, and the diagnostic importance of information from carers. *Irish Journal of Psychology* **14**(1): 110–29

Neugebauer R (1996) Mental handicap in Medieval and early modern England: Criteria, measurement and care. In: Wright D, Digby A (eds) *From Idiocy to Mental Deficiency: Historical Perspectives on People with Learning Disabilities*. Routledge, London

Nirje B (1972) The right to self determination. In: Wolfensberger W (ed) *The Principle of Normalisation in Human Services*. National Institute on Mental Retardation, Toronto

Northfield J, Turnbull J (2001) Experiences from cancer services. In: Hogg J, Northfield J, Turnbull J (eds) *Cancer and People with Learning Disabilities*. BILD, Kidderminster

O'Brien J (1987) A guide to life-style planning: Using the activities catalogue to integrate services and natural support systems. In: Wilson BM, Bellamy GT (eds) *The Activities Catalogue: An Alternative Curriculum for Youth and Adults with Severe Disabilities*. Brookes, Baltimore, MD

O'Brien J, Lyle C (1987) *Framework for Accomplishment*. Responsive Systems Associates, Decatur, GA

O'Brien J, Tyne A (1981) *The Principle of Normalisation: A Foundation for Effective Services*. CMH, London

O'Callaghan A, Murphy G, Clare ICH (2003) The impact of abuse on men and women with severe learning disabilities and their families. *British Journal of Learning Disabilities* 31(4): 175–80

Oliver M (1990) *The Politics of Disablement*. Macmillan, Basingstoke

Parkes N, Hodges N (2006) Working with and supporting men with a learning disability who are gay, bisexual or attracted to the same sex. In: Jukes M, Aldridge J (eds) *Person-Centred Practices: A Therapeutic Perspective*. Quay Books, London

Pearson K, Jaederholm GA (0000) *Mendelism and the Problem of Mental Deficiency II: On the Continuity of Mental Defect*. Department of Applied Statistics, University of London

Petersen A (1997) Risk, governance and the new public health. In:Petersen A, Bunton R (eds) *Foucault: Health and Medicine*. Routledge, London: 189–206

Petersen A, Bunton R (2002) *The New Genetics and the Public's Health*. Routledge, London

Potter J (1996) *Representing Reality: Discourse, Rhetoric and Social Construction*. Sage, London

Powell M, Flynn M (2005) Promoting independence through work. In: Grant G, Goward P, Richardson M, Ramcharan P (eds) *Learning Disability: A Life Cycle Approach*. Open University Press. Buckingham

Race D (1999) Hearts and minds: Social role valorization, UK academia and services for people with a learning disability. *Disability and Society* 14(4): 519–38

Race D, Boxall K, Carson I (2005) Towards a dialogue for practice: Reconciling social role valorization and the social model of disability.

Disability and Society **20**(5): 507–21

Rapley M, Ridgway J (1998) 'Quality of life' talk and the corporatisation of intellectual disability. *Disability and Society* **13**(3): 451–71

Richardson M (2005) Critiques of segregation and eugenics. In: Grant G, Goward P, Richardson M, Ramcharan P (eds) *Learning Disability: A Life Cycle Approach*. Open University Press, Buckingham

Riley D (1992) Citizenship and the Welfare State. In: Allen J, Braham P, Lewis P (eds) *Political and Economic Forms of Modernity*. Polity Press in association with the Open University, Cambridge

Rogers R, Mills L, Buckle J (1999) Providing equal access to primary care services. *Learning Disability Practice* **2**(1): 24–5

Rose N (1996) The death of the social? Re-figuring the territory of Government. *Economy and Society* **25**(3): 327–56

Rose N (1999) *Powers of Freedom: Reframing Political Thought*. Cambridge University Press, Cambridge

Rose S (1993) Social policy: A perspective on service developments and inter-agency working. In: Brigden P, Todd M (eds) *Concepts in Community Care for People with a Learning Difficulty*. Macmillan, Basingstoke

Rushton P (1996) Idiocy, the family and the community in early modern North-East England. In: Wright D, Digby A (eds) *From Idiocy to Mental Deficiency: Historical Perspectives on People with Learning Disabilities*. Routledge, London

Ryan J, Thomas F (1980) *The Politics of Mental Handicap*. Penguin, Harmondsworth

Sachs J (1997) *The Politics of Hope*. Jonathon Cape, London

Sanderson H, Duffy S, Poll C, Hatton C (2006b) In control: The story so far. *Journal of Integrated Care* **14**(4): 3–13

Sanderson H, Thomson J, Kilbane J (2006a) The emergence of person centred planning as evidence based practice. *Journal of Integrated Care* **14**(2): 18–25

Scheerenberger RC (1987) *A History of Mental Retardation: A Quarter Century of Promise*. Brookes, Baltimore

Scott G (2000) New Labour and the restructuring of welfare – what's in it for women? *International Journal of Sociology and Social Policy* **20**(6): 51–65

Scottish Executive (2002) *Promoting Health, Supporting Inclusion: The National Review of the Contribution of All Nurses and Midwives to the Care and Support of People with Learning Disabilities*. Scottish

Executive, Edinburgh

Seebohm F (1968) *Report of the Committee on Local Authority and Allied Personal Social Services*. HMSO, London

Seguin E (1866) *Idiocy and Its Treatment by the Physiological Method*. William Wood, New York

Sham S (1996) Reaching Chinese children with learning disability in greater Manchester. *British Journal of Learning disability 24:* 104–9

Sines D (1993) *Opportunities for Change: A new direction for nursing for people with learning disabilities*. Department of Health, London

Skull A (1984). *Decarceration: Community Treatment and the Deviant: A Radical View*. 2nd edn. Polity Press, Cambridge

Smiley E, Cooper SA, Miller SM, Robertson P, Simpson N (2002) Specialist health services for people with intellectual disability in Scotland. *Journal of Intellectual Disability Research* **46:** 585–93

Spiker P (1990) Mental handicap and citizenship. *Journal of Applied Philosophy* **2**(7): 139–51

Steele B, Sergison M (2001) *Improving the Quality of Life of Ethnic Minority Children with Learning Disability*. Huddersfield NHS Trust, Huddersfield

Taylor D (1996) Citizenship and social power. In: Taylor D (ed) *Critical Social Policy – A Reader, Social Policy and Social Relations*. Sage, London

Taylor Gooby P (1993) Citizenship, dependency and the welfare mix: Problems of inclusion and exclusion. *International Journal of Health Services* **23**(3): 455–74

Thompson D, Wright S (2001) *Misplaced and Forgotten: People With Learning Disabilities in Residential Services for Older People*. Foundation for People with Learning Disabilities, London

Thomson M (1996) Family, community and the State: The micro-politics of mental deficiency. In: Wright D, Digby A (eds) *From Idiocy to Mental Deficiency: Historical Perspectives on People With Learning Disabilities*. Routledge, London

Tizard J (1954) Institutional defectives. *American Journal on Mental Deficiency*, **59**: 158–65

Turner BS (1990) Outline of a theory of citizenship. *Sociology* **24**(2): 189–217

Tyler S (1997) The use of psychotropic drugs. In: Oliver R (ed) *Seminars in the Psychiatry of Learning Disabilities*. Bell and Bain, Glasgow

Van Steenbergen B (1994) The condition of citizenship: An introduction.

In: van Steenbergen B (ed) *The Condition of Citizenship*. Sage, London

Walmsley J (1993) Talking to top people: Some issues relating to the Citizenship of people with learning disabilities. In: Swain J, Finklestein V, Oliver M (eds) *Disabling Barriers – Enabling Environments*. Sage, London

Walmsley J (2001) Normalisation, emancipatory research and inclusive research in learning disability. *Disability and Society* **16**(2): 187–205

Walsh PN, Heller T, Schuph N, van Schrojenstein Latman-de Valk H (2000) Healthy *Ageing – Adults with Intellectual Disabilities: Women's Health Issues*. World Health Organization, Geneva, Switzerland

Weeks J (1985) *Sexuality and Its Discontents: Meaning, Myths and Modern Sexualities*. Routledge and Kegan Paul, London

Wertheimer A (1996) *Changing Days: Developing New Day Opportunities for People Who Have Learning Difficulties*. Kings Fund, London

Wertheimer A (2005) *Today and Tomorrow: Findings of the Growing Older with Learning Disabilities Programme*. Foundation for People with Learning Disabilities, London

Wetherell M (2001) Debates in Discourse Research. In: Wetherell M, Taylor S, Yates SJ (eds) *Discourse Theory and Practice: A Reader*. Sage, London: 380–99

Whittaker A, McIntosh B (2000) Changing days. *British Journal of Learning Disability* **28**(1): 3–8

Williams A, Phillips L, Ahmed Z (2002) Assessment and management of auto-erotic asphyxiation in a young man with learning disability: A multidisciplinary approach to intervention. *British Journal of Learning Disability* **28**(3): 109–12

Williams D (1979a) Why I would not sign the Jay Report. *Nursing Mirror* **148**(11): 6–7

Williams D (1979b) Jay Report: What chance implementation? *Nursing Times* **75**(11): 429

Williams V, Hoadley S (2005) *Linking Up: Emotional Support for Young People with Learning Disability*. Foundation for People with Learning Disability. London

Williams A, Phillips L, Ahmed Z (2000) Assessment and management of auto-erotic asphyxiation in a young man with learning disability: A multidisciplinary approach to intervention. *British Journal of Learning Disabilities*, **28**(3):109–12

Wistow G (2003) The future aims and objectives of social care. In: Kendall I, Harker L (eds) *From Welfare to Wellbeing: The Future of Social*

Care. Institute of Public Policy Research, London

Wistow G (2005) *Developing Social Care: The Past, the Present and the Future*. Social Care Institute for Excellence: Adult Services Position Paper 04. Bristol: Policy Press

Wolfensberger W (1972) *The Principle of Normalisation in Human Services*. National Institute on Mental Retardation, Toronto

Wolfensberger W (1977) *A Balanced Multi-Component Advocacy Protection Schema*. Canadian Association for the Mentally Retarded, Toronto

Wolfensberger W (1983a) Social role valorisation: A proposed new term for the principle of normalisation. *Mental Retardation* **21**(6): 234–9

Wolfensberger W, Thomas S (1983b) *PASSING (Programme Analysis of Service Systems Implementing Normalisation Goals)*. Canadian National Institute of Mental Retardation, Ontario

Wood Committee (1929). *Report of the Joint Departmental Committee on Mental Deficiency*. Board of Education and Board of Control, London

World Health Organization (2000) *Ageing and Intellectual Disabilities – Improving Longevity and Promoting Healthy Ageing: Summative Report*. World Health Organization, Geneva

Wright D (1996) 'Childlike in his Innocence': Lay attitudes to 'Idiots' and 'Imbeciles' in Victorian England. In: Wright D, Digby A (eds.) *From Idiocy to Mental Deficiency: Historical Perspectives on People With Learning Disabilities*. Routledge, London

CHAPTER 5

Researching learning disability nursing

Ruth Northway

Introduction

Recent years have seen an increase in the number of textbooks focusing on learning disability nursing practice. However, the inclusion of a chapter devoted to research within such texts remains relatively rare. The opportunity to write this chapter is, therefore, a significant and rare privilege.

The starting point for research is a question that needs addressing. From this flow a number of further questions, such as: Why is this an important issue? How can the question best be addressed? What methods will provide the relevant information? How can we make sense of the information that is gathered? Who needs to know the findings of the research? In keeping with this questioning approach the chapter focuses on the following in order to explore research in the context of learning disability nursing:

- Why do we need research?
- What is the current situation in learning disability nursing research?
- What challenges do we face in developing learning disability nursing research?
- How can we respond to these challenges?

The aims of the chapter are thus to provide an overview of learning disability nursing research, to provide some practical suggestions as to how this can be further developed, and hence to encourage readers to actively engage in this process of development. Given the breadth of the subject and the constraints of chapter length every effort has been made to support the discussion with reference to appropriate literature so that readers can follow up areas of particular interest if they so wish.

Underpinning these aims is the belief that while not all learning disability nurses will undertake original research, all learning disability nurses have a responsibility to engage with and to promote research. It is thus hoped that readers will find this chapter relevant to their practice and that it will provide a framework for the development of learning disability nursing research.

Why do we need research?

Parahoo (2006) suggests that nursing can achieve parity with other professions by the creation of a body of knowledge and that research is the means by which such knowledge can be both developed and validated. While this is an important reason to undertake nursing research, professional advancement, however, cannot be the sole driving force.

Abbott (2002: 17) argues that nursing research '…is essential for improving the standards and quality of patient care'. Indeed, as Burton and Chapman (2004) note, the decisions made by practitioners based upon such research have key implications both for clients and for those who support them. Accordingly the Nursing and Midwifery Council (NMC) have identified in their Code (NMC, 2008) that all nurses '…must deliver care based on the best available evidence or best practice'. Similarly, in the *Good Practice in Learning Disability Nursing* document (Department of Health, 2007) Benchmark 11 states that 'Learning disability nurses are able to base their practice on sound evidence and contribute to the development of the local and national evidence base regarding the health needs of people with learning disabilities'. While research is only one form of evidence, there is thus a clear professional responsibility placed upon all nurses to utilise research to inform their practice where such research is available. This requires not only that nurses have knowledge and skills in relation to research awareness, critical appraisal, reflection and decision making (McSherry et al, 2002) but also that research which is relevant to practice is both accessible and available. However, since research is one of the 'main tools' available to assist in the questioning of practice and the development of answers to such questions (Parahoo, 2006), all practitioners have a role to play in the identification of research questions. All nurses therefore need to be research minded where this quality is defined as '…an attitude and an ability to ask questions of one's practice which can be answered through the process of research' (Parahoo, 2006:13).

In addition to professional reasons for undertaking research and using research to inform practice other motivating factors can also be found within the literature. McConkey (1998) reminds us of the link between evidence-based practice and 'value for money' services referring to these two factors as 'twin forces'. There is thus an economic dimension to evidence-based practice that cannot be ignored: where services have limited financial resources there may be a reluctance to use such resources to support interventions if evidence of effectiveness is not available. It is of concern that a decade later Griffiths et al (2007) note the continued lack of an adequate evidence base for learning disability nursing.

This may have particular implications for learning disability nurses since

Turnbull (1997) pointed to the lack of evidence of effectiveness in relation to learning disability nursing practice. He further argued that the absence of such evidence may be interpreted as a lack of evidence of a sound basis for nursing practice.

In seeking to develop research-based evidence and to use it within practice it is essential that we focus not only on what we do but also upon how the evidence base is both developed and applied. For example Jukes (2003) notes the importance of tailoring the application of theory to practice so that the needs of the individual are met rather than application at a global level, and Burton and Chapman (2004) remind us that the practitioner and the client can have differing views as to the effectiveness of an intervention. Gates and Atherton (2001) thus argue that, within the context of learning disabilities, the issue of evidence-based practice has to be considered alongside other key issues such as empowerment and the involvement of service users. They further argue that if we are to establish evidence for the use of any intervention in practice then this process needs to include seeking the views and wishes of people with learning disabilities.

It can thus be seen that there are a number of compelling reasons as to why learning disability nurses need to engage with research. Indeed a failure to do so may pose a significant threat to the development of learning disability nursing practice and the extent to which it is able effectively to meet the needs of people with learning disabilities. The current position in relation to learning disability nursing research thus needs to be explored.

The current situation in learning disability nursing

It has been suggested that learning disability nursing draws upon a number of other academic disciplines for its evidence base (Kay, 1995; Gates and Atherton, 2001; Mitchell, 2004). Indeed learning disability nursing research operates at the interface between wider nursing research and wider learning disability research (*Figure 5.1*). Before considering learning disability nursing research it is thus necessary to examine the context within which it exists and hence each of these two fields of research require some consideration.

Nursing research

Nursing research has been defined as '...the systematic investigation of nursing practice and the effects of this practice on patient care, on individual, family or community health' (Abbott, 2002:15). Parahoo (2006) suggests that defining nursing research can be difficult both due to a lack of consensus with regard to the definition of nursing and also due to the fact that nursing roles are constantly evolving and expanding. Accordingly he

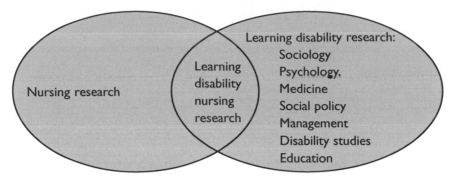

Figure 5.1. The position of learning disability nursing research (Northway et al, 2006).

offers a somewhat more inclusive definition than Abbott suggesting that it also encompasses research that focuses on the training and education of nurses, on organisational delivery of services, on the conditions in which nurses work, the way in which they influence such work environments, and the impact of their work on themselves.

Nursing has been viewed as a young academic discipline and hence nursing research has been described as being at 'a relatively early stage of development' (Task Group 3, 2001). This means that, compared to other healthcare professions, such as medicine and psychology, nursing does not have such a long tradition of undertaking research.

In 2001 the Centre for Policy in Nursing Research et al reported that while there had been an increase in published nursing and midwifery nursing research over the previous 10 years it had not increased since 1995. In addition almost three quarters of the research which had been published did not indicate a funding source, suggesting that such studies had been self-funded. The need to improve the funding for nursing research has thus been noted (Task Group 3, 2001).

Another measure of the progress which has been made in relation to nursing research is the research assessment exercise that is undertaken periodicially in all subject areas within the UK. The 2001 report of the Nursing and Midwifery RAE Panel (HEFCE, 2001) noted an increase in the number of nursing departments submitting their work for assessment, an improvement in the number of submissions achieving a higher grade, and an increase in the number of staff submitted. These are all positive developments which suggest an expansion in nursing research. Nonetheless, the report also noted difficulties due to low funding levels and sources of funding, and to the underdevelopment of collaboration in relation to topic areas and research programmes, which were fragile due to high levels of staff movement. In addition while they noted some 'relatively solid' areas of research (which included care of older people, mental health, and pain management) learning disability was not identified as one such area. The overall picture which emerged was, therefore, of nursing as a discipline that is growing in research strength but which still faced considerable challenges in developing further.

The subject overview report of the RAE 2008 Sub Panel 11 (Nursing and Midwifery) (HEFCE, 2009) notes that fewer nursing departments submitted themselves for assessment than did so in 2001 (35 as opposed to 43). Nonetheless some positive developments are noted such as strengths in research focused on patient benefit and the development of service user involvement. It is concluded that monies invested in nursing research since 2001 have led to capacity building and the development of research leaders. However, it is stressed that such investment needs to be 'sustained and enhanced'. Specific subject areas are not commented upon within the report so it is not possible to assess the performance of learning disability nursing research in this context.

In developing their practice, learning disability nurses need to draw not only upon learning disability-specific nursing research but also upon wider nursing research while understanding the need for critical appraisal and careful monitoring of its impact upon individual clients. For example, it is important to access the research concerning the assessment and management of pain in order that people with learning disabilities have access to the most effective treatments. However, it is also important to acknowledge that some people with learning disabilities may express pain in different ways, thus making some standard assessments difficult, and that some interventions designed to reduce pain can have differing levels of effectiveness with clients who have pre-existing neurological damage.

Learning disability research

There appear to be differing views regarding the current situation in relation to learning disability research. Recently, McKenzie et al (2006:10) have argued that 'the field of learning disabilities as a whole has a relatively robust evidence base'. However, Parmenter (2001:191) suggested that many of the interventions used in the field of learning disabilities are 'of uncertain value and ... have never been tested'. It seems unlikely, however, that the situation would have changed so dramatically in the five years between publication of these two comments. Indeed Dalton and McVilly (2004) argue that one of the major ethical issues that needs to be addressed by both the scientific community and Governments is the lack of research in the field of learning disabilities. It would seem more likely, therefore, that while there is a relatively strong body of research in relation to some aspects of learning disability, deficits exist in other areas.

To understand this situation it is important to understand the historical context of learning disability research. In 1958 Clarke and Clarke observed that learning disabilities had been a neglected area of study and 26 years later Digby (1996) suggested that the 'social marginality' of people with learning disabilities had been mirrored by their 'academic marginality'. This suggests that learning disability had not, traditionally been viewed as a key area of academic interest and hence research in this field has been slower to develop. A lack of political interest might also explain this situation since Turnbull (1997) argues that learning disability research has not been viewed as a Government priority despite the fact that significant Government resources are spent on supporting this client group. Funding for research in this area can thus limit the extent of research in this field, as acknowledged at an international level by Dalton and McVilly (2004).

Allen (1997) undertook a review of research in the field of learning disabilities and identified three main types of research – local investigations or evaluations of service developments, epidemiological research, and large-scale studies. In commenting upon the quality of such research she suggests that there are often 'tenuous relationships' between the needs of the researcher and those of people with learning disabilities; information is often not provided as to how the consent of people with learning disabilities was obtained when they acted as research subjects; and there was duplication of work. In relation to this last point she distinguishes between 'duplication' and 'replication', arguing that the latter is a valid scientific process.

The overall conclusion that Allen draws is that 'research into learning disability is, by and large, not co-ordinated, work is disparate and therefore fails to address the immediate health needs in the lives of people with learning disabilities in a focused way' (1997:360). While research in this field should obviously be concerned with more than just the health needs of people with learning disabilities, and while even if good quality research exists it may not be translated into practice, the picture which emerges is one of research studies often being undertaken in isolation from each other and failing to have an impact on the lives of people with learning disabilities.

It has been suggested that research in relation to learning disabilities can pose methodological challenges. McConkey (1998), for example, identifies three key areas of difficulty in relation to such research. The first relates to difficulties that arise due to imprecise definitions and the heterogeneity of the population to whom the label 'learning disabilities' is applied. For example, the needs of someone with profound and multiple disabilities will differ greatly from those of someone with mild learning disabilities. This means that there can be difficulties both in obtaining an adequate sample and in generalising from the findings of research. Second, he suggests that few of the measures used in studies have been tested in relation to reliability and validity. Finally, he notes that few longitudinal studies have been undertaken which means that both changes over time and the sustainability of any gains made due to interventions may be difficult to determine.

Burton and Chapman (2004) have also identified some key difficulties with undertaking and utilising research in the field of learning disability. First they argue that the context in which many interventions are delivered is an 'open system' and hence they are influenced by many factors. Second, they argue that meanings are both individually and collectively created and thus, as has previously been noted, client and practitioner views regarding interventions and their impact can differ. Finally the contexts in which interventions are delivered vary considerably and hence interventions developed within a well-resourced research centre may not be as effective when utilised by staff in an under-resourced service.

Nonetheless, when considered in an international context, research in this field has developed, as witnessed by organisations such as the International Association for the Scientific Study of Intellectual Disability (IASSID). Furthermore, if presentations at the quadrennial IASSID World Congresses are considered then it can also be seen that over a 33-year period the focus of the research shifted somewhat, with a decline in biomedical papers and an increase in the proportion of papers that focus on social or behavioural research (Parmenter, 2004). The proportion of papers focusing on epidemiology, policy, early intervention and vocational issues remained relatively constant over the same period (Parmenter, 2004).

As with nursing research it can thus be seen that research in relation to learning disabilities is also very much at a developmental stage and shares some common challenges such as access to funding and the development of sustainable lines of inquiry.

Learning disability nursing research

Research undertaken by Parahoo et al (2000) found that only a quarter of their sample of 87 learning disability nurses in Northern Ireland reported using research frequently or all of the time in their practice. Some of the reasons for this lack of use were given as being a lack of awareness and a lack of access to research. However, it was also suggested by the authors that proportionally less research has been carried out in learning disability nursing when compared with other branches of nursing: the nurses cannot therefore use what is not available.

While learning disability nurses can (and do) draw upon research undertaken by other branches of nursing and also upon wider learning disability research there is a need for research that focuses upon their specific contribution and upon the effectiveness of their interventions. As Parahoo et al (2000:608) comment, 'there appears to be a lack of research providing the necessary evidence for practice in the field of learning disability in general and learning disability nursing in particular'.

The limited extent of this research has been noted by a number of authors. For example Kay (1995:96) commented that as part of the nursing profession learning disability nursing requires an 'adequate research-based resource'. However, he also argued that 'it is still some way from achieving this' and suggested that what research there was had tended to focus upon staffing issues, training and resource issues rather than upon clinical nursing practice. Turnbull (1997) also points to limited research in this field and Moulster and Turnbull (2004:65) similarly comment upon 'the little research into the area of learning disability nursing practice'.

These observations are perhaps not surprising given the discussion in preceding sections: both nursing research and learning disability research are at relatively early developmental stages and they both share common challenges such as difficulties with accessing funding. In addition, problems of definition have been noted both within nursing research (Parahoo, 2006) and within learning disability research (McConkey, 1998). Furthermore since learning disability nurses form both a small part of the wider nursing profession and also a small part of the wider group of professionals involved in supporting people with a learning disability, they may face additional challenges in developing research since learning disability nursing-specific research may not be viewed as a priority in the context of competing demands.

It is important to note, however, that each of the above observations regarding the limited research in this field was made in the absence of a systematic literature review of research undertaken by, or concerning, learning disability nurses. In order to address this deficit the author of this chapter, along with colleagues, thus sought and obtained funding to undertake such a review focusing on research published by learning disability nurses or concerning learning disability nursing in the UK and Ireland during the years 1995 to 2003 (Northway et al, 2006). (NB while some non-UK and Ireland studies were included in this review they were considered separately since specialist learning disability nursing does not exist in all countries and, where it does, the training, preparation, and roles of such nurses differ. It was not possible, therefore, to compare like with like).

This review adopted a systematic approach to searching the literature using a variety of terms to interrogate a range of electronic databases, undertaking a hand search of key journals, and also using a snowball technique in which the reference lists of papers obtained were scanned for further papers (see Northway et al, 2006 for further information). In total 142 papers meeting the inclusion criteria were identified and it was possible to identify learning disability nurses as authors in 129 of these. It should be noted, however, that this does not equate to 142 different studies since some papers reported different aspects of the same study. The papers included in the review were categorised in the following way:

- Educational and professional developments (*n* = 35)
- Healthcare experiences (*n* = 28)
- Service development and delivery (*n* = 23)
- Challenging behaviour (*n* = 18)
- Methodology (*n* = 15)
- Role of the learning disability nurse (*n* = 10)
- Historical research (*n* = 7)
- Therapeutic interventions (*n* = 6)

Difficulties were encountered with assigning papers to a single category since some focused on more than one area. For example, some of the papers that focused on challenging behaviour inevitably touched upon the role of the nurse in delivering interventions. Papers were thus assigned on the basis of their predominant focus. While each of these areas can be seen to meet the definition of nursing research offered by Parahoo (2006) it is interesting to note that, as observed by Kay (1995), a significant number of papers focused on educational and professional issues as well as on service development and delivery rather than on clinical nursing practice. This is of concern in the context previously discussed whereby an absence of evidence of effectiveness is likely to be viewed negatively.

A range of methodologies was used within the studies reported. Forty two used a qualitative approach, 50 a quantitative approach, 25 mixed methods and 25 other approaches (including methodological papers, historical research and systematic reviews of the literature).

The year in which the papers were published was noted and from this it was evident that while there had been a big increase in the number of papers published in 1998 (from 7 in the previous year to 20) the number published per year had remained relatively stable since then (range 19–23). While occurring some three years later (1998 as opposed to 1995) this 'plateau effect' may be seen to reflect the wider situation in nursing research whereby the number of papers published per annum had not increased since 1995 (Centre for Policy in Nursing Research et al, 2001).

The two journals publishing the greatest number of papers included in the study were the *Journal of Learning Disabilities* (previously the *Journal of Learning Disabilities for Nursing, Health and Social Care* and now the *Journal of Intellectual Disabilities*), which published 35 papers during the period, and *Learning Disability Practice,* which published 19. This is particularly worthy of note since the former was first published in 1997 and the latter in 1998 meaning that they were not in existence for the entire period which formed the focus of the review.

In drawing conclusions from this review it is important to note its limitations, particularly the fact that it focused only on published research. Accordingly there will be other research undertaken by, or concerning, learning disability nursing which has not been included (for example, that undertaken as part of master's programmes or local evaluation studies). In addition it was, of necessity, limited to a particular time period and further research is required to determine whether the trends detected have been maintained. However, some positive developments were noted such as the increase in papers published, the number of papers in which a learning disability nurse is an author and the range of journals in which the papers were published.

Nonetheless some areas for development were also identified, most notably the need to extend the range of research designs used, the need to address those areas of research identified as requiring attention within existing studies, the need for action in relation to funding, the need to develop collaboration, and the need to actively involve people with learning disabilities in the research process. This latter recommendation is also evident in the publication by the UK Learning Disability Consultant Nurse Network (UKLDCNN, 2006: 16) in which they argue that involving people with learning disabilities is 'a matter for any learning disability nurse researcher'.

Subsequent to the Northway et al review a further review was undertaken by a team of researchers at King's College London (Griffiths et al, 2007). They used a broader definition of learning disability nursing research, utilised a different search strategy and encompassed a wider range of years (1996–2006); 180 papers were identified as meeting the criteria for inclusion in the review. This includes non-UK papers. The overall conclusion drawn by the researchers makes uncomfortable reading:

The extent of learning disability nursing research is limited in quantity and its ability to provide reliable, generalisable or trustworthy insights. Much of what exists is fragmented and consists of small scale evaluations which may provide guidance and inspiration for service development but do not, in themselves, constitute robust research evidence...We conclude that the current body of learning disability research is not fit for purpose in terms of its extent, quantity or quality.

In order to change this situation a number of recommendations are made which include prioritising research which focuses on determining the

Table 5.1. Challenges facing the development of learning disability nursing research

The challenge of relevance	The challenge of ethics
The challenge of coherence	The challenge of inclusion
The challenge of priority setting	The challenge of funding

impact of nursing interventions. Other recommendations include greater programmatic research, valuing of replication studies and greater attention to the quality of studies. The need to form 'strategic alliances' either with the wider nursing research community and/or disciplines such as psychology and social work is proposed.

Generating the research is, however, only one aspect of evidence-based practice: the link with practice also needs to be explored. While the study undertaken by Parahoo et al (2000) provides some insight into the extent of research used within practice, the authors also note a 'paucity' of data concerning the research activities of learning disability nurses (including the extent to which they use research). The need for further studies concerning the extent to which learning disability nurses access and utilise research has thus been identified (Northway et al, 2006).

Challenges faced in developing learning disability nursing research

The current situation in relation to learning disability nursing research has been discussed above and the need to both undertake more research in this field (Griffiths et al 2007; Northway et al, 2006; UKLDCNN, 2006) and to ensure that research is utilised to inform practice (UKLDCNN, 2006) have been noted. The UKLDCNN (2006:16) have suggested that:

The challenge for learning disability nurses is to understand research as a way to answer day-to-day clinical questions either through networking, accessing evidence, or conducting research. These activities should not be seen as the domain of a few but as one part of each nurse's broader role.

If learning disability nurses are to respond to this challenge, however, it is important that they recognise other challenges that need to be addressed in order that learning disability nursing research can develop. Accordingly six key challenges will be explored here (*Table 5.1*). It should be noted that all are important and they are inter-related, hence they are not presented in any order of priority.

The challenge of relevance

Relevance in the context of learning disability nursing research can mean a number of different things. For example, if research is to be used in practice by learning disability nurses then they need to see it as relevant to their practice. Without such relevance it is unlikely that practitioners will be motivated to access existing research and critically appraise it let alone seek to develop research of their own. Questions thus need to arise from practice, and dissemination of findings needs to stress the relevance to and implications for practice.

Most importantly, if learning disability nursing practice is concerned with enhancing the quality of life experienced by people with learning disabilities then the research undertaken must be relevant to the needs of people with learning disabilities. This in turn raises the question of how such relevance may be determined and requires that we actively engage with those whom we support in order to determine the issues that are relevant to them. We need to better understand how our interventions impact on their lives and it is suggested that this can best be determined by investigation of the lived experiences of people with learning disabilities (Jukes, 2003). This has implications not only for what we research but also for the methodologies and methods we select to address the identified questions. It also requires that strategies are developed to ensure that people with learning disabilities are able to access learning disability nursing research (UKLDCNN, 2006). Careful attention must thus be given to how research findings can be disseminated in a meaningful way.

It is also important to remember that people with learning disabilities are often living with their families. While family needs may differ from those of the client, learning disability nurses often work within the context of the family and support the family as well as the client. This being the case then research also needs to be relevant to their needs and they need to be able to access learning disability nursing research.

Finally learning disability nurses also need to consider how best to ensure that the research undertaken is relevant to the service, to the research funders and to the policy makers, since each of these groups may be key to providing the support required in order to undertake research.

The challenge of coherence

Just as the challenge of relevance has a number of dimensions so does the challenge of coherence. First there is the need to ensure that there is coherence between values, research questions and methods used to address such questions. For example both learning disability policy documents (such as

Scottish Executive, 2000; Department of Health, 2001; National Assembly for Wales, 2002a; Department of Health Social Services and Public Safety, 2004) and nursing policy documents (such as the National Assembly for Wales, 2002b; Scottish Executive, 2002) stress the importance of inclusion. This philosophy thus needs to inform the value base of learning disability nursing research hence the challenges of inclusive research practice will be discussed further below.

Coherence does, however, also need to operate at another level and if we are to develop learning disability nursing research then we need to ensure that there is coherence between research, practice and education. Whereas it is normally the relationship between research and practice which is discussed, it is also essential that we consider the ways in which education plays an integral and important role. Education must be relevant to practice and must be informed by research. It must also serve to sow the seeds of research mindedness among nurses.

Pre-registration nurse training has the potential to develop student interest in research, to help them understand its relevance to their practice, to develop confidence in accessing and appraising research evidence and to begin to develop the knowledge and skills needed to undertake original research. Use of the word 'potential' is deliberate here since the absence of current research concerning the impact of pre-registration nurse training on the development of research mindedness among learning disability nurses means that it is difficult to determine the extent to which this potential is met. The research undertaken by Parahoo et al (2000), however, suggests that this potential may not be fully realised given the small number of nurses reporting use of research in their day-to-day practice.

Post-registration nurse education needs to build upon the work undertaken within pre-registration education, and learning disability nurses need to be supported to develop their research skills further. This should include support up to post-doctoral level where appropriate. However, a challenge which is presented at all stages of nurse education is for those facilitating such education to help students see the relevance of research to their practice.

The challenge of priority setting

Setting priorities is always a difficult process. In the context of learning disability nursing research this is true for a number of reasons. First, there is the question of whose priorities should take precedence. For example the priorities of people with learning disabilities may not be the same as those of their families and these may differ from the views of nurses, service provider organisations and policy makers. A further important party that requires careful consideration are the funders of research who will each have their own priorities for allocation of their monies. Second, given that research in this area is limited, it means that much remains to be done. Selecting the most appropriate priority can, therefore, be difficult since there are many pressing areas that require investigation.

Finally, as has previously been noted, learning disability nursing will always be a small part of the wider family of nursing and also a small part of the range of professionals involved in supporting people with learning disabilities. It is thus important to note that supporting learning disability nursing research may not always be viewed as a priority by others. The challenge for learning disability nurses thus lies in recognising these tensions and in developing ways by which they can most effectively be managed.

The challenge of ethics

The limited research in the learning disability field has previously been noted (Dalton and McVilly, 2004) and elsewhere it is suggested that the ethical issues involved in undertaking research with this client group have contributed to difficulties in researching this area (Kay, 1995; Fisher, 2004). Such ethical challenges can arise both from action (undertaking research) and inaction (failing to undertake research). The nature of these ethical challenges thus needs to be better understood.

People with learning disabilities may be considered to be one of the 'vulnerable groups' in relation to research. This means that they can be vulnerable to abuse and exploitation in the context of research as witnessed by some examples from history. For example, Friedlander (1995) recounts details of the 'scientific experiments' undertaken in Nazi Germany which sought to devise ways of killing certain groups of humans 'cheaply and expeditiously'. Accordingly, disabled people (including those with a learning disability) were locked in a pillbox which was then dynamited, locked in a sealed room and subjected to exhaust fumes. More recently, in Willowbrook Hospital in the US a policy was implemented as late as 1972 in which children with learning disabilities could not be admitted to the facility unless their parents consented to them taking part in a study which sought to examine the natural history of infectious hepatitis and the effect of gamma globulin. In the study children were deliberately infected with hepatitis but only some received gamma globulin: it was withheld from others (Haber, 2002). These examples demonstrate that the ethical principles of non-maleficence (to do no harm) and autonomy (ensuring valid consent which is free from coercion) were violated.

One possible response to such violations is to argue that undertaking research involving people with learning disabilities raises too many ethical issues and that the best way to safeguard them is to exclude them from research wherever possible. However, such a position also has ethical implications as it can serve to marginalise the views and experiences of people with learning disabilities, it can exclude them from access to potentially beneficial treatments and interventions, and it could lead to an unfair and unjust distribution of resources. The ethical principle of justice (ensuring that everyone has an equal chance of benefiting from the research) would thus be violated.

While it might be expected that ethics committees would serve to ensure that appropriate decisions are made concerning the conduct of research in this field concerns have been expressed in relation to inconsistency of decision making among such committees (Lai et al, 2006). Personal experience has shown that while some ethics committees can be supportive and welcome the inclusion of people with learning disabilities in research both as participants and as researchers (see Ham et al, 2004) others can have negative views concerning the capacity of people with learning disabilities. The challenge that needs to be addressed is how the inclusion of people with learning disabilities can be facilitated in a way that is ethical and which promotes and preserves their dignity, autonomy and rights. Furthermore how can ethics committees best be made aware of such ethical methods of promoting such inclusion?

The challenge of inclusion

The need for research to be relevant to the lives of people with learning disabilities and their families has been noted above, as has the need to ensure that research is congruent with important values and principles, such as inclusion. In the context of developing research this means that the challenge lies first in identifying those barriers that have traditionally excluded key groups of people from the research process (other than their acting as passive subjects in other people's research).

To promote inclusion it is, however, necessary to change those systems and structures that have traditionally served to exclude (Northway, 1997). This requires that attitudes concerning the ability of people with learning disabilities to engage in research are challenged along with existing ways of undertaking research, that new ways of approaching it are explored and that the experience of engaging in this process is shared so that others can learn from our experiences. It is also essential that support is provided for people with learning disabilities to understand more about research and that they have the opportunity to develop their skills in this area if this is something which they wish to do. Such support may be financial (paying people with learning disabilities for their time and other expenses), educational (providing support to develop knowledge and skills concerning research) or practical (for example, the provision of easy-to-read information or transport).

In considering inclusion, however, it is also important to remember that practitioners have, traditionally, also often been excluded from the research process. Indeed Beresford (2005:7) argues that both service users and practitioners are at 'high risk of being overlooked, devalued and ignored'. A further challenge thus lies in developing ways of including those practitioners who have not viewed research as a key part of their role and in supporting them to actively engage in the process whether as a critical user of research in their day-to-day practice, as part of a research team, or in developing the knowledge and skills necessary to undertake original research.

The challenge of funding

The limited funding available for both nursing research and for learning disability research has already been noted. For researchers wishing to undertake learning disability nursing research the challenge is, therefore, self-evident. If further evidence is needed then it can be seen in the review of learning disability nursing research (Northway et al, 2006) where only 10% of the studies reviewed cited a funding source compared with 27% of studies in a review of wider nursing research (Centre for Policy in Nursing Research et al, 2001). This suggests that learning disability nursing research is less well funded than other areas of nursing research and that, as a consequence, many of the studies undertaken are self-funded. In addition, if sources of funding are considered, it can be seen that none of the studies reviewed by Northway et al (2006) cited funding from major charitable bodies or from the Research Councils.

Such difficulties with funding can limit the research that takes place in the field since self-funding means that studies are often small-scale, localised, and do not form part of a coherent programme of research. These factors may serve to limit the extent to which it is possible to generalise from the findings. Furthermore it can affect the way in which the research is viewed by others since the source of research funding is viewed as one indicator of quality (Higher Education Funding Council et al, 2006).

The challenge for learning disability nurses thus lies in developing mechanisms through which more research funding may be secured from a wider range of sources (to include 'quality' monies secured on a competitive basis). This is not to argue that small-scale local studies should not continue but rather to suggest that the range of funding sources needs to be extended and that learning disability nurses need to develop the knowledge, skills and confidence to seek funding from some of the larger, prestigious funding bodies.

Responding to the challenges

Having identified the key challenges that need to be addressed if learning disability nursing research is to be developed it is important that consideration is given as to how such challenges may best be addressed. Accordingly four key developments are discussed below. While they are presented separately here it will be noted that, as with the challenges, they are inter-related.

The development of participative research approaches

There has been considerable discussion over the past decade regarding the development of participatory, emancipatory and inclusive approaches to research with people with learning disabilities. It is beyond the scope of this chapter to explore the similarities and differences between these approaches but these can be accessed elsewhere (see, for example, Kiernan, 1999; Chappell, 2000; Northway, 2003; Walmsley and Johnson, 2003). In this context the term 'participative approaches' will be used to encompass the range of approaches that seek to promote the active participation of people with learning disabilities in research and, where possible, to support them in taking control over the decision making processes involved in research. This includes the identification of research questions, determining methodologies and methods, seeking research funding, gathering and analysing data and reporting and disseminating findings.

By definition, participative approaches to research seek to promote the active involvement of groups who were previously excluded or who were in danger of being excluded. Seeking to develop such research is thus a key step towards meeting the challenge of inclusion, previously identified, as well as promoting coherence between values, research questions and methods. In addition it is suggested that participatory research is a process that combines research, education and action (practice) (Khanlou and Peter, 2005) it thus also promotes coherence between these different elements. Moreover, since it seeks to address questions of relevance to the community (Macaulay et al, 1999) it addresses the challenge of relevance. Finally it has been suggested that participatory research can promote greater 'ethical acceptability' by giving people greater control over the research process (Thomas and O'Kane, 1998).

There is some evidence of the development of participative research approaches within the context of learning disability nursing research (see for example, Richardson, 1997, 2000; McClimmens, 1999; Northway 2000, 2003; Ham et al, 2004). It is viewed as having much to offer research in this field since it enables learning disability nurse researchers to work with people with learning disabilities to ensure that their views are central to the process of practice, policy and research development. It promotes a reflexive approach towards both research and practice and it brings research and practice closer together (Northway, 2003). Thus while not all learning disability nursing research will be participative in nature there is a need to ensure that it does form an integral part of the expansion of research in this area (Northway, 2003), particularly since it has the potential to address many of the challenges previously identified.

In discussing the challenge of inclusion, however, it was noted that practitioners as well as service users have often been excluded from active participation in the research process (Beresford, 2005). It is thus important to note that participative approaches have also been used to promote the participation of practitioners in research. For example Koch et al (2002) worked with nurses to develop research projects that arose from practice concerns, which sought to investigate these areas of practice and which used the findings of research to enhance and improve practice. Such an approach would also appear to have potential in the context of learning disability nursing research.

The development of a supportive culture

Parahoo et al (2000:611) argue that:

> *Without an environment which encourages questioning, supports innovation, provides adequate resources and in which individuals are valued, evidence-based practice will be a difficult and arduous journey to achieve.*

If research is thus to develop within the context of learning disability nursing then there needs to be a culture that encourages and nurtures such development. This culture needs to be developed and maintained in both practice and educational settings (thus addressing the challenge of coherence).

Jukes (2003) suggests that in order to do this we need to move beyond the positions of 'elitism' and 'anti-intellectualism'. The former refers to an academic culture in which theory is perceived as being superior to the 'real world' of learning disability practice and the latter does not value theory since it is perceived as 'not only irrelevant but also a barrier to existing practice'. We have all encountered examples of people taking up such positions but neither is helpful in this context since, as has already been argued, both research and practice, coupled with education, are essential in the development of learning disability nursing research. Practitioners working in practice, educational and research settings thus need to work together in a collaborative manner.

Jukes goes on to suggest a number of ways in which a shared and supportive culture can be developed. The first of these is the development of learning sets in which people come together with the focus on a particular issue, the aim being to narrow the theory–practice gap. In this context such a development could bring together practitioners, academics and researchers to focus upon a particular issue and to draw upon each others' experience and expertise in order to use research to inform practice development.

A second suggestion put forward by Jukes is the development and use of research networks. One such network has been established in the north of England – the Yorkshire Universities Learning Disability Nursing Research and Development Forum. This is a joint venture between the Universities of Leeds, Huddersfield, Bradford, Hull and York, its terms of reference being:

- To provide a regular and accessible medium through which research and good practice initiatives can be shared across the region.
- To provide support to service colleagues to enable them to share examples of their work with others.
- To facilitate networking opportunities.
- To create opportunities for research collaboration between individual universities and practice areas.
- To boost the national profile of Yorkshire universities and associated service providers in the delivery of high quality education and practice in the field of learning disabilities. (Atherton, personal communication, 2006)

It can thus be seen that the emphasis is on bringing together learning disability nurses from a variety of backgrounds in order to disseminate research and encourage its use in practice as well as providing a forum through which service- and university-based staff can come together to develop collaborative research. Meetings are held approximately once every three months and attendance has reached over 70 with both qualified and student nurses attending. Some of the areas that have already been explored within this forum are health, palliative care and working with families.

The third means of bringing together theory and practice, as identified by Jukes (2003), is the development of 'communities of practice'. Such communities are said to provide a context for both the acquisition and creation of knowledge (Wenger, 1998). In the context of learning disability nursing research they can thus provide the opportunity for acquiring new knowledge either concerning the research process or the findings of existing research, as well as providing a context in which new knowledge can be created through the development of research. Three dimensions are viewed as essential to the development of such communities:

- Mutual engagement – this is a defining feature of a community since practice 'does not exist in the abstract' and meanings are negotiated through interactions with others.

- Joint enterprise – this includes the collective process of negotiation, it is defined by the participants and hence belongs to them, and it involves mutual accountability.
- Shared repertoire – the routines and ways of working become part of the community practice and act as a resource. (Wenger, 1998)

Communities of practice have been developed in a range of nursing contexts (see, for example, Lathlean and Le May, 2002; Moule, 2006). According to Lathlean and Le May the factors that influence the development, functioning and maintenance of communities of practice include membership, commitment (both from within the community and from outside it), relevance (to local communities and existing services), enthusiasm, infrastructure, skills (in accessing and appraising evidence) and resources for achieving the desired changes. At the time of writing the authors noted, however, that it was not possible to comment on the sustainability of the communities once facilitation was withdrawn.

The 'incidental' development of a community of practice has been reported in the context of developing learning disability nursing research (McKenzie et al, 2006). This initiative arose from a recognition that academic as well as clinical staff can face barriers to the development of research since there are many demands on their time and other resources and the culture within which they work may not support such development. In order to change this they established a group that met initially once every six weeks the aims being:

- To share research ideas and skills.
- To develop confidence in using research methodologies which were unfamiliar.
- To undertake clinically relevant research.
- To explore ways of encouraging nursing students to undertake research both before and after qualification. (McKenzie et al, 2006)

It was recognised, however, that such a development required the commitment of resources and hence a 'research buddy' role was created and funded. Essentially the focus of this role was to provide dedicated time to facilitate the translation of ideas into research proposals and to write up the research results for publication. As a result of this initiative a number of papers have been published and clinical staff and students have also become involved in making presentations at conferences and writing up research for publication.

It can thus be seen that the development of communities of practice has the potential to assist in the development of a culture that supports research in the context of learning disability nursing by bringing together those with a shared interest and by bringing theory and practice closer together. However, since learning through engagement with others is a key element, they also have the potential to respond to the challenge of coherence: research, practice and education develop together. Moreover, while Jukes (2003) suggests that such communities bring together research and practice-based communities, there is also the potential to include people with learning disabilities and their families, hence responding to the challenge of inclusion as well.

One final area that requires some discussion in relation to the development of a supportive culture is the role that nurse education can play in this process. Nursing students need to be encouraged to value the contribution of research from the early stages of their training and an educational programme designed to do this is viewed as important (Parahoo et al, 2000). The following are suggested as possible strategies by which this might be achieved:

- Research (where it is available) should underpin all teaching, thus demonstrating clear links between theory and practice.
- Teaching strategies should encourage a questioning approach among students and enable them to highlight areas of concern or interest within practice, to formulate research questions, and to identify potential ways of addressing such questions.
- Students must be supported not only to critically appraise research but also to consider the implications for practice arising from the research in the light of their appraisal.
- Where possible, teaching of research methods should draw upon real examples of learning disability nursing research and should enable students to hear about current research from those engaged in undertaking such research. This might, for example, include lecturers, practitioners and people with learning disabilities.
- Students should be encouraged to engage in networking activities and to attend seminars and conferences.

The development of ethical awareness

Dalton and McVilly (2004) argue that 'rigorous ethical safeguards' are needed in the context of research if people with learning disabilities are to be protected from vulnerability to exploitation and abuse. Accordingly they have developed some guidelines that can be used in the context of international, multicentre research. However, Lai et al (2006) argue that the need to weigh up conflicting ethical principles in the context of learning disability research makes it hard to apply a fixed set of guidelines to decision making processes.

Learning disability nurses thus need to be aware of the strategies that may be used to promote autonomy when seeking the consent of people with learning disabilities to participate in research. For example, in addition to the need to promote understanding via the use of accessible information, Dalton and McVilly (2004) also advocate the use of 'process consent' in which each new stage of the research involves explanation of what is involved and the involvement of participants is renegotiated. Information is thus presented at regular intervals and participants are given the opportunity to withdraw at any stage.

Lai et al (2006) argue that while it is unethical to expose people with learning disabilities to greater risks than the rest of society it is also unethical to deny them access to the potential benefits of research. Careful consideration thus needs to be given to the risk–benefit ratio in which the potential benefits of participation in the research need to be weighed against the possible risks that may result. Benefits may be direct or indirect where the former means that benefits of participation may be experienced directly by participants. For example, people with learning disabilities taking part in a drugs trial may benefit from access to newer forms of treatment or those taking part in an evaluation of a service that they use may benefit directly from changes being made to that service. However, in much research the benefits may be more indirect in that the participants may not experience personal gains although they may potentially benefit from longer-term changes that aim to improve service provision for all people with learning disabilities.

Risks that can occur in the context of research include the risk of physical or psychological harm but can also include the risk to personal reputation (as a consequence of either taking part or failing to take part) and the risk of exploitation. Dalton and McVilly (2004:63) argue that the risks involved should not normally exceed those involved in '…the provision of routine support or therapy, medical or psychological treatments'. Where risks do exceed this then safeguards should be in place that minimise the effects of such risks should they occur.

Learning disability nurses wishing to undertake research must thus be able to engage in ethical debates, to select from a range of possible actions and to justify their decisions. However, it is not just those nurses who undertake research who need to develop ethical awareness since those who wish to utilise research to inform their practice also need to be able critically to appraise its ethical aspects: if the research was not undertaken in an ethical manner then its quality and appropriateness for practice must be questioned.

The development of strategic thinking

Strategic thinking requires not only a clear idea of your aims but also a plan for how you will achieve such aims and an awareness of the difficulties that may be experienced in the process. If learning disability nursing research is to develop there is a need for the development of such strategic thinking since, without it, research in this field will be slow to develop and there is the danger that we perpetuate the situation in which research undertaken duplicates (rather than replicates) existing research, that it is uncoordinated and that its relevance to the needs of people with learning disabilities is open to question (Allen, 1997).

At present there is no definitive strategic document regarding the development of research in the context of learning disability nursing. Such a development would, however, be helpful for the reasons outlined above and it is hoped that the discussion set out in this chapter can assist in this process. Nonetheless, in the absence of such a document, it is possible to determine from existing literature some possible priority areas for inclusion.

The UKLDCNN (2006) have called upon individual practitioners to undertake more research, in particular stressing the need to focus upon research that addresses the health and behavioural needs of people with a learning disability. A similar view was put forward by Manthorpe et al (2003:133) who identified the need for evidence that learning disability nursing interventions work '…in terms of positive outcomes in health and well being' and also by Griffiths et al (2007) who recommend the development of studies which determine the effectiveness of nursing interventions with a specific focus on access to healthcare and behavioural problems.

Northway et al (2006), based on their review of research undertaken between 1995 and 2003, also make a number of recommendations that could inform the strategic direction of learning disability nursing research. For example, they highlight the need to extend the range of research methodologies, to act upon recommendations for further research within studies already published, to promote the wider inclusion of people with learning disabilities in research and to develop national and international research collaborations. This latter point is important since few multi-centre studies and no international comparative studies were found in the review. With the advent of devolution within the UK, and the consequent development of different learning disability policies and nursing policies within each of the four countries it is essential that the impact of such policies on practice are explored and lessons learnt. In addition, since there is world wide evidence of the health disparities experienced by people with learning disabilities, and since nurses have a key role to play in identifying and addressing such disparities, there would seem to be a pressing need for some international nursing studies. Northway et al (2006) also argue that the issue of funding for learning disability nursing research needs to be explored as a matter of priority.

At a strategic level, UKLDCNN (2006) call for the development and dissemination of standards for learning disability nursing research and for user involvement in education, practice development and research to be promoted more widely. They also note that further work is needed to build upon their document and that research (along with other areas) should be considered in more depth.

Taken together these recommendations might usefully form the starting point for the development of a more strategic approach to learning disability nursing research. However, alongside these there would appear to be the need for some work to be undertaken in relation to priority setting since (given the limited research base in this field) there would appear to be many areas to address. Such a process would need to involve all key stakeholders if it is to be inclusive and if the resulting agenda is to be viewed as relevant. This means that people with learning disabilities, their families, practitioners, academics, service providers, policy makers and research funders would need to be involved, the aim being to try to identify some areas of consensus regarding priorities.

A clear strategic approach to learning disability nursing research may take some time to develop but in the meantime there are some strategies that can be used by individuals and groups wishing to develop research in this area. These include:

- The development of strategic alliances – such alliances might be with (for example) people with learning disabilities, with other learning disability nurses, with other professionals, or with nurses working in other fields of nursing. By working together and pooling expertise then wider opportunities may become accessible.
- The development of policy awareness – research funding can often be tied to policy objectives. By ensuring that we have a good awareness of these we can anticipate priorities and be ready to respond to them. In addition we can seek to influence policy in order to promote issues of concern to people with a learning disability, their families and learning disability nurses.
- The use of lateral thinking – a number of times in this chapter difficulties with accessing funding for learning disability nursing research have been highlighted. It is unlikely that this will change in the short term and hence it is necessary that we take a different approach. If, for example, monies are available for research in relation to the management of chronic health problems then we need to make the case for undertaking such research in the context of learning disabilities. If funding is available for the study of nurse leadership then we need to be able to argue that such research could be undertaken in the context of learning disability nursing.

Conclusions

This chapter has sought to explore the current situation in relation to learning disability nursing research, to identify the challenges that must be addressed when seeking to expand research in this field, and to suggest some strategies that can be used in order to address these challenges. It has been argued that while the extent of learning disability nursing research currently is limited it is a developing area that has the potential to expand further. Indeed there are pressing reasons as to why such development must take place. However, if this is to happen effectively then a strategic and co-ordinated approach needs to be developed. Practitioners, researchers and academics need to work together at local, national and international levels, they need to adopt an inclusive approach, they need to ensure that research is relevant, that it is conducted ethically, and that it impacts on practice. Most importantly they need to ensure that any research undertaken impacts positively on the lives of people with learning disabilities.

References

Abbott P (2002) Implementing evidence-informed nursing. Research awareness. In: McSherry R, Simmons M, Abbott P (eds) *Evidence-Informed Nursing. A Guide for Clinical Nurses*. Routledge, London: 14–40

Allen J (1997) Contemporary and new horizons in learning disability research. In: Gates B, Beacock C (eds) *Dimensions of Learning Disability*. Bailliere Tindall, Edinburgh: 343–64

Beresford P (2005) Theory and practice of user involvement in research. Making the connection with public policy and practice. In: Lowes L, Hulatt I (eds) *Involving Service Users in Health and Social Care Research*. Routledge, London: 6–17

Burton M, Chapman MJ (2004) Problems of evidence based practice in community based services. *Journal of Learning Disabilities* **8**(1): 56–70

Centre for Policy in Nursing Research, CHEMS Consulting, Higher Education Consultancy Group and the Research Forum for Allied Health Professions (2001) *Promoting Research in Nursing and the Allied Health Professions*. Centre for Policy in Nursing Research, London

Chappell A. (2000) Emergence of participatory methodology in learning difficulty research: Understanding the context. *British Journal of Learning Disabilities* **28**(1): 38–43

Clarke AM, Clarke ADB (1958) Foreword. In: Clarke AM, Clarke AB (eds) *Mental Deficiency: The Changing Outlook* (2nd edn). Methuen London: xiii - xiv

Dalton AJ, McVilly KR (2004) Ethics guidelines for international multicenter research involving people with intellectual disabilities. *Journal of Policy and Practice in Intellectual Disabilities* **1**(2): 57–70

Department of Health (2001) *Valuing People: A New Strategy for Learning Disability for the 21st Century.* Department of Health, London

Department of Health (2007) *Good Practice in Learning Disability Nursing.* Department of Health, London

Department of Health, Social Services and Public Safety (2004) *Equal Lives: Review of Policy and Services for People with Learning Disabilities in Northern Ireland,* Stormont: Belfast

Digby A (1996) Contexts and perspectives. In: Wright D, Digby A (eds) *From Idiocy to Mental Deficiency. Historical Perspectives in People with Learning Disabilities,* Routledge London: 1–21

Fisher K (2004) Health disparities and mental retardation. *Journal of Nursing Scholarship* **36**(1): 48–53

Friedlander H (1995) *The Origins of Nazi Genocide. From Euthanasia to the Final Solution.* University of North Carolina Press, Chapel Hill

Gates B, Atherton H (2001) The challenge of evidence-based practice for learning disabilities. *British Journal of Nursing* **10**(8): 517–22

Griffiths P, Bennett J, Smith E (2007) *The Research Base for Learning Disability Nursing: A Rapid Scoping Review*, King's College, London

Haber J (2002) Legal and ethical issues. In: LoBiondo-Wood G, Haber J (eds) *Nursing Research. Methods, Critical Appraisal and Utilization.* Mosby, St Louis: 265–91

Ham M, Jones N, Mansell I, Northway R, Price L, Walker G (2004) 'I'm a researcher!' Working together to gain ethical approval for a participatory research study. *Journal of Learning Disabilities* **8**(4): 397–407

Higher Education Funding Council for England (2001) *RAE Unit of Assessment 10 – Nursing Overall Assessment of the Sector.* Available from: www.hero.ac.uk/rae/overview/docs/UoA10.pdf [Accessed 5th February 2009]

Higher Education Funding Council for England (2009) *RAE 2008 Unit of Assessment 11 Subject Overview Report*, Bristol : HEFCE. Available from: http://www.rae.ac.uk/pubs/2009/ov/ [accessed 5th February 2009]

Higher Education Funding Council for England, Scottish Funding
Council, Higher Education Funding Council for Wales, Department
for Employment and Learning (2006) *RAE 2008. Panel Criteria and
Working Methods. Panel C.* Higher Education Funding Council for
England, Bristol

Jukes M (2003) Towards practice development in contemporary learning
disability nursing. In: Jukes M, Bollard M (eds) *Contemporary
Learning Disability Practice.* Quay Books, Salisbury: 3–19

Kay B (1995) Grasping the research nettle in learning disabilities nursing.
British Journal of Nursing **4**(2): 96–8

Khanlou N, Peter E (2005) Participatory action research: Considerations
for ethical review. *Social Sciences and Medicine* **60:** 2333–40

Kiernan C (1999) Participation in research by people with learning
disability: Origins and issues. *British Journal of Learning Disabilities*
27(2): 43–7

Koch T, Selim P, Kralik D (2002) Enhancing lives through the
development of a community-based participatory action research
programme. *Journal of Clinical Nursing* **11:** 109–17

Lai R, Elliot D, Ouellette-Kuntz H (2006) Attitudes of research ethics
committee members towards individuals with intellectual disabilities:
The need for more research. *Journal of Policy and Practice in
Intellectual Disabilities* **2**: 114–118

Lathlean J, Le May A (2002) Communities of practice: an opportunity for
interagency working. *Journal of Advanced Nursing* **11:** 394–8

Macaulay A, Commanda LE, Freeman WL, Gibson N, McCabe ML,
Robbins CM, Twohig PL (1999) Participatory research maximises
community and lay involvement, *British Medical Journal* 319: 7748

Manthorpe J, Alaszewski A, Gates B, Ayer S, Motherby E (2003) Learning
disability nursing: User and carer perceptions. *Journal of Learning
Disabilities* **7**(2): 119–35

McClimmens A (1999) Participatory research with people who have a
learning difficulty: Journeys without a road map. *Journal of Learning
Disabilities for Nursing, Health and Social Care* **4**: 219–28

McConkey R (1998) Matching services to client needs: A research agenda
for the new century. *Journal of Learning Disabilities for Nursing,
Health and Social Care* **2**(2): 57–9

McKenzie K, Kwaitek E, Loads D, MacGregor L, Powell H (2006)
Encouraging learning disability nursing research, *Learning Disability
Practice* **9**(5): 10-4

McSherry R, Simmons M, Pearce P (2002) An introduction to evidence informed nursing. In: McSherry R, Simmons M, Abbott P (eds) *Evidence-Informed Nursing. A Guide for Clinical Nurses*. Routledge, London: 1–13

Mitchell D (2004) Learning disability nursing. *British Journal of Learning Disabilities* 32(3): 115–8

Moule P (2006) E-learning for healthcare students: Development of the communities of practice framework. *Journal of Advanced Nursing* 54(3): 370–80

Moulster G, Turnbull J (2004) The purpose and practice of learning disability nursing. In: Turnbull J (ed) *Learning Disability Nursing*. Blackwell, Oxford: 57–72

National Assembly for Wales (2002a) *Fulfilling the Promises: Proposals for Services for People with Learning Disabilities. Consultation Documents*. National Assembly for Wales, Cardiff

National Assembly for Wales (2002b) *Inclusion, Partnership and Innovation*. National Assembly for Wales, Cardiff

Northway R (1997) Integration and inclusion: Illusion or progress in services for disabled people? *Social Policy and Administration* 31(2): 157–72

Northway R (2000) Finding out together: Lessons in participatory research for the learning disability nurse. *Mental Healthcare* 3(7): 229–32

Northway R (2003) Participatory research. In: Jukes M, Bollard M (eds) *Contemporary Learning Disability Practice*. Quay Books, Salisbury: 165–74

Northway R, Mitchell D, Kaur-Mann K (2006) *Review of Learning Disability Nursing Research 1995–2003*. University of Glamorgan, Pontypridd

Nursing and Midwifery Council (2008) *The Code. Standards of Conduct, Performance and Ethics for Nurses and Midwives*, London: NMC

Parahoo K (2006) *Nursing Research. Principles, Process and Issues*. 2nd edn. Palgrave MacMillan, Basingstoke

Parahoo K, Barr O, McCaughan E (2000) Research utilisation and attitudes towards research among learning disabilities nurses in Ireland. *Journal of Advanced Nursing* 31(3): 607–13

Parmenter T (2001) The contribution of science in facilitating the inclusion of people with intellectual disability in the community. *Journal of Intellectual Disability Research* 45(3): 183–93

Parmenter T (2004) Contributions of IASSID to the scientific study of intellectual disability: The past, the present and the future. *Journal of Policy and Practice in Intellectual Disabilities* **1**(2): 71–8

Richardson M (1997) Participatory research methods: People with learning disabilities. *British Journal of Nursing* **6**(9): 1114–21

Richardson M (2000) How we live: Participatory research with six people with learning difficulties. *Journal of Advanced Nursing* **32**(6): 1383–95

Scottish Executive (2000) *The Same as You? A Review of Services for People with Learning Disabilities.* The Stationary Office, Edinburgh

Scottish Executive (2002) *Promoting Health Supporting Inclusion.* The Stationary Office, Edinburgh

Task Group 3 (2001) *Research in Nursing and Allied Health Professions.* Higher Education Funding Council for England, Bristol

Thomas N, O'Kane C (1998) The ethics of participatory research with children. *Children and Society* **12:** 336–48

Turnbull J (1997) Learning disability nursing: A position paper. *Journal of Learning Disabilities for Nursing, Health and Social Care* **1**(4): 186–190

United Kingdom Learning Disability Consultant Nurse Network (2006) *Shaping the Future: A Vision for Learning Disability Nursing.* UKLDCNN, United Kingdom

Walmsley J, Johnson K (2003) *Inclusive Research with People with Learning Disabilities. Past, Present and Futures.* Jessica Kingsley, London

Wenger E (1998) *Communities of Practice. Learning, Meaning and Identity.* Cambridge University Press, Cambridge:

Section Three:

Practices

CHAPTER 6

Community learning disability nursing

Mark Jukes and Simon Jones

Introduction

Community learning disability nursing (CLDN) is a term that perhaps only 50 years ago would have been meaningless. Prefixing either an organisation, facility or service with the term 'community' is relatively recent. 'Learning disability' is a term that has only recently replaced an ever-changing lexicon of terminology commencing, in recent history, with the Mental Deficiency Act of 1913 using the nowadays highly derogatory terms of 'idiot', 'imbecile' and 'feeble-minded' The Mental Deficiency Act of 1927 focused on the term 'defective' and the Mental Health Act of 1983 used the term 'mental impairment'. Based on this progression of language it is reasonable to assume that even the expression 'learning disability' as a descriptor, is fading and now intellectual disability is becoming more conventional.

The only common theme in the title CLDN is 'nursing' and it could be argued that, for most of the general population, the work of a CLDN does not fit easily into the stereotype of a nurse who is perceived as wearing a uniform and working in a hospital, surgery or primary healthcare centre.

The manner in which the terminology has changed illustrates very well how the whole concept of CLDN has been developed as a rather muddled reaction to social change and political events rather than following a pre-chartered and evolutionary pathway towards contemporary practice.

This semantic use of terms permeates every aspect of CLDN. For community learning disability nurses, this seemingly endless argument over what nomenclature to use is as potentially tedious as the accompanying arguments over what is the role of the CLDN. This chapter however, seeks to provide some explanation, and hopefully provide further focus and clarity to the discussion.

Mobbs et al (2002) observe that CLDN 'is a continually evolving discipline and defining the role is far from easy'. Turnbull (2004) however, makes the crucial and seminal point that 'although many health and social care and educational professionals work with people with learning disabilities, learning disability nurses are the sole professional group who have been educated to work with them'.

This chapter considers how CLDN has evolved over the last 30 years since its inception from the point where the long-stay hospital model began to wane in popularity, firstly with theoreticians, psychologists and sociologists (e.g. Kurtz and Wolfensberger), society and politicians and finally, and probably more fundamentally some would argue, with Government economists.

Consideration is given to how CLDN has refined its role and how the different regions within the UK and Ireland have developed services, and the question of whether learning disability services should plan to become more specialist or more generalist or whether in fact they can do both is explored.

Community learning disability nursing

The essential question has always been, 'What is the need that learning disability nurses meet?' When in the not so distant past, and certainly right up to the end of the 20th century, society confined those with a learning disability in a long-stay specialist hospital, this question was easy: the simplistic answer would be 'all'. However, as soon as learning disability nurses led (or followed) their clients out into the community there was immediately a multiplicity of care providers consisting, as noted by Clifton et al (1992) of:

- Primary carers
- Social workers
- Educationalists
- Voluntary workers
- And, probably most significantly, family and informal carers.

Establishing which of these roles fits best with the classification of CLDN has been convoluted, and for many, is still unresolved (Jukes, 2003; Brittle, 2004).

Cullen (Department of Health, 1991), maintained that the distinction between health and social care is largely artificial and that all people, including those with a learning disability, have a mixture of needs. However, the National Health Service and Community Care Act (1990) required a clear distinction to be drawn between social and health responsibilities.

The speed of the move into the community for people with learning disability has been slow (Glasby, 2000). It would seem that as society's collective consciousness moved more and more towards a philosophy that sought to value humanity equally, then the rationale for treating learning disabled people differently and keeping them 'out of sight and out of mind' in long-stay hospitals was no longer valid or appropriate (Gates, 1997). Equally, as identified earlier, past economics of such a change were compelling: long-stay hospitals were funded exclusively by the NHS, whereas people living in the community could live at home or in residential or supported housing, where they could also claim social security and housing benefits. In a community-based model, and with existing primary care services largely supporting health needs, the huge costs to the NHS of the long-stay hospitals could be almost completely avoided (with the possible exception of the cost of retained units and paying for placements for a few in independent hospitals).

It was even worth the NHS financing and subsidising the change and supporting many of the community-based residential services as the long-term savings were potentially considerable. (Since 2006 this funding of social and residential care has been extensively reviewed as the Strategic Health Authorities, who are the commissioning bodies, seek to claw back much of the financial support. They are seeking to achieve this further saving by the simple strategy of revisiting the question of whether the funding of residential care in the community is not more correctly termed a social care need rather than a healthcare one. Therefore, as such, it does not represent an appropriate or justifiable use of already stretched health services monies, the current ethos being supported or independent living driven by direct independent payments, where service users are tenants.)

Whatever conclusion one draws as to motivation for change the move to a community-based model of care was inevitable and accordingly community-based specialist services began to be established throughout the UK as described by Meehan et al (1995).

However, almost from inception, not all the commissioning authorities were convinced of the need for such specialists. The Jay Report (1979) was perhaps the most candid in recommending that learning disability nurses should see themselves remaining in their original role as residential care workers and advocated that mainstream primary and secondary health services ought to be tasked with providing healthcare to those with a learning disability. It is against this background of debate about patient needs and roles that the community learning disability nurse has developed. (The discomfort with which learning disability nurses see their role is illustrated further through defining this population, in that how do learning disability community nurses refer to the people they are working with; are they 'patients, clients, residents or service users'? These semantics seem to achieve nothing, but do waste an inordinate amount of valuable time and interest some academics, but very few 'patients, clients, residents or service users'.)

The policy framework

There have been numerous Government guidance documents and reports, such as Briggs (1972), Jay (1979) and policy statements, such as *Continuing the Commitment* (Kay et al, 1995) and, more recently, the White Paper *Valuing People* (Department of Health, 2001) which have all sought to define who has both the responsibility and the expertise to promote the health and well-being of people with a learning disability. Other regions have also produced their own strategy policy frameworks where Scotland has the *The Same as You?* (Scottish Executive, 2000), Northern Ireland has *Equal Lives* (Department of Health, Social Services and Public Safety, 2005) and Wales *Fulfilling the Promise* (Welsh Office, 2001).

Included within England's *Valuing People* is a section entitled 'Improving health for people with a learning disability'. This chapter opens by stating that the Government's objective is to 'Enable people with a learning disability to access a health service designed around their individual needs, with fast and convenient care delivered to a consistently high standard, and with additional support where necessary'. Since *Valuing People* (Department of Health, 2001),and six years later *Valuing People Now: From Progress to Transformation*, a consultation document, was released (Department of Health, 2007a).This review recognised that targets and objectives in relation to health action planning have not been achieved, and although a framework for commissioning more effective primary care is identified, no explicit reference is made towards the value of CLDN's or community learning disability teams in this process, apart from investing in liaison nurses between mainstream and specialist learning disability services.

Valuing People Now: A New Three Year Strategy for People with Learning Disabilities (Department of Health, 2009) places emphasis on healthcare training for all, and within Recommendation 8 explicitly refers to how strategic health facilitators/or local community learning disability teams can provide training to general practitioners and general practice staff.

Clifton et al (1992) were commissioned to investigate the transferability of learning disability nurses' skills from hospital to community and the uniqueness of those skills. Their research concluded that there were no explicit or individual skills that were unique to learning disability nurses. However, they did conclude that there was a generality of skills, the so-called 'skills plus' factor that were of value. Clooby (2000) asserts the view that healthcare for people with a learning disability could be provided by trained practitioners who are not necessarily specialist learning disability nurses. Bollard (1999) and Hames and Carlson (2006) identify that primary healthcare nurses who have contact with people with learning disabilities need to recognise when they need to seek help from specialist services and community learning disability nurses and teams when providing health checks. The Chief Nursing Officer, in 1985, stated that 'the (learning disability) nurse's role is one of providing individualised care to people with a learning disability and their families and collaborating with others to create alternatives to hospital care'. Mitchell (2000) suggests that learning disability nurses may have been one of the major contributors to the confusion regarding their role, in that they have continually advocated that people with a learning disability are not ill, and therefore do not need nursing. Mitchell (2004) similarly comments that community learning disability nursing has been traditionally marginalised within the 'family' of nursing due to its failure to be part of the 'sickness' model of care.

The role

In terms of role application specific issues require pursuing in relation to the focus of working practices for the CLDN namely:

- Multi-tasking health and/or social care agent.
- Care management.
- Health role.
- Specialist practice.
- Adoption of specialist/community learning disability nursing.
- Contemporary perspectives.

Multi-tasking health or social care agent

Barr (2006) provides an overview of the changes in the caseload and working practices of community nurses in learning disabilities over an 11 year period in Northern Ireland. However, in terms of a historical developmental perspective, the origins for community learning disability nursing with community psychiatric nursing as a post-qualifying specialty, first emerged in 1974 under the auspices of the Joint Board in Clinical Nursing Studies.

Also at this time, Strong and Sandland (1974) conducted the first survey about the work of community nurses among senior officers in 53 hospitals in England. *Table 6.1* shows findings from this survey which found that the role was an extension of nurses' role from the hospital base and as such was perceived as part of the community. The purpose of the role was broad and was focused around helping to provide the learning disabled person with the range of skills they needed to either remain in or be able to reintegrate into society.

Table 6.1. Role of the community nurse in 1974

Finding employment and accommodation	Liaising with employers. Assessing performance Providing a follow-up service for client Landlady counselling
Social education	Teaching clients at home, e.g. domestic skills
Pre-admission visits	Allaying anxiety in the family over admission. Following up client on discharge, advising on social training and management
Home visiting of inpatients	Visiting families of children who are not visited in hospital. Performing follow-up visits requested by local authorities.
Outpatient clinics	Assisting with clinical investigations
Community liaison officer	Not yet fully established as role from survey

Data from Strong and Sandland (1974)

Table 6.2. Role of the community nurse in 1981

Professional advisor	Genetic factors. Normal and abnormal development Physiological and nutritional care Employment and housing
Counsellor	Psychological adjustment to life stressors within and outside the family
Practical helper	Transport. Temporary relief for family
Clinical practitioner	Injections and medications Special treatments
Benefits informant	Advice, e.g. Mobility and Attendance Allowance
General information bank	Voluntary and statutory organisations Legal rights
Arranger	Short-term care and day care Laundry services/aids and adaptations
Coordinator	Link person, e.g. adult training centre/school
Teacher	Sex education/behaviour therapy
Trainer	Feeding, toileting, occupational therapy and simple physiotherapy

Data from Elliot-Cannon (1981)

In 1981 the role was further articulated as having a comprehensive social and healthcare focus by Elliot-Cannon (1981). This broad spectrum approach is shown in *Table 6.2*.

However, unlike Strong and Sandland (1974), Elliot-Cannon's descriptors were not based upon empirical data, but rather from a personal professional observation. The emphasis was on an all-encompassing supportive role for maintaining clients in the community. In 1985 the accelerating movement of services and people towards the community also brought continued criticisms of the role of nursing and nurses during the 1980s. This wave of uncertainty was fuelled by the House of Commons Select Committee's (1985) second report which recommended that

> '...the Department gather information on the tasks of community mental handicap nurses, and produce an agreed statement on their role and functions.'

The Royal College of Nursing (1985) responded with role descriptors (*Table 6.3*) that focused on the practitioner working within a multi-disciplinary team.

The Royal College of Nursing Learning Disability Forum (1992) produced yet further role descriptors, identifying that the role of the CLDN encompassed and adopted a nursing process framework (see *Table 6.4*).

With the development of such role descriptors from the Royal College of Nursing, acknowledgment is made that such descriptors were articulated more through forum discussion than through research, as identified by the Royal College of Nursing as being of necessity to pursue in order to secure an evidence-based approach to practice.

Since 1992, a number of studies have concentrated on the development of this specialist practitioner. In these studies approaches to understanding the role of the CLDN has been largely through small-scale research on the analysis of caseloads, and from research into qualified and unqualified CLDN's perceptions on practice during the late 1980s and 1990s (Jukes, 1994 a,b; Mansell and Harris, 1998; Barr, 2006). More recently, Slevin et al (2007) have examined the effectiveness of community learning disability teams, in the context of being either of a multi or uni-disciplinary configuration, and have once more called for more evidence/research into the efficacy of such teams.

Care management

From the mid to late 1990s through to the present there has been another twist in the application of CLDN practice in the form of care management

---

Table 6.3. Role of the community nurse in 1985

Advising on	Prevention and developmental needs
	Behaviour management
	Benefits and national resources.
	Education
Monitoring and evaluation of	Planned intervention
	Administration of medication
	Health-related needs
Promoting	Self-help groups
	Workshops regarding self-help skills
Liaising with	Voluntary groups
	Primary healthcare and community
	Mental health teams
	Private organisations
Counselling	Individuals and families
	School, work and leisure centre staff
Researching	Promotion of further research within community nursing
Reporting	Service deficits and future requirements for service provision

Data from Royal College of Nursing (1985)

Table 6.4. Role of the community nurse in 1992

- Advising on such things as developmental needs, social and interpersonal skills, benefits, care and medical conditions
- Assessment of skills, physical and emotional health, domestic aids and adaptations
- Implementing counselling, psychotherapy and therapeutic approaches
- Monitoring and evaluating physical and mental health care plans and treatment, and also own care delivery and service provision
- Promoting such things as self-help groups, local initiatives and generic services
- Liaising with private and voluntary organisations, professional and generic services
- Educating both service users and carers
- Researching to ensure evidence-based practice

Data from Royal College of Nursing (1992)

functions, forced upon CLDNs through the NHS and Community Care Act (1989). There are nuances in how the health and social care divide has been interpreted,where learning disability, as an area of work, has been perceived by many as a social care phenomenon. The result of this is that in some areas CLDN nurses have been amalgamated/subsumed into social care teams, as opposed to them maintaining specialist clinical practice through an individual case management and person-centred approach.

The role of the CLDN therefore, in these arrangements, is to provide a needs assessment and prescribe care management packages of care alongside their social work colleagues, which, from a professional nursing perspective, has created a dissonance due to care management being perceived, and in many cases operationalised, to provide a rationing of resources rather than defining and providing individual and person-centred approaches. Additionally, CLDNs are used to providing clinical interventions based on specialist education within the context of working with families and clients, and carrying caseloads that have been determined through community learning disability team referrals and based upon a defined level of need.

Alasewski et al (2000), in their final report to the ENB on learning disability nursing education, found that nurses tended to gravitate towards specialisation so as to maintain their clinical role, as opposed to being coerced into management and administrative roles. Community nursing and behaviour therapy are illustrated as examples of such areas of specialisation, which illustrates in part nurses' frustration of where professional and service developments are impacting upon where they feel practice should be focused. Messant and Caan (2000) have suggested that few social service managers have the experience to appreciate the value of CLDNs, and that the skills of the latter are being ignored, diluted or required to adopt a quasi-care management function rather than a 'hands-on' approach.

Greig and Peck (1998) have also discussed this aspect of work by community nurses in the context of the community learning disability team, and have recommended that the best use of the community nurse is, in practice, working with people and their families, and infer this also should apply to social workers for what constitutes 'real' social work as opposed to care management.

Health role

Since *Valuing People* (Department of Health, 2001) the CLDN role has evolved into one that has a more pronounced health focus, although the role is still extremely wide-ranging. Part of the impetus for this change was that previously published research (Howells, 1986; Barker and Howells, 1990; Holland and Young, 1990; Meehan et al, 1995; Matthews, 1996) had identified that the healthcare needs of the learning disabled population were not being met due to a multiplicity of reasons most notably poor communication skills, inability to access facilities (due to either physical disability or an awareness of what was available) and primary healthcare teams lacking knowledge about working with individuals with learning disabilities.

Additionally, people with a learning disability, as Williamson and Johnson (2004) observe, have in fact greater health needs than the general population in that they are significantly more likely to have problems related to genetic conditions such as coronary heart disease, respiratory disease, sensory impairments, epilepsy, dementia and thyroid problems. Additionally, they are more prone to mental health issues, osteoporosis and risk factors associated with poor health and a sedentary lifestyle such as being underweight or obese.

Research by Boarder (2002) and Mobbs et al (2002) has identified, respectively, views from community nurses themselves about their role and practice, and views of service managers as identified in *Table 6.5* as priorities for clinical practice. This continues to present a crystallising of roles with a multiplicity of roles and interventions.

Table 6.5. Service managers' views of priorities for clinical practice

Boarder (2002)	*Mobbs et al. (2002)*
• Emphasis on interdisciplinary work	• Assessment
• Teamwork	• Advice and support
• Service development	• Ongoing health monitoring
• Staff and carer training	• Nursing care
• Supporting community living	• Counselling
• Increase in health focus	• Health promotion
• Working with people with	• Clinical procedures
learning difficulties in areas of:	• Health screening (assessment)
• Health maintenance/promotion	• Crisis intervention
• Physical and mental health difficulties	• Client reviews
• Bereavement counselling	
• Sex education and counselling	
• Playgroups and work with schools	
• Assessment	
• Research	
• Advocacy	
• Maintenance in the community	
• Challenging behaviour	
• Skills development	
• Personal development and relationships	

Specialist practice

An area for continued debate is whether the CLDN should only deal with specific areas of health practice which have a high correlation with the presence of a learning disability. Mobbs et al (2002), in their research, suggest such areas as epilepsy, mental health (in learning disabilities) and challenging behaviour. More recently, health promotion and health screening have come to the forefront as research has continually highlighted the health divide that exists between people with a learning disability and the general population, as particularly highlighted in *Valuing People* and more recently in the Healthcare Commission report into learning disabilities (2005) entitled *Draft Three Year Strategic Plan for Adults with Learning Disabilities 2006-2009:Consultation November 2005*.

Specialist health and nursing texts with 'Community nursing' as a title, are intended for primary care community nurses such as public health nurses, practice nurses, district nurses, school nurses and midwives. While these texts devote a significant component to all aspects of community nursing such as assessment, treatment, public health and health promotion, carers needs, mental health and community psychiatric nursing, conspicuous by its absence, in a majority of cases, is learning disability nursing. Many texts do not have a single paragraph about learning disabilities let alone a chapter, which all the other subjects appear to warrant. This graphically illustrates the position that, although CLDNs may see themselves as part of a primary healthcare workforce, at the forefront of innovative health provision, education and health promotion, and working to achieve a greater integration of services, it is clear that other nursing professions, academics, practitioners and commentators do not.

Glasby (2000) citing Mitchell (1998) observes that learning disability nurses have remained marginalised within the wider nursing profession. Hunt (2001) and Hames and Carlson (2006) identify that primary healthcare teams have little knowledge of the needs of people with a learning disability and the role of CLDNs/teams in health promotion and health facilitation, suggesting that communication difficulties were the principal stumbling block. Hannon (2003) claims that all health professionals in every aspect of the health services are expected to have a greater awareness of the needs of people with a learning disability and to adapt their services accordingly. However, when the Royal College of Physicians published its Charter and Guidelines, entitled *Disabled People Using Hospital* in 1998, very few health professionals in Hannon's experience were either aware of it or familiar with its contents.

Bollard and Jukes (1999) have observed that learning disability nursing as a profession is particularly vulnerable to the influences of philosophical, theoretical and policy changes. This is, in part, due to the very nature of the role, not being ill defined, but defined in the absence of rigorous research. This has meant that the influences on the development of practice have been due to various health and social care policy reforms, and not through the impact of practice and research determinants of how such nurses can influence and benefit people and their families. Slevin et al (2008) reassert this call for further research into effectiveness and the practice base of community learning disability teams.

Mobbs et al (2002) found that CLDNs have 'specialised', and that many teams have prioritised or, rather, had to prioritise due to scarcity of nursing resources, and to concentrate on the following:

- Hospital liaison (including admissions and discharges).
- Challenging behaviour management.
- Mental health issues, especially if this involved admission to a mental health acute unit, inpatient care plans and discharges, and, increasingly significant, dementia care.
- Epilepsy care and support, carer/staff training and nurse-led prescribing clinics.
- Dementia care and support.
- Carer support and advice.
- Advice to fellow community-based professionals regarding:
  - Consent
  - Admissions and discharges to general hospitals
  - Learning disability syndromes and autistic spectrum disorders.
- Signposting to services provided elsewhere such as continence, communication, occupational, family and psychological therapy, advocacy, sensory impairment support, diabetes management, and primary and secondary health services.
- Health action planning and health needs assessments.
- Signposting and advising around general health issues.
- Care staff training, especially epilepsy and medication administration.
- Medication advice.
- Depot injections.
- Continuing care monies applications.
- Transition from child to adult services liaison.
- Specifically excluded for some CLDNs, and specifically included for others, was care management. Additionally most CLDNs avoid or refer elsewhere for benefits advice, employment, housing and education.
- The overwhelming majority of CLDN's have a service criterion which expressly defines that a service can only to be provided to those with a clinically determined learning disability (Typically an IQ below 70 or where intellectual function was demonstrably significantly impaired as a result of genetic abnormalities).

Even a cursory examination of the list immediately challenges the assertion that such a wide-ranging list of tasks can be termed 'specialisation'. Nevertheless, the theory is that although the list is long it excludes work that can very adequately be provided by generic health professionals such as district nurses, practice nurses and continence and diabetic nurses, to name but a few. One particularly disappointing aspect of the above list is that, with the possible exception of health action planning, the work is all reactive rather than proactive. Although *Valuing People* stressed the need to promote healthy living and accessing health screening, much of the work of colleagues in community teams is still very much around dealing with a continuous stream of referrals for pre-existing or acute health-related problems.

In order to consider more widely the evolution of the role of the CLDN, the way services have developed within the UK and Ireland can be compared to how the same issue has been dealt with by different health authorities.

Adoption of specialist/community learning disability nursing across the UK

As might be anticipated within England different Health Authorities have adopted different models. Somerset distinguished itself in 1993, as reported by Carlisle (1993), through making all its community mental handicap nurses (as they were then known) redundant as they felt they would not (or perhaps should not) be needed, with other services being expected to take up the various roles required. This decision was reversed in 2001 and currently the number of community nurses is being steadily expanded.

Mobbs et al (2002) analysed the working practices of CLDNs across England. They identified that there were 194 managers of CLDN in England and that many teams had CLDNs specialising in particular fields of practice, such as challenging behaviour (27%), epilepsy (20%), forensic issues (20%) and mental health (18%). Training of care staff was also a significant part of the workload with training being offered in such areas as epilepsy (95%), challenging behaviour (88%), drug administration (82%) and skills development (81%). Some nurses also trained in control and restraint techniques (41%) and just under a quarter (23%) dealt with both adults and children.

Mobbs et al (2002) concluded 'the fears expressed by commentators in the early 1990s that the days of CLDNs were numbered have not been borne out. Indeed, CLDNs appear to be developing new and varied roles, and this trend is predicted to continue.'

In 1973 (Swamm, 1997) services for people with learning disabilities in Northern Ireland were reorganised and integrated into the general health and personal social services structures. In 1978 there were 1337 people in long-stay hospitals, and, according to Dixon et al (2004), this number has reduced drastically, although even to the present day Northern Ireland has not been able to close all its long-stay units, with approximately 390 individuals still being housed in this manner.

Parahoo and Barr (1996) researched the work of CLDNs in Northern Ireland and noted that their work was principally related to, in order of time spent: physical care, epilepsy, aggression and mental health. However, when asked which areas learning disability nurses would wish to develop the service in, these were identified as: specialisation, early intervention, more client-centred than administrative, increased use of clinics, public education and greater input into service planning. These sentiments echo those expressed by the author in the previous section and perhaps reflect a common lack of resources, in that learning disability nurses have insufficient time to meet current workloads let alone to be able work proactively.

In October 2002 the Department of Health and Children, Eire published the *Proposed Framework for the Development of Clinical Specialism and Advanced Practice in Mental Handicap Nursing*. This 46 page document comprehensively recommended how services should be developed by ensuring learning disability nurses are both trained and facilitated to work and have expertise in the following key areas of support for a person with a learning disability:

- Sensory development.
- Management of behaviour.
- Multiple and complex disabilities.
- Assistive technology (principally in the area of communication).
- Health promotion.
- Respite assessment and intervention.
- Training and employment.
- Community nursing.
- Palliative care.
- Mental health and intellectual disability.
- Advocacy and activation (community participation).
- Communication: speech and language.
- Developmental education.
- Care of the older person.
- Interpersonal relationships and counselling.
- Early intervention.

This ambitious list highlights how anomalous it is to describe learning disability nursing as specialised when it can potentially be so wide ranging.

A more recent Position Paper by the National Council for the

Professional Development of Nursing and Midwifery (NCPDNM, 2006), has further focused upon the clinical nurse specialist (CNS) and advanced nurse practitioner (ANP) role in terms of health inequalities, social inclusion and whether in fact intellectual disability practitioners could be set up as a joint appointment with another service and act as an agent of social change. As from September 2006 the Council had approved CNS posts in intellectual disability services, and included:

- Challenging behaviour (26).
- Community nursing (26).
- Early intervention (16).
- Creative, recreational and diversional activation (9).
- Autism spectrum conditions (6).
- Health promotion (6).
- Older people (4).

The 'All Wales Strategy' was launched in 1983 and one of its aims was to develop community-based support (Gates, 1997), to ensure access to the same healthcare as others living in the community, with additional support to meet those with learning disability's special needs. In 1992 the Welsh Health planning Forum devised a 'Protocol for investment in health gain' specifically for those with learning disability and, when taken into account with the 'All Wales Strategy', enabled a harmonising advancement to the improvement of services.

This strategy focused on the integration of health services for those with a learning disability. They used the World Health Organization holistic definition of health rather than a biophysiological one (Turnbull, 2004), thus their aim was to work towards 'health gain' for those with a learning disability. This policy fits well with the broader aims of promoting anti-oppressive practices through participation, community presence and empowerment as espoused by Wolfensberger (2002). In 2002, *Inclusion, Partnership and Innovation* (Welsh Assembly Government) was published as part of the *Realising the Potential Initiative* (National Assembly for Wales, 1999) for nursing and from this report a framework was established which identified the key areas of learning disability nursing in which community nursing was included (*Box 6.1*).

In 2002 the Scottish Health Authority published *Promoting Health, Supporting People*, which McKenzie and Powell (2004) argue gave out a clear message 'that the care and support of people with a learning disability is the business of all nurses and each must play a part in promoting health'. The reports advocates that 'NHS boards should ensure that there are learning disability community nurses based in, and working collaboratively as integrated members of primary care teams'. The Scottish Executive

---

Box 6.1. Key areas of learning disability nursing

- All registered learning disability nurses will have a theoretical and clinical base to their practice, which will enable them to create environments of care that promote health, growth and opportunity for the individual client.
- In partnership, all learning disability nurses will work effectively with their clients and their clients' families to provide high quality, inclusive and measurable care.
- All learning disability nurses will develop their practice in a reflective and evidence-based manner. Their practice will be founded upon a standard of education which enables them to function as equal partners with other health care professionals, supported by continued professional development and clinical supervision.
- Existing career paths for learning disability nurses in Wales will be enhanced, and new ones developed. Such career paths should allow senior staff to remain clinically involved if they so wish. They should also break down unhelpful barriers between education, research and practice, as well as between learning disability nursing and the wider health and social care context.
- The unique value of the learning disability nurse will be recognised and appropriately utilised to meet the holistic needs of people with a learning disability.

Welsh Assembly Government (2002:7–11)

---

envisaged a 'tiered' approach to services with the lower tier meeting the needs of the majority of the learning disability population with higher tiers, up to tier 4, being increasingly specialised and meeting the needs of a smaller group with highly complex needs

This was followed by *Health Needs Assessment* (NHS Scotland, 2004) which highlighted the health inequalities prevalent between the general population and those with a learning disability in Scotland.

Thus Scotland, like Wales, was striving to develop an integrated model of healthcare with individuals with learning disability accessing mainstream services and mainstream services being urged to ensure they were equipped to meet this client group's needs.

Contemporary perspectives

Challenging behaviour

A recent innovation within community teams is the creation of specialist rapid intervention teams. Other localities have similar teams variously termed intensive therapy teams, behavioural nurse teams, and crisis intervention teams.

These teams exist to meet the needs of those individuals with a learning disability whose behaviour is seen as extremely challenging. This might typically be due to a mental health problem, such as a personality disorder, or to very severe autism. Alternatively they may have a forensic history or be highly self-injurious. Whatever the nature of their behaviour they will inevitable pose a considerable challenge to community-based services. For many of these people local services are inadequate to meet their needs and they may have had to access out-of-county specialist services, which characteristically are extremely expensive and necessitate the individual involved having to move away from family, friends and familiar surroundings.

Accordingly, these specialist teams have been created to support people with challenging behaviour to stay within local services and to re-assess those placed out of the county with a view to supporting their return. As in the move out of long-stay hospitals the rationale for keeping people within the county is arguably highly beneficial for the individuals well-being and for maintaining local connections. Equally, it is likely to prove highly cost effective in that the health authority will no longer have to pay for psychiatric, psychology and other therapies from a third party but can provide these from within existing services at projected/actual lower costs.

Health facilitation and health action plans

Valuing People requires services to establish enhanced services around health action plans. The NHS Plan (Department of Health, 2000) stated that 'inequalities in health cannot be tackled without dealing with the fundamental causes; including poverty, low educational attainment, unemployment, discrimination and social exclusion. These factors affect many people with a learning disability'.

Previously published research by Howells (1986), Barker and Howells (1990), Holland and Young (1990), Meehan et al (1995), Matthews (1996), and Ruddick (2005) had identified that the healthcare needs of the learning disabled population were not being met due to a variety of reasons, including poor communication skills, inability to access facilities, primary healthcare teams lacking knowledge about learning disabilities and an emphasis on social and residential aspects of life being emphasised within a quality of life framework.

Additionally, people with a learning disability, as Williamson and Johnson (2004) identify, have greater health needs than the general population.

Therefore the Government initiated a range of health-related initiatives as proposed in *Valuing People* (Department of Health, 2001), including:

- All people with a learning disability should have an individual health facilitator.
- All people with a learning disability should be registered with a general practitioner.
- All people with a learning disability should have a health action plan.
- NHS should ensure that all mainstream hospitals services are accessible to people with a learning disability.
- There should be a new role for specialist learning disability services.

As well as published research influencing the Government's thinking there was also the work of the various learning disability charities such as Mencap, the Down's Syndrome Society and the National Autistic Society (Matthews, 2002). Mencap particularly have had ongoing campaigns and its current publications, *Treat Me Right* (Mencap, 2005) and *Death by Indifference* (Mencap, 2007), aim to raise awareness of the health and treatment inequalities suffered by people with a learning disability.

The implementation of the *Valuing People* White Paper policy has had a significant influence on the role the various health and social care professionals involved in the care of people with a learning disability (Matthews, 2005). A Health Inequalities Report from a London Borough (Barking and Dagenham, 2001: 56) recommended that in order for the health needs for people with learning disabilities to be addressed appropriately, 'Partnership Boards, PCT's and Social Services (the community learning disability team), need to decide what is the best and most effective way for community learning disability nurses to link with primary care.' This is a clear indicator for community learning disability teams to take the lead to implement health action planning with service users. Many different models have evolved which inevitably require each area to dedicate clinical time to the development of an implementation plan and a health action plan tool (Mackenzie, 2004). In England, *Healthcare for All* (Michael, 2008), is a far-reaching document which furthers the agenda for creating a health system whereby access to healthcare for people with learning disabilities is achieved through education across all sectors. This report pivots around 10 principal recommendations which embrace annual health checks, support in general hospitals, communication and tighter inspections and regulation in the support of people gaining more effective access and treatment.

CLDN's in many areas have taken the lead for implementation of health facilitation and health action planning. As elsewhere in the UK this has had a fundamental effect in shifting priorities so that health action planning is principally a proactive strategy whereas previously community learning disability services had tended to work largely reactively (Hannon, 2003).

Other health professionals' roles altered as well. General practitioners were required to be able to identify who on their lists had a learning disability and Primary Care Trusts were required to financially support the general practitioners to offer extended consultation times for those with an identified learning disability. Equally, as Kerr and Lennox (1997) have observed, general practitioners did not perceive that part of their role was as a provider of health promotion for people with a learning disability.

Scott et al (2005) observe that social care staff were also expected to take on the role of health facilitator. This is a far more proactive approach to positive healthcare and health promotion than had previously been required under the Commission for Social Care Inspection Care Standards legislation (2005). Previously, residential carers had been expected to meet national minimum standards by 'monitoring and attending to health needs' as they arose (Thompson and Cobb, 2004).

The funding for the health action plan initiative was provided by the Government as part of the £50 million per annum funding for all the various initiatives included in the *Valuing People* White Paper (Department of Health, 2001) such as housing, day services, employment, etc. The health-related elements of this provision was allocated via strategic health authorities to Primary Care Trusts.

However, responsibility for overseeing the implementation of the various initiatives contained in the White Paper was allocated to separate regional bodies, the regional Learning Disability Partnership Boards (LDPB) as described in the British Institute for Learning Disabilities (2005) factsheet. Thus although the LDPB were not budget holders per se they have considerable influence as to how funding is allocated. This has meant that community learning disability teams have had to compete for resources to implement health action plans against other bodies applying for funding for other projects for learning disabled people. The LDPB have therefore determined the allocation of funding based on their own assessment of the priorities contained in the White Paper (Scott et al, 2005). The net effect is that community learning disability teams are mandated to implement health action plans for all service users but are not guaranteed funding for resources to do this work.

The implications for resources however go deeper (Williamson and Johnson, 2004), as a health action plan is only an initial step; once it has been completed then the expectation is, based on the research that prompted the initiative, that further work will be required to implement the action plan. The health action plan will create a much greater need for health services than previously existed to meet the unrecognised health needs of the learning disabled person. Even in the event of the individual having no current health issues, part of the health action plan is to increase the uptake of screening services, which for most people with a learning disability will require the support of a carer or health facilitator.

The provision of a health facilitator for every service user is a further resource issue (Thompson and Cobb, 2004). The *Valuing People* White Paper stipulates that every individual with a learning disability will need the support of a 'health facilitator' to enable him or her to have and implement a health action plan. For those living at home or in community care this role would probably fall by default to their principal carer (although the expectation of the White Paper was that people would be able to exercise a choice). However, for many people living independently or semi-independently there is no one at present to fulfil this role.

Community learning disability nurses are grasping the nettle in terms of assimilating this role into either a specialist role, or as part of the existing repertoire of roles within the scope of community learning disability practice. For some nurses they will be expected to support this additional role as well, again with potentially no extra funding available to enable them to do so. In terms of levels of health facilitation, some nurses are operating from a strategic operational level, where the expectancy is to act as a change agent to lead the political calling for health facilitation to primary healthcare services. Here practitioners are required to effect change by:

- Influencing social inclusion into mainstream primary healthcare services.
- Developing collaborative working relationships.
- Developing educational resources.
- Developing systems and protocols for primary healthcare staff to meet the needs of the person with learning disability.

Community learning disability nurses in this role usually represent nurses who have undertaken specialist practitioner education, or are acting in the capacity of specialist/advanced practitioner/consultant status, as exemplified in *Chapter 7* where Susan Brady illustrates this strategic application in both practice and research.

Community learning disability nurses, who assimilate health facilitation as an extension to their existing role, are usually acting on an individual case finding level where they act as 'empowerment agents' and advocate when supporting people with a learning disability to:
- Navigate their way around primary healthcare services.
- Build bridges with primary, acute and specialist services.
- Develop educational resources for individuals with learning disability, and their unpaid/paid carers.

At another level community nurses can also act as educators and 'empowerment agents' to assist unpaid/paid carers to:

- Recognise deterioration in health.
- Help people with learning disabilities to recognise ill-health and access primary health care services.

As Johnson et al (1995) assert, 'political systems have the power to redefine boundaries between occupational groups and to shape relationships between professionals and their clients'. This policy has required the involvement of not just the whole of the community learning disability team (therapists, social workers and psychologists), but also inter-professional working across general practices, Primary Care Trusts and acute services in that they are all involved in actioning the health action plan (Matthews, 2005).

As Matthews (2005) says, there has been a resistance from some general practitioners and Primary Care Trusts as this work is not currently part of their accountability agreement. *Valuing People* was a White Paper and is not a National Service Framework and therefore seems to carry less weight with Primary Care Trusts. However, elements of the White Paper have subsequently been incorporated in the National Service Framework such as the Mental Health Older People Services and Long-Term Conditions as described by the Department of Health (2005). This should, as McConkey (2002) suggests, assist in encouragement and stimulate the involvement of those health professionals not currently directly involved in the care of those with a learning disability.

Conclusion

As stated in the introduction to this chapter the development of the role of the community learning disability nurse has been one of meeting the needs of this marginalised client group,while also recognising that as community integration has progressed, those needs have broadened to an extent that a whole panoply of services is required. For individuals to function in the community they need housing, employment, financial advice, community facilities, social networks, education and healthcare.

People with learning disabilities will have additional communication and intellectual issues, that will inhibit their needs being met without some additional level of support. Community learning disability nurses have recognised, through practice and from the research identified in this chapter, that it is not feasible for them to provide specialist support in all these areas, especially as each area requires specialist knowledge and application of specialist interventions. Therefore, the role of the community learning disability nurse has become further defined and specific,while still retaining a broad range of skills.

It is quite clear from a cursory examination that the value of community learning disability nursing for people with a learning disability and their families is in the area of promoting social inclusion.

Problems of identity and communication across seamless services is still a major quest for the community learning disability nurse to pursue as an agenda for practice, so as to make access to mainstream services more transparent and responsive to the needs of marginalised groups.

The recent Healthcare Commission findings in Cornwall and Sutton and Merton Primary Healthcare Trusts (2006, 2007) are indicative of the fact that a gradual decay in services and resources occurs over time. This will inevitably include an absence of investment in specialists and specialist provision in training for learning disability nursing. Absence of such specialist nurses results in an inability of such nurses to emerge as leaders to manage change and to promote innovative approaches to working within a variety of settings. Services, as identified within the Healthcare Commission Reports, will continue to be in a state of decay without an investment in the education for specialist learning disability nurses. The recent *Good Practice in Learning Disability Nursing Report* (Department of Health, 2007: 34) identifies the necessity to strengthen the competency base of those nurses who currently work in specialist in-patient settings.

In terms of community nursing, this report (Department of Health, 2007:38) also identifies the current tensions with the care management role and makes the recommendation that although care management is important, community nurses should take on the role only when it is to the benefit of the service user.

To enhance person-centred practices, community learning disability nurses are critical agents of change who promote inclusion, facilitate and 'plug the gaps' in mainstream services for people with a learning disability and 'bridge the gaps' of communication and understanding between mainstream and specialist services for those people and families with a learning disability.

However, as identified earlier in this chapter continued research into community learning disability nursing is still a requirement in today's changing landscape of services, although specialist areas such as health facilitation is beginning to impact on how the role is reconfiguring mainstream services.

References

Alaszewski A, Gates B, Ayer S, et al (2000) *Education for Diversity and Change :Final Report of the ENB Funded Project on Educational Preparation for Learning Disability Nursing.* University of Hull, UK

All Wales Nursing Group (1992) *A Strategy for Mental Handicap Nursing in Wales.* Cardiff, All Wales Nursing Group

Barker M, Howells G (1990) *The Medical Needs of Adults, Primary Care for People with a Mental Handicap.* Occasional Paper 47. Royal College of General Practitioners, London

Barking and Dagenham PCT (2001) *Health Inequalities, Annual Public Health Report. Chapter 4. Improving access and health outcomes for disadvantaged communities.* Barking and Dagenham PCT

Barr O (2006) The evolving role of community nurses for people with learning disabilities: Changes over an 11 year period. *Journal of Clinical Nursing* **15:** 72–82

Boarder J (2002) Perceptions of experienced Community Learning Disability Nurses of their roles and ways of working: An Exploratory study. Report for Welsh National Board Training Research Fellowship. Cardiff, Welsh National Board

Bollard M (1999) Improving primary healthcare for people with learning disabilities. *British Journal of Nursing* **8**(18): 1216–21

Bollard M, Jukes MJD (1999) Specialist Practitioner within Community Learning Disability Nursing and the Primary Healthcare Team. *Journal of Intellectual Disabilities* **3**(1): 11–19

Briggs A (1972) *Report of the Committee of Nursing.* HMSO, London Cmnd 5115

British Institute of Learning Disabilities (BILD) (2005) *Factsheet – Partnership Boards.* Available from: www.bild.org.uk/pdfs/05faqs/pb.pdf. [accessed 10 March 2009

Brittle R (2004) Managing the needs of people who have a learning disability. *Nursing Times* **100**(10):

Carlisle D (1993) Somerset Unit makes last of Community RNMHs Redundant. *Nursing Times* **89**(6): 10

Clifton M, Shaw I, Brown J (1992) *Transferability of Mental Handicap Nursing Skills from Hospital to Community.* University of York Department of Social Policy and Social Work, York

Commission for Social Care Inspection (2005) Available from: http://www.csci.org.uk/15/6/05

Cullen C (1991) *Community Care in the Next Decade and Beyond. Mental Handicap Nursing. Report Commissioned by the Four Chief Nursing Officers.* HMSO, London

Department of Health (2000) *NHS Plan: A Plan for Investment. A Plan for Reform.* Department of Health, London

Department of Health (2001) *Valuing People: A New Strategy for Learning Disability in the 21st Century.* Department of Health, London

Department of Health (2002) *Action for Health. Health Action Plans and Health Facilitation*. HMSO, London

Department of Health. (2005).*The National Service Framework for Long Term Conditions*. HMSO, Leeds

Department of Health (2007a) *Valuing People Now - From Progress to Transformation*. HMSO, London

Department of Health (2007b) *Good Practice in Learning Disability Nursing*. Department of Health, London.

Department of Health (2009) *Valuing People Now: A New Three Year Strategy for People with Learning Disabilities*. HMSO, London

Department of Health and Children (2002) *Proposed Framework for the Development of Clinical Specialism and Advanced Practice in Mental Handicap Nursing*. Stationary Office.Dublin

Department of Health, Social Services and Public Safety (2005) *Equal Lives: Review of Policy and Services for People with a Learning Disability in Northern Ireland*. The Stationery Office, Belfast.

Dixon P, Spollen M, McConkey R, Jamison J (2004) *Modelling the distribution of services for people with learning disabilities in Northern Ireland*. Available from: www.dhsspsni.gov.uk/learning-disability-report. pdf. [last accessed 10 March 2009]

Elliot-Cannon C (1981) Do the mentally handicapped need specialist community nursing care? *Nursing Times* **77**(27): 77–80

Gates B (1997) *Learning Disabilities*. Churchill Livingstone, Edinburgh

Glasby J (2000) An eye to the future. *Learning Disability Practice* **3**(3):

Greig R, Peck E (1998) Is there a future for the Community Learning Disability Team? *Tizard Learning Disability Review* **3**(1): 35–41

Hames A, Carlson T (2006) Are primary healthcare staff aware of the role of community learning disability teams in relation to health promotion and health facilitation? *British Journal of Learning Disabilities* **34**(1): 6–10

Hannon L (2003) Secondary healthcare for people with learning disabilities. *Nursing Standard* **17**(46): 39–42

Healthcare Commission (2007) *Investigation into the Service for People with Learning Disabilities Provided by Sutton and Merton Primary Care Trust*. Commission for Healthcare Audit & Inspection, London

Healthcare Commission AND Commission for Social Care Inspection (2006) *Joint Investigation Into the Provision of Services for People with Learning Disabilities at Cornwall Partnership NHS Trust*. Commission for Healthcare Audit & Inspection, London

Holland M, Young C (1990) *Mental Handicap. Primary Care for People with a Mental Handicap*. Occasional Paper 47. Royal College of General Practitioners, London

House of Commons Social Services Select Committee (1985) *Community Care with Special Reference to Adult Mentally Ill and Mentally Handicapped People*.HMSO.London

Howells (1986) Are the medical needs of mentally handicapped adults being met? *Journal of the Royal College of General Practitioners* **36**(291): 449–53

Hunt C (2001) Community nurse, learning disabilities: A case study of the use of evidence based screening tool to identify and meet the health needs of people with a learning disability. *Journal of Learning Disabilities* **5**(1): 9–18

Jay P (1979) *Report of the Committee of Enquiry into Mental Handicap Nursing and Care*. HMSO, London Cmnd 7468-1

Joint Board of Clinical Nursing Studies (1974) *Course No. 800.Outline Curriculum in Community Psychiatric Nursing for Registered Nurses*. Joint Board of Clinical Nursing Studies, London

Johnson T, Larkin G, Saks M (1995) *Health Professions and the State in Europe*. Routledge, London

Jukes M (1994a) Development of the community nurse in learning disability 1. *British Journal of Nursing* **3**(15): 779–83

Jukes M (1994b) Development of the community nurse in learning disability 2. *British Journal of Nursing* **3**(16): 848–53

Jukes M (2003) Towards practice development in contemporary learning disability nursing. In: Jukes M, Bollard M (eds) *Contemporary Learning Disability Practice*. Quay Books, Salisbury

Kay B, Rose S, Turnbull J (1995) *Continuing the Commitment. The report of the learning disability nursing project*. Department of Health, London

Kerr M, Lennox NG (1997) Primary healthcare and people with an intellectual disability: The evidence base. *Journal of Intellectual Disability Research* 41(5): 365–72

Mackenzie K (2004) Health screening. *Learning Disability Practice* **7**(10)

Mansell I, Harris P (1998) Role of the registered nurse learning disability within community support teams for people with learning disabilities. *Journal of Learning Disabilities for Nursing, Health and Social Care* **2**(4): 190–4

Matthews DR (1996) Learning disabilities: The challenge for nursing. *Nursing Times* **92**(27): 35–8

Matthews DR (2002) Learning disabilities: The need for better healthcare.

Nursing Standard **16**(39): 2002

Matthews DR (2005) Healthcare and learning disability. *Learning Disability Practice* **8**(5):

McConkey R (2002) Changes in the attitudes of GPs to the health screening of patients with learning disabilities. *Journal of Learning Disabilities* **6**(4): 373–84

McKenzie K, Powell H (2004) Health Screening. *Learning Disability Practice* **7:** 10 Dec 2004

Meehan S, Moore G, Barr O (1995) Specialist services for people with a learning disability. *Nursing Times* **91**(13): 33–5

Michael J (2008) *Healthcare for All. Independent Inquiry into access to healthcare for people with learning disabilities.* Available from: www. iahpld.org.uk/Healthcare_final.pdf

Mitchell D (2000) Parallel stigma? Nurses and people with learning disabilities. *British Journal of Learning Disabilities* **28:** 78–81

Mencap (2005) *Treat Me Right! Better Healthcare for People with a Learning Disability.*Mencap.London

Mencap (2007) *Death by Indifference! Following up the Treat Me Right! Report* Mencap, London

Messent P, Caan W (2000) Learning disability nurses must stay linked to the NHS. *British Journal of Nursing.* **9**(19): 2062

Mitchell D (2004) Learning disability nursing. *British Journal of Learning Disabilities* **32:** 115–8

Mobbs C, Hadley S, Wittering R, Bailey N (2002) An exploration of the role of community nurse, learning disability, in England. *British Journal of Learning Disabilities* **30:** 13–8

National Assembly for Wales (1999) *'Realising the Potential' A Strategic Framework for Nursing, Midwifery and Health Visiting in Wales into the 21st Century.* National Assembly for Wales, Cardiff

NHS Scotland (2004) *Health Needs Assessment Report. People with learning disabilities in Scotland.* NHS Scotland – Public Health Institute of Scotland, Glasgow

Parahoo K, Barr O (1996) Community Mental Handicap Nursing Services in Northern Ireland: A profile of clients and selected working practices. *Journal of Clinical Nursing* **5**: 211–28

Royal College of Nursing (1985) *The Role and Function of the Domiciliary Nurse in Mental Handicap.* Royal College of Nursing, London

Royal College of Nursing (1992) *The Role of the Community Nurse.* Royal College of Nursing, London

Royal College of Physicians (1998) *Disabled People Using Hospital: A Charter and Guidelines.* Royal College of Physicians, London

Ruddick L (2005) Health of people with intellectual disabilities: A review of factors influencing access to healthcare. *British Journal of Health Psychology* **10**(4): 559–70

Scott E, Elvish J, Luft L, Wilson M (2005) The development and use of a personal health resource. *Learning Disability Practice* **8**(2): 27–31

Scottish Executive (2000) *The Same as You?* The Stationery Office, Edinburgh

Scottish Health Authority (2002) *Promoting Health, Supporting People.* The Stationery Office, Edinburgh

Slevin E, McConkey R, Truesdale-Kennedy M, Barr O, Taggart L (2007) Community Learning Disability Teams:Perceived effectiveness,multi-disciplinary working and service user satisfaction. *Journal of Intellectual Disabilities* **11**(4): 329–42

Slevin E, Truesdale-Kennedy M, McConkey R, Barr O, Taggart L (2008) Community Learning Disability Teams: Developments, composition and good practice. *Journal of Intellectual Disabilities* **12**(1): 59–79

Strong PG, Sandland ET (1974). Subnormality nursing in the community. *Nursing Times* **70**(10): 354–6

Swaann C (1997) Development of services. In: Gates B (ed) *Learning Disabilities.* Churchill Livingstone, Edinburgh

Thompson J, Cobb J (2004) Person centred health action planning. *Learning Disability Practice* **7**(5): 12–5

Turnbull J (2004) *Learning Disability Nursing.* Blackwell Publishing, Oxford

Welsh Assembly Government (2002) *'Realising the Potential' Briefing Paper 3.Inclusion,Partnership and Innovation; A Framework for Realising Potential of Learning Disability Nursing in Wales.* Welsh Assembly Government, Cardiff

Welsh Office (2001) *Fulfilling the Promises.*Cardiff.Welsh Assembly

Wheeler P (2003) Patients rights: Consent to treatment for men and women with a learning disability or who are otherwise mentally incapacitated. *Learning Disability Practice* **6**(5): 29–37

Williamson A, Johnson J (2004) Improving services for people with learning disabilities. *Nursing Standard* **18**(24): 43–51

Wolfensberger W (2002) Social Role Valorisation and/or/versus, "Empowerment". *Mental Retardation* **40**: 252–8

CHAPTER 7

Health facilitation

Susan Brady

Introduction

According to the Department of Health (2006) and NHS Quality Improvement Scotland (2006), outcomes for people with learning disabilities fall short when compared with outcomes for the non-disabled population. People with learning disabilities are known, as a group, to access health screening services less than the rest of the population, in particular breast and cervical screening. There is often inadequate diagnosis and treatment for heart disease, hypothyroidism and osteoporosis. The Department of Health (2006) also report that people with learning disabilities have an over-dependence on psychotropic medication. Studies have found a high prevalence of health problems whether in institutional or community care. Improvement in public health has resulted in improved life expectancy for people with learning disabilities, but it is still less than the rest of the population. Continuing inequalities in the distribution of health services has led to inequality in access, putting people with learning disabilities at risk.

History of the development of community care policy

Komaromy (2001), suggests that since the 1980s three dimensions have structured the debate about community care policy.

- A shift in location.
- A shift in perspective.
- A shift in power.

Institutional care only began in the middle of the 19th century, where local parishes made provision for care of the 'sick poor'. These people were looked after in their own homes often by local poor people who were paid to do so. During the Victorian period there was a significant growth of institutions, workhouses and asylums. Then, as we entered the early part of the 20th century, there was a focus and backwards turn towards some form of community care and a real shift in mental healthcare provision. In 1961 the Health Minister, Enoch Powell, announced the future plans for closure of the 'mental hospital'. Over the next 30 years further developments saw the closure of large hospitals for learning disabilities and mental health, in order to provide people with the opportunities to live a more independent and 'normal' life within smaller homes in the community. Initial closures in the 1970s were slow but the 1980s and 1990s saw a majority of them close down with an emphasis on the provision of community care. In 1970 a lobby was formed from which a new philosophy of normalisation began. This focused on the rights of people with a learning disability to have an ordinary life, including the right to live in the community and participate in community life, introducing a more social model of disability (Komaromy, 2001). This philosophy of care directed community services to provide care in a way that empowered individuals with a learning disability. Normalisation as a strategy is sufficiently general to apply to other groups covered by the policy of community care, such as older people. Despite the positive approach of normalisation, it has been criticised for its tendency to make the experiences of people with disabilities invisible, in that, if everyone is treated the same, ignoring specific needs, then the environment within which they live will be inflexible and inadaptable. The basic needs of the individual may be overlooked. Central to access is the necessity for good communication and awareness of others so that people with learning disabilities are supported to understand, express needs, feelings and choices. In a recent publication by the NHS Quality Improvement in Scotland (2006) reference was made to the fact that people with a learning disability are more likely to have an impairment of communication than the rest of the population and therefore require specialist consideration. Also highlighted in this document was that heightened awareness of the distinct needs of people with a learning disability could do much to reduce what is often unintentional discrimination and to enhance access. What people with learning disabilities want is to have equal access to services that they require with additional support to use them as indicated (Department of Health, 2001).

Public funding

The NHS Community Care Act was introduced in 1990 and implemented in 1993. Local authorities were given the freedom to spend money on either institutional or non-institutional care. The Act suggested that 85% of the money was to be given to providers in the independent sector. This made social services responsible for the organisation and funding of community care. The shift in location from institutions to communities was to result in the change to social security payments. The intention was to supply incentives for greater responsiveness to the needs of consumers while being attentive to cost and quality. However, at the same time both health and social care boundaries were becoming blurred.

Partnerships in community care

The White Paper *Modernising Social Services* (Department of Health, 1998a), proposed a new statutory duty of partnership requiring the NHS and local authorities to work together in order to offer a seamless service. The Government announced its proposals for changes to the NHS and organisation of social care. Demands for health and social-care agencies to work in an integrated way did not take into account the reality that they are very different organisations. The main barriers to working across boundaries are the potential difficulties in how the relationship of power is shared between health and social services. The problem of who does what and who pays the cost, and establishing systems of effective communication act as further barriers to effective working.

Developments in primary care

Developments in primary care were also continuing during this time. However services to meet the needs of people with learning disabilities were not incorporated effectively into the planning process. The last 15 years has seen a move from GP fundholding in 1990, through Primary Care Groups (PCGs) to the newly formed Primary Care Trusts (PCTs) in 2002. Government strategies, *Signposts to Success* (Department of Health, 1998b), *Once a Day* (Department of Health, 1999) and *Valuing People* (Department of Health, 2001), all give guidance for primary care when providing services for people with learning disabilities. The provision of healthcare to individuals is increasingly the remit of primary care teams. It has been evident that this vulnerable group of people have high levels of hidden morbidity, low levels of health promotion and low rates of consultation allied to deficits in communication and understanding (Kerr, 1998). Despite this, primary care providers are still unclear how to meet the needs of people with learning disabilities. Many are unaware of the developments since the Community Care Act (1990). The model of integrated health and social care is fundamental to the provision of quality healthcare. Comprehensive health surveillance should include all aspects of social care provision. Health professionals working within multi-agency support teams can be utilised to help manage the interface between the services and enhance communication. Primary healthcare teams should be viewed as significant members of those support teams. A comprehensive health check could be integrated within the holistic assessment processes of case management or other planning initiatives. The relationship between learning disability services and primary care needs to be enhanced. At the very least, GPs should have an awareness of the individual's key worker or point of contact in the specialist team. Comprehensive registers should be set up within primary care teams providing key information with regards to the health and social needs of individuals (Department of Health, 2001). If GPs do not provide positive patient-centred approaches, people with learning disabilities will be less satisfied, less enabled and may have a greater symptom burden with higher rates of referral (Little et al, 2001). This could have additional implications for cost.

Primary care trust infrastructure

Primary care trusts provide a structure within which the internal market can be exercised with objectives, controls, procedures, budgets and information flows. They are subject to external control, evaluation and assessment. They are monitored by the NHS incorporating performance management to ensure compliance with standards and policies. The organisation of PCTs provides extra resources and influence over healthcare. The focus of PCTs is to provide population and needs-led services by incorporating collaborative partnership working. However, there are problems with this system. There is a need to reorganise boundaries but there remain complexities of maintaining partnership arrangements. The role of provider/purchaser of healthcare that PCTs take on could threaten managers' relationships of trust with patients. Also PCGs/PCTs, as commissioners, may have to make potentially difficult or unpopular decisions.

Moving forward for better access

There has been recent national and international moves to improve user satisfaction and equality of access to primary care services (Stein, 2000; Lennox et al, 2001; Powrie, 2003). This has placed responsibility upon services that provide healthcare to people with learning disabilities to improve the care they provide. This presents major challenges to primary care services (Cumella et al, 1992; Evans et al, 1994; Howells, 1996). To address this issue the Government have introduced the concept of health facilitation, (Department of Health, 2001). Health facilitation involves both casework to help people access mainstream services and also development work within mainstream services to help all parts of the NHS to develop necessary skills. It has emerged from the wishes of people with learning disabilities, their carers and support workers, who requested support to help them navigate their way through the health service in order to access the best and most appropriate healthcare (Department of Health, 2002). Community learning disability teams are expected to take on the role of health facilitators in order to meet these targets.

Health facilitation

Health facilitation is a key concept in an increasingly sophisticated service. Together with the Patient Advocacy Service (PALS) and Partnership Boards, new opportunities exist to improve the health needs of people with learning disabilities. What is apparent is the need for additional support for people with learning disabilities, as primary care will not be able to provide appropriate care in isolation. The Department of Health (2001) suggested that by appointing health facilitators by spring 2003 and developing health action plans for people with learning disabilities by 2005 they would meet their targets. This process has started to happen, although no additional funds have been allocated to support this process and guidance given to the PCTs has been patchy. Annual joint health checks can not only benefit the individuals with learning disabilities but can help providers of services by generating valuable information on demography needs and provide clinical information to the PCTs. By identifying problems early, costly, more serious or chronic illnesses may well be avoided. Providing joint annual health checks is one way in which primary and specialist services can work together, supported by the concept of health facilitation. It is important that the outcomes from the identification of health needs within a population of people with learning disabilities informs the decision making process for the provision of future services and policies.

Background

The healthcare needs of people with learning disabilities has, within the past 20 years come, under the spotlight. Both community-based studies (Singh, 1997) and general practice surveys (Kerr et al, 1996; Thornton, 1997) show deficiencies in the provision of healthcare for people with learning disabilities. The current policy agenda has put the development of sound and effective partnerships across agencies at the very heart of service delivery (Department of Health, 1997; 1998b; 1999; 2001; 2006). In response to the World Health Organisation (WHO) call for better services, Government initiatives, *Health of the Nation* (Department of Health, 1995), *Once a Day* (Department of Health, 1998), *Signposts for Success* (Department of Health, 1999), *Valuing People* (Department of Health, 2001), *Our Health, Our Care, Our Say* (Department of Health, 2006) have highlighted the inequalities faced by people with learning disabilities in accessing primary healthcare and provide guidance on effective delivery of that care. Despite these initiatives however, there is little doubt that people with learning disabilities and their carers remain vulnerable members of society (Singh, 1997). The equitable inclusion of people with learning disabilities into a primary care framework presents an important challenge to providers. Primary care may need to change the focus of its work in order to support communities to actively promote public health in its area. There is still wide recognition that the primary care team has very little knowledge of the health needs of people with learning disabilities (Hunt et al, 2001). Communication difficulties often mean that people with learning disabilities and primary care services are unable to establish an effective interface, creating problems with understanding at a most basic level (Lawrie, 1995). Research into how GPs offer primary healthcare to people with learning disabilities highlights their difficulties in effectively meeting their needs. Authors such as Minihan et al (1993) and Garrard (1983) emphasise the special challenges made to GPs and their lack of experience and training with this client group (Stein, 2000; Meehan et al, 1995; Lawrie,1995). Various studies and reviews make recommendations for further training for medical students and GPs, with the need for specialists to inform them of the particular health needs of people with learning disabilities (Kerr et al, 1996; Singh, 1997; Lennox & Kerr, 1997; Martin and Martin, 1999; Beck, 2002; Jukes and Bollard, 2002). Kerr et al (1996) argue that 'integration of people with a learning disability into a primary care system, will not occur by relying on generic primary healthcare systems to develop this care in isolation'. This is supported by the fact that GPs and primary care staff are confused over what constitutes a learning disability. Rodgers (1993) argues for the need for greater cooperation between primary and specialist services in order to deliver equitable healthcare.

Summary of literature review

The literature review conducted has, in general, revealed that few studies have focused on the effectiveness of support offered by health facilitators. This is possibly due to the fact that health facilitation is still a developing concept. Some areas in the UK may not have health facilitators in place as yet. Many studies are still focusing on what needs to be done to promote partnership working. There also remains limited published surveys of GP attitudes towards people with learning disability (Ineichen & Russell, 1980; Langan et al, 1993; Hilderbrand, 1995; Kerr et al, 1996; Bond et al, 1997; Stein, 2000). The outcome of these studies suggests the continued need for specialist input to support primary care services. Current initiatives to develop health facilitators and health action plans is seen as an excellent opportunity to make an enormous difference to the health and subsequent quality of life for people with learning disabilities (Matthews, 2002).

Introduction to the present study

There have been continuing inequalities in the distribution of health services and therefore inequality in access (Allsop, 1992). People with learning disabilities are particularly at risk (Department of Health, 1999). Healthcare has been criticised for being bureaucratically organised and alienating for the individual. People with learning disabilities expressed anxiety and confusion when faced with the medical profession (Department of Health, 2001).

Various studies and reviews make recommendations for further training for medical students and GPs, with the need for specialists to inform them of the particular health needs of people with learning disabilities. However integration of people with a learning disability into a primary care system will not occur by relying on generic primary healthcare systems to develop this care in isolation. This is supported by the fact that GPs and primary care staff are confused over what constitutes a learning disability. There is a need for greater cooperation between primary and specialist services in order to deliver equitable healthcare. To address these barriers, the Department of Health has set various targets. One of these targets is for health facilitators to be in place to support people with learning disabilities. This study examines the developing role of the health facilitator and existing health facilitation strategies that aim to improve access to primary care for people with learning disabilities. Building on the findings and recommendations of previous research studies and Government policy, the project facilitator conducted an evaluation study within a large city utilising a qualitative postal questionnaire. The aim of the study was to determine if an electronic learning disability health screening template was useful in supporting GPs to offer annual health checks to their patients with learning disabilities. The findings of the study have shown that the majority of GPs value the support of the health facilitator. The electronic health screening template has been described by GPs as an inventory of information shared between services. It has highlighted health risks to patients with learning disabilities and has supported a referral process enabling people with learning disabilities to access appropriate healthcare services that meet their needs. Further training needs of GPs are also highlighted in the study in particular issues with consent, the health action planning process and the evidence base behind annual health checks for people with a learning disability.

Health access pilot study

Over the past seven years, various pilot projects in Birmingham have examined the health needs of people with learning disabilities and the inequality in access to health services. Local research shows that in the inner city areas of Birmingham the incidence of learning disability was double the national average, at around 6.3%. A high proportion of people living within these areas were from black and minority ethnic groups. Learning disability is more likely to occur in some ethnic minority groups (Department of Health, 1999)

In order to facilitate better access to primary care services for people with learning disabilities, a proposal was put forward to conduct a pilot for a health screening project. Ethical approval and funding were sought and approval for the study to be conducted was agreed. The aim of the pilot was to develop and implement a health screening tool and improve access to primary and secondary care services for people with learning disabilities living within the inner city areas. The Access to Primary Care Project (Brady, 2004) commenced in September 1999 and a sample group of adults with learning disabilities were offered a comprehensive health check with follow up approximately one year afterwards. The pilot project was conducted over a two year period.

The project nurse initially developed a database for two PCG areas. She identified a total of 537 people with learning disability within the area. This was not an exhaustive list, but was gathered over a six-month period at the beginning of the project in order to identify the local population within the inner city areas of Birmingham. A total of 189 people with learning disabilities were offered a health check. Of these, 113 were male and 76 female. The total number of people receiving a health check was 175. These checks were conducted by either the project facilitator, a community development worker, a support worker or a community nurse/ health facilitator working within the Heart of Birmingham PCT area. They used a health screening questionnaire developed by the project facilitator. An additional 21 primary health checks were completed by the primary healthcare team using the Cardiff Health Check health screening tool. A total of four GP practices agreed to facilitate health checks for their patients with learning disability. Fourteen people in total chose not to take up the offer to have a health check. This suggests that the approach taken to implement the health checks was an effective one as only 7% of those invited for a health check refrained. The majority of people receiving input for the first phase of health checks had referrals made as a result of their health check. Thirty different and previously undiagnosed health problems were identified in total. See *Table 7.1.*

Table 7.1. Health problems identified as a result of the primary healthcare check

Behaviour difficulties	70
Incontinence	53
Visual impairment	51
Skin problems	41
Epilepsy	38
Psychiatric disorder	36
Dental problems	31
Hearing impairment	30
Obesity	22
Cardiovascular problems	20
Eating disorder	20
Respiratory problems	19
Gynaecological problems	17
Impacted ear wax	15
Eye infection	13
Constipation	12
Thyroid disorder	11
Underweight	11
Osteoarthritis	7
Gastric problems	6
Diabetes	5
Kidney problems	5
Alcohol or drug dependency	3
Sickle cell anaemia	3
Alzheimer's/dementia	2
Cancer	2
Thalassaemia	1
Umbilical hernia	1
Migraine	1

Medication

Of those that received a health check, 76% were taking medication for health conditions, predominately for epilepsy and behaviour management. Those receiving medication for epilepsy were commonly prescribed drugs such as: phenobarbitone, sodium valproate, phenytoin and carbamazepine as first line drugs in the management of epilepsy, despite national recommendations for these drugs to be used with caution. There was evidence that women were also prescribed carbamazepine and sodium valproate despite national guidance that these should not be drugs of choice for women, due to the fact that they are hepatic enzyme inducing drugs. These affect a woman's menstrual cycle, hormone balance, and interact with other drugs such as the contraceptive pill. Sodium valproate, in particular, can also cause an increased risk of deformity/brain damage to the unborn foetus if these drugs are taken during pregnancy (National Institute for Clinical Excellence, 2004).

Risk factors identified

Several risk factors for type 2 diabetes were revealed as a result of the health checks. At least 20 people were suffering from eating disorders, skin problems and cardiovascular disease, all risk factors for type 2 diabetes. A significant number also suffered from visual disturbances that can also be attributed to diabetes in some people. Diabetes is up to four times more common in some ethnic minority groups. This is also a risk factor for the Heart of Birmingham area. Active diabetes screening is not routinely offered by the GPs or practice nurses. Primary healthcare practitioners are dependant on individuals to report any symptoms or changes in their health to help them make a diagnosis. This in itself serves as a barrier for access to primary care services for any individual with communication difficulties. This is concerning to the sample group as 57% were identified as having communication difficulties.

Sexual health screening

The sample group were asked if they had ever received any sexual health counselling regarding relationships, contraception, sexually transmitted diseases or pregnancy. Of the respondents 96% reported that they had never received counselling. This is a significant number indicating that structures need to be developed to enable people with learning disabilities to access sexual health promotion opportunities. Cervical screening opportunities were also poor. Only 24% of women were offered cervical screening. Similar poor results were also shown in women eligible for breast examination and screening (17%). This compares to the screening opportunities for non-learning disabled population within the Heart of Birmingham where uptake is much higher at around 73%.

Follow up health checks

The health checks were repeated approximately 12 months later to review the individual's health status and to monitor any referrals made. The referrals generated from the health check identified the need for input by 13 different agencies. In total 103 referrals were generated.

Incidence of follow up as a result of the initial health check

Of those participants that responded, a significant number (69%) reported that they had been contacted or received follow up as a result of the referral made from the initial health check. When asked if the service was appropriate to meet their needs, the majority (87%) of people with learning disability said that it was.

Follow up annual health check as a result of the project

A total of 34% reported that they had been offered an annual health check by either the practice nurse or GP. Other qualitative studies using semi-structured interviews, questionnaires and focus groups were used to measure the attitudes of people with learning disabilities, their carers and primary care staff in relation to access to primary care. These studies all highlighted the training and communication needs of service users and healthcare providers.

Collaborative practice

Collaboration between primary, secondary and acute services has been suggested as the way forward to promote better services (Martin and Martin, 1999; Brady et al, 2002; Glasby, 2002). Although the pilot study showed that there had been a positive influence on primary care staff offering annual health checks for people with learning disabilities, it also highlighted the need to adapt the health screening tool so that it would be compatible with the existing computer systems used within primary care surgeries in Birmingham. It was identified that there were five computer systems commonly used by the GPs within their surgeries. To address this issue, the project facilitator established a working group made up of clinical system facilitators from the PCT, GP, practice nurses, learning disability community nurses, practice managers and administration staff to develop an appropriate tool. Initially a screening tool compatible with the Emis LV system was developed and then piloted within one GP surgery in South Birmingham PCT. Following some minor adaptations it gained approval from the four PCTs and the template was distributed to all practices across the city. Other templates were developed so that other existing computer systems could accommodate the learning disability template. Six community nurse/health facilitators were seconded for an 18 month period to support primary care surgeries across the city to implement learning disability practice registers and annual health screening and facilitate the development of health action plans for people with learning disabilities. They worked closely with individual GP surgeries to develop good partnerships with primary care staff. They offered advice on issues concerning learning disability and acted as a liaison point for the specialist service. GPs' attitudes towards offering the annual health screening using the template was mixed. Many felt that it fell outside their general medical services contract and that they should be reimbursed for any additional work that was conducted. However despite this issue 37% of GPs continued to work collaboratively with the health facilitators in developing practice registers of their patients with learning disabilities, performing annual health checks and supporting referrals for follow up interventions.

Gaining consensus from primary care

In order to address the barrier of reimbursement, the project facilitator forwarded proposals to all four PCT areas in the city for a locally enhanced service for learning disabilities. The enhanced service proposal provided various options for primary care services, identifying how they could be supported to meet the needs of their patients with learning disabilities.

The National Plan (Department of Health, 2000) reinforces the importance of getting the basics right and highlights an approach to managing the health needs of people with learning disabilities which provides quality outcomes for service users, carers and staff alike. This looks at improving the patient's journey and experience. The wishes of service users and staff were acknowledged and training needs addressed. It was anticipated that the approach would enable all practice registers to be completed in readiness to commence health screening and health action planning for people with learning disabilities from 2005 onwards. Information from the health check was also used to support statistics for the National Service Framework (NSF) targets and the Quality Outcome Framework (QOF). This approach has been recognised by the Department of Health as an example to partnership boards on how best they can meet the needs of their learning disabled population (Department of Health, 2002). This option enables the targets set by the Government in *Valuing*

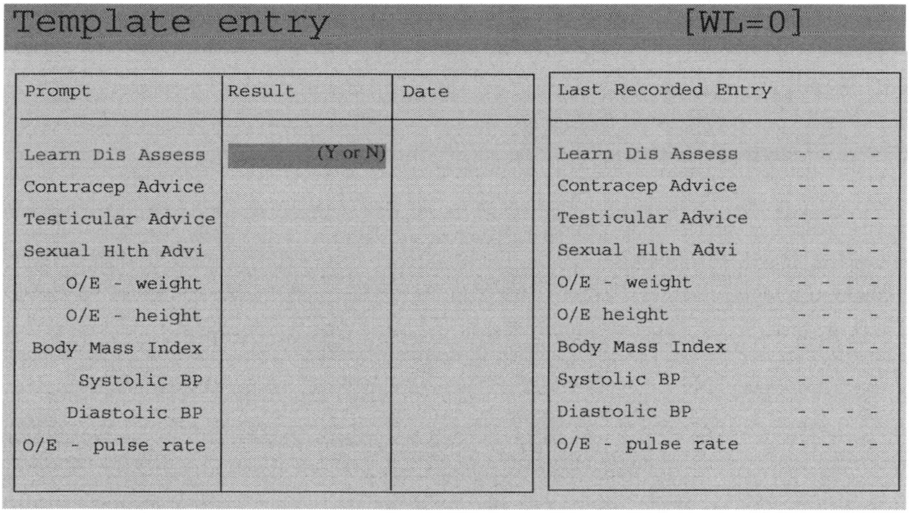

```
Template entry                              [WL=0]
```

Prompt	Result	Date	Last Recorded Entry
Learn Dis Assess	(Y or N)		Learn Dis Assess - - - -
Contracep Advice			Contracep Advice - - - -
Testicular Advice			Testicular Advice - - - -
Sexual Hlth Advi			Sexual Hlth Advi - - - -
O/E - weight			O/E - weight - - - -
O/E - height			O/E height - - - -
Body Mass Index			Body Mass Index - - - -
Systolic BP			Systolic BP - - - -
Diastolic BP			Diastolic BP - - - -
O/E - pulse rate			O/E - pulse rate - - - -

Figure 7.1. Electronic learning disability health screening template (SBPCT, 2004)

People to be met. People with learning disabilities will have access to health services they require and additional support from an advocate/ health facilitator. Accessible information will be made available via a personal health action plan. Joint information systems have been developed at no additional cost to either service with resources being managed more effectively.

The learning disability health screening template

An electronic learning disability health screening template has been developed to enable primary care to identify the health status of their patients with learning disabilities and their additional risk factors with a protocol for its use. See *Figure 7.1*.

Training opportunities have been provided for staff, service users and their carers. Barriers have started to come down but there is still a long way to go if an inclusive and equitable health service is to be offered to people with learning disabilities across the city. All primary care teams need to support the Government objectives for meeting the health needs of people with learning disabilities. The learning disability service cannot meet the needs of people with learning disabilities without their input.

Evaluating effectiveness

It was appropriate and timely therefore that an evaluation was conducted to establish the effectiveness of the new electronic learning disability template in practice.The findings of the project will support the evaluation of the health facilitation model in the city including the locally enhanced service for learning disabilities within one PCT area. The results will influence the future use of any joint electronic information systems. This will enable the learning disability service to build upon good practice and to develop appropriate strategies for future policy planning. It is envisaged that this will influence the changing role of the community learning disability nurse and the advanced practitioner/nurse consultant for learning disabilities. The project facilitator will disseminate the findings of the study by presenting to local and national forums and through various publications.

Title of project

The project was titled: How effective is an electronic health screening template in assisting GPs to address the health needs of people with learning disabilities?

Aim of study

The aim of the study is to conduct an evaluation on the effectiveness of the current health screening tool that has been incorporated into the locally enhanced service for learning disabilities. The project facilitator will determine how effective the electronic learning disability health screening template has been in supporting GPs to meet the health needs of their patients with learning disabilities.

Objectives of the study

The objectives of the study were:

- To identify outcomes for the health facilitation model in Birmingham.
- To develop a qualitative questionnaire to measure GPs' experience when utilising the template as part of an annual health check for their patients with learning disabilities.
- To establish support required by GPs in providing a service to people with learning disabilities.
- To identify service barriers to service provision for people with learning disabilities.
- To promote partnership working and communication between learning disability and primary care services.
- To establish whether GPs value the support of identified health facilitators.
- To make recommendations for future nursing practice.

Methodology

The project facilitator has incorporated evaluative research (Weiss, 1998) in this study. This method was chosen to determine the impact and effectiveness of the health facilitation model in Birmingham. A systematic assessment of the operation of the current initiative was undertaken and the impact of the program documented. This was compared to a set of explicit standards as a means of contributing to future health facilitation program and nursing policy. A qualitative approach was used to identify specific attitudes, feelings and experiences of the participants.

Study design

Data collection method

Postal self-completed questionnaires were used in the study. The advantage of this method is that large numbers of the population can be sampled at relatively low cost over a wide geographical area.

Design of instrument

Open-ended questions were used in the questionnaires. The project facilitator created the questionnaire with the intention of gathering a range of possible data where no previous data already existed. The purpose was to extract the personal views and experiences of the GPs using the health screening template in everyday practice. Instructions were provided with the questionnaire stating its purpose.

Piloting data collecting instrument

The project facilitator worked alongside a GP advisor, academic supervisor and clinical managers to determine the appropriateness of the format of the questionnaire and to identify any ambiguities. Once the content was agreed it was piloted with a GP within a PCT area prior to the implementation of the study.

Testing validity

The project facilitator's aim was to examine the full scope of the research question in a balanced way. As there had been no previous studies that examined the effectiveness of an electronic health screening tool the project facilitator designed the questionnaire in order to evaluate current practice and to make recommendations for future policy within nursing. Prior to distribution of the postal questionnaire, identified GPs were contacted via the telephone and face to face to explain that the questionnaire would be forwarded to them. The purpose of the evaluation was also discussed. This was done to encourage participation in the study. The questionnaire was utilised in order to evaluate an existing initiative that was due for review. It was timely therefore that the questionnaire was sent out at this time as the PCT was already undertaking an internal audit of the locally enhanced service. This potentially avoided wasting time and cost as participants responded quickly, possibly due to the association with the PCT audit. Consent forms and stamped addressed envelopes were also sent out with the questionnaire to aid a fast response from participants.

Sample

The evaluation study was conducted in one PCT area in a large city. Registered and practising GPs were identified within this PCT area. Those GPs that had signed up to the enhanced service for learning disabilities were selected for the target group. A random sample of eight GPs were selected to take part in the study.

Data analysis

Several techniques are available for data analysis when using the phenomenological method (LoBiondo-Wood & Haber, 2002). Content analysis (Cavanagh, 1997) was performed on the data collated from the open-ended questions. This systematic approach confirms the applicability of clinical strategies for health facilitation already developed from single qualitative studies. This analysis allowed the facilitator to evaluate clinical outcomes and implement future interventions based on the experience of the clinical phenomenon identified. A statistical package was also used in the evaluation (Gen Stat Student Release 8.1 PC Windows XP) incorporating the Fisher's exact test. This test procedure calculates an exact probability value for the relationship between two dichotomous variables, as found in a two by two crossover design. The program calculates the difference between the data observed and the data expected. This was utilised so that combinations of data results, which had the same marginal totals, could be listed and probabilities attached to them. This enabled the project facilitator to work out the probability of an observed result and its significance.

Ethical issues

Prior to the implementation of this study ethical approval was sought. The Chief Executive, Research and Development Team and service managers for South Birmingham PCT were informed about the proposed study in their area via letter. The project facilitator submitted an ethics application form to the PCT Research and Development Team and Local Ethics Committee for approval. Approval was given and the facilitator approached the sample group for their consent to participate in the study. This was obtained via consent slip on a standard GP letter providing details of the proposed study to all GP participants. This letter had a tear off slip at the bottom to be returned by GPs wishing to participate. All data generated was anonymised and kept confidentially in a locked cupboard in accordance with the Data Protection Act (1998). Only the project facilitator had access to the information. Following the analysis of the data, the returned questionnaires were shredded. The project facilitator recorded any feelings of bias during the data gathering process to ensure that an accurate account of the participants' attitudes and experiences were documented.

Results/findings

The qualitative questionnaires were posted out to eight GPs in the PCT area. One GP did not participate due to being on holiday at the time but five agreed to participate in the study and completed the questionnaires. This shows a good response rate (64%). The questionnaire was made up of 11 open-ended questions relating to the implementation of the electronic health screening template. The questions and responses are discussed below.

Participants were initially asked about when they were first made aware of the template. All had received correspondence from the health facilitator ranging over a 2 year period. The average (mean) time GPs had been aware of the template was 16 months. In addition to this they were asked to comment on how long they had been using the template within their surgery. The time span ranged from 12 to 24 months; the average (mean) time GPs had been utilising the template was 13 months.

Support offered to primary care

When asked to comment about their initial thoughts when first using the template 80% expressed some uncertainty as to why the template was needed in the first place. Twenty per cent felt that they should be reimbursed for additional screening whereas the remaining 80% assumed that this fell within existing general medical services. Despite some initial reservations 60% were happy to use the template in order to manage the needs of their patients with learning disabilities more effectively. Whilst using the template in practice, 60% felt that they were supported effectively to carry out the screening. Support that was valued by GPs ranged from IT support to load the template to assistance in identifying patients with learning disabilities on practice lists prior to screening. This support was offered by the health facilitator in conjunction with PCT clinical systems facilitators. The sample group did identify some areas that caused difficulties when offering the health checks. These areas focused on:

- The time it took to complete the health check was longer than a single appointment.
- There was some uncertainty about what to do with issues of consent.
- Lack of clarity about what primary care's role was in relation to the health action planning process. The majority of GPs felt that health action planning should be the role of the specialist service. Difficulties that were experienced were resolved for all four GPs that requested it (80%). The support offered to GPs was valued by them. In particular reference was made to the benefits of accessible information/letters, information provided on health needs of people with learning disability, support with initiating practice registers and having a named contact with the specialist service.

Benefits of the health screening template

The sample group were asked to comment on how they felt that the template had supported them to manage the health needs of their patients with learning disabilities. Responses documented included:

- 'Brought patients to our attention. One of our patients hadn't been to the surgery for nearly 12 years. We didn't realise until the practice list of patients with learning disabilities was completed.'
- 'The template highlights current health risks that may not be communicated by the patient with learning disabilities or who has communication difficulties.'
- 'The template identified specific investigations that should be conducted for people with learning disabilities. We wouldn't normally offer such a detailed health check. This is improving the service we offer to our patients.'
- 'The template acted as an inventory of information to share between primary care and the learning disability service.'

Table 7.2. Results of Fisher Exact Test

Supported	Yes/possibly	No
Helpful/useful	4	I
One-tailed significance level	.200	
Mid-*P* value	.100	
Two-tailed significance level		
Two times one-tailed significance level	.400	
Mid-*P* value	.200	
Sum of all outcomes with prob ≤ observed	.200	
Mid-*P* value	.100	

- 'This template is easy to use and compatible with existing primary care systems. It supports the Quality Outcome Framework (QOF) as well as National Framework Targets for our patients with learning disabilities.'

When asked to comment on whether or not they felt the health screening tool was useful in meeting the health needs of their patients, 80% agreed it was. No suggestions were made to improve upon the existing template.

Encouraging collaboration

Some ways in which the implementation of the template has influenced the GPs to work in collaboration is through joint health promotion clinics, liaison with an identified health facilitator on a regular basis, appropriate referrals and the health action planning process.

Training needs of GPs highlighted

Training needs of GPs that were highlighted related to four main areas:

- Issues with consent.
- Health action planning process.
- IT skills competence.
- Understanding the need for some aspects of the template (evidence base).

Fisher Exact Test

To further support the evaluation of the data the Fisher Exact Test was used to determine statistical relevance of the usefulness of the support offered to the GPs by the health facilitators. A statistical package was utilised (GenStat Student Release 8.1 for PC/Windows XP). This test did not show any statistical relevance, possibly due to the small sample size. The results are shown in *Table 7.2*.

The health facilitators have addressed the GPs' specific training needs. The GPs found the template easy to use and felt supported to overcome any difficulties experienced. Those responses that were less positive were expressed from GPs that had been using the template for the shortest period of time (between 6 and 12 months); those who had been using it longer had a positive view of its usefulness. The template was seen to be effective in practice at identifying specific health needs of people with learning disabilities. It supports partnership working/collaboration across different organisations whilst addressing current barriers to health access. Specific training needs of primary care have been highlighted. Evidence supports the fact that GPs value the support offered by health facilitators and do utilise their skills.

Critique of project

In order for health facilitation and health action planning to be successful it is essential that all professionals working with people with learning disabilities communicate and collaborate effectively. It is important to make connections between primary care and learning disability services, whilst acknowledging the challenges involved in working across traditional boundaries and service cultures (Giraud-Saunders, 2000).

This study involved GPs practising within one large PCT in the UK. Therefore the findings of the study may only reflect their views from a local context and should not be generalised. Due to the fact that the project facilitator is known to many of the GPs as the clinical lead for health facilitation, the way in which the participants answer questions on the questionnaire may be affected, introducing bias. In order to address this issue the project facilitator made note of any eventualities in the evaluation of the study. She also considered her own views on health facilitation to ensure that these did not influence the outcome of the study.

In an attempt to strengthen the evaluation the project facilitator used a triangulation of methods, incorporating the Fisher Exact Test. However this test did not show any statistical significance when used against the data generated in the evaluation. This is likely to be due to the small sample size of the study. Time limitations of the study and limited resources have determined the sample size and content. Therefore it has only been possible to incorporate content analysis of the data provided. Ideally the sample size should have been larger to enable a wider range of responses to be recorded.

In addition, it is important to acknowledge that service users and their carers should also have the opportunity to comment on the effectiveness of the service provided to them by the health facilitators if their needs are to be met. This should be a priority for future research, not only in Birmingham but also in other areas across the UK where health facilitators are currently providing a service.

Conclusion

This study has shown that support offered to GPs during the implementation of the health screening template was valued and any training needs highlighted were addressed either by the health facilitator or the clinical systems facilitator for the PCT area. Partnership working is now in place across learning disability and primary care services. Health facilitators continue to support and manage any problems experienced to enable a positive working relationship between services to continue. GPs' attitudes have changed since the implementation of the template. In the main, attitudes have been positive and, despite any reservations in initially using the template, all eight GPs have continued to use the template in their everyday practice even post-pilot. Barriers are starting to come down.

The health screening template, if it continues to be used in the future will assist PCTs in achieving clinical governance standards within their learning disabilities population. PCTs have the responsibility for improving the health of their community by developing primary and community services and commissioning high quality secondary care services (Department of Health, 1998). The template will provide a useful tool in:

- Preventing illness and assisting in early diagnosis.
- Identifying previously unrecognised health problems in people with learning disabilities.
- Early identification of health problems, which can prevent the development of more serious problems.
- Reducing risks to those suffering from mental illness and challenging behaviour by early detection and treatment.
- Providing health promotion to prevent coronary heart disease and to assist in smoking cessation.
- Potential for reduced prescribing as a result of medication reviews.
- Assist in continuing professional development of primary health staff.
- Assist in building up a register of all people with learning disabilities within each practice.
- Addressing inequalities in health by facilitating improvement in access to primary care services in order to achieve health improvement.

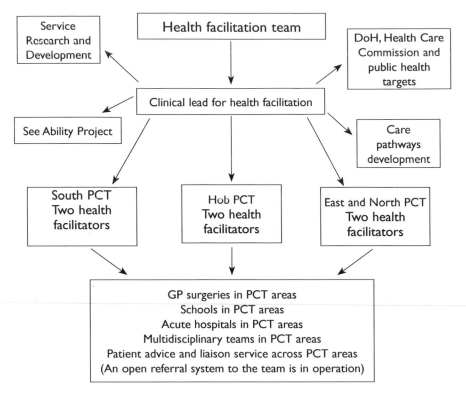

Figure 7.3. Structure of the health facilitation team.

- Improving communication between people with learning disabilities, their carers and healthcare professionals.

Recommendations

The findings of the study need to be disseminated so that they can support the development of future health policy. A model for health facilitation has been provided in this study which can be adapted within other PCT areas. As an advanced nurse practitioner the project facilitator must now seek to influence the national agenda to ensure that strategies across the country target the best health outcomes for people with learning disabilities and ensure that resources are focused on these. The NHS Plan (Department of Health, 2000) promotes the role of nurses in taking a lead in influencing how local services are organised and run. The health facilitator is now in an ideal position to influence commissioners of PCTs and services.

Taking a health facilitation model forward

Now that an effective health facilitation model has been implemented across the city resources have been redirected to this area. This has led to the establishment of a citywide health facilitation team which is line managed by the project facilitator. See *Figure 7.3*.

Role development and advanced nursing practice

Over the last seven years the project facilitator has moved through four role stages as shown in *Figure 7.4*.

The project facilitator's transition from community nurse to advanced nurse practitioner has not only supported the development of more accessible

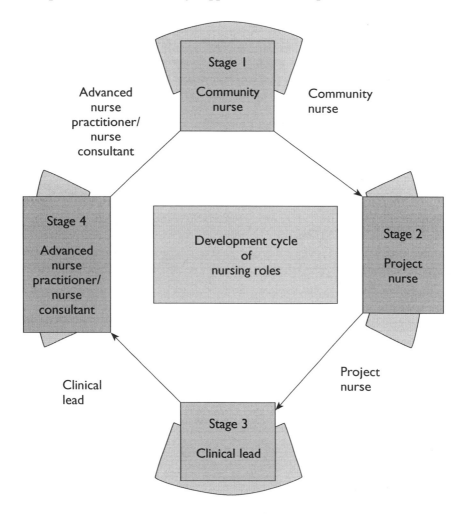

Figure 7.4. Development cycle of nursing roles.

health services for people with learning disabilities but also her own professional development. The introduction of advanced nurse practitioners, nurse consultants and modern matrons into the community continues to show improvements in the delivery of care for service users as intended. This evidence contained within this study further supports this concept.

Wider influence

Influencing policy makers at national level is, according to McGee and Castledine (2003), dependent on advanced practitioners being able to identify the degree of risk to a population of a particular health problem or disease and the factors that contribute to its development. The project facilitator has identified the risks to the target population of people with learning disabilities as a result of various pilot studies. Through collaboration with public health colleagues, primary care and policy makers it has been possible to critically appraise and synthesise the evidence from relevant research and this evaluation study. A picture of the national situation has been provided in this evaluation and despite the small size of the study it is likely to have a significant impact on the development of future national policy relating to meeting the health needs of people with learning disabilities. National and international interest has been generated around the learning disability health screening template since its development. Twenty four PCT areas across the country are using the template and interest has also been shown by the Welsh Centre for Learning Disabilities and the Centre for Research and Development in Australia.

Progress in Birmingham

Work in Birmingham continues. Since the initial pilot there has been an increased uptake of learning disability health checks, health action plans and health promotion opportunities (Brady, 2007):

- Individuals not registered with GPs supported to access GP within local area = 31.
- Patients with learning disability registered on practice lists = 8000+.
- Health checks completed = 1500+.
- Health action plans completed = 472.
- Training and support offered to residential homes to meet Commission for Social Care Inspection requirements = 205.
- Number of people facilitated to have an eye test = 97.
- Number of people facilitated to have eye surgery = 9.
- Number of people facilitated to receive eye treatment = 13.

Department of Health, London

Department of Health (2003) *Building on the Best*. HMSO, London

Department of Health (2006) *Our Health, Our Care, Our Say*. NHS Executive, London

Evans G, Todd S, Beyer S, Felce D, Perry J (1994) Assessing the impact of the All-Wales Mental Handicap Strategy: A survey of four districts. *Journal of Intellectual Disability Research* **38**:109–33

Garrard SD (1983) Community health issues. In: Watson JL, Mulick JA (eds.) *Handbook of Mental Retardation*. Pergamon Press, New York: 289–305

Giraud-Saunders A (2000) Making connections: Learning disability services and primary care groups/trusts. *Managing Community Care* **8:** 30–4

Glasby AM (2002) Meeting the needs of people with learning disabilities in acute care. *British Journal of Nursing* **11**(21): 1389–92

Hilderbrand J (1995) *The Views of General Practitioners in Merton, Sutton and Wandsworth on Primary Care for People with Learning Disabilities*. Dissertation for MSc in Public Health: St.Georges Medical School, London

Howells G (1996) Situations vacant: Doctors required to provide care for people with learning disability. *British Journal of Learning Disability* **Feb 24**: 104–9

Hunt C, Wakefield S, Hunt G (2001) Community nurse for learning disabilities: A case study of the use of an evidence-based screening tool to identify and meet the health needs of people with learning disabilities. *Journal of Learning Disabilities* **5**(1): 9–18

Ineichen B, Russell JAO (1980) *Mental Handicap and Community Care - The Viewpoint of the General Practitioner*. Bristol University, Bristol

Jukes M, Bollard M (2002) Health facilitators in learning disability are important roles. *British Journal of Nursing* **11:** 297

Kerr M (1998) *Innovations in Health Care for People with Intellectual Disabilities*. Lisieux Hall Publications, Lancashire

Kerr M, Dunstan F, Thapar A (1996). Attitudes of general practitioners to people with a learning disability. *British Journal of General Practice* **46:** 2–4

Komaromy C (2001) *Dilemmas in UK Health Care*. Buckingham, Open University Press

Langan J, Russell O, Whitfield M (1993) *Community Care and the General Practitioner: Primary Health Care for People with Learning Disabilities. Report to the Department of Health*. Norah Fry Research Centre, University of Bristol

Lawrie K (1995) Better health care for people with learning disabilities. *Nursing Times* **91**(19): 32–4

Lennox NG, Green M, Diggens J, Ugoni A (2001) Audit and comprehensive health assessment programme in the primary healthcare of adults with intellectual disability: A pilot study. *Journal Intellectual Disability Research* **45**: 226–32

Lennox NG, Kerr MP (1997) Primary health care and people with an intellectual disability: The evidence base. *Journal of Intellectual Disability Research* **41**(5): 365–72

Little P, Everitt H, Williamson I, Warner G, Moore M, Gould C, Ferrier K, Payne S. (2001) Preferences of patients for patient centred approach to consultation in primary care: Observational study. *British Medical Journal* **322**: 468

LoBiondo-Wood G, Haber J (2002) *Nursing Research. Methods, Critical Appraisal and Utilization* (5th edn.) Mosby, St Louis

Martin GHB, Martin DH (1999) *A register for patients with learning disabilities in general practice reveals increasing prevalence and associated needs*. Personal communication

Matthews D (2002) Learning disabilities: The need for better health care. *Nursing Standard* **16**: 40–2

McGee P, Castledine G (2003) *Advanced Nursing Practice*. Wiley, Chichester

Meehan S, Moore G, Barr O (1995) Specialist services for people with learning disabilities. *Nursing Times* **91**(13): 33–5

Minihan PM, Dean DH, Lyons CM (1993) Managing the care of patients with mental retardation: A survey of physicians. *Mental Retardation* **31**: 239–46

NHS Quality Improvement Scotland (2006) Best Practice Statement – February 2006. Promoting access to healthcare for people with a learning disability- A guide for frontline NHS staff. NHS Quality Improvement Scotland, Edinburgh

National Institute for Clinical Excellence (2004) *The Epilepsies and Management of the Epilepsies in Adults and Children in Primary and Secondary Care (CG20)*. guidance.nice.org.uk/CG20

Powrie E (2003) Primary health care provision for adults with a learning disability. *Journal of Advanced Nursing* **42**(4): 413–23

Rodgers J (1993) Primary health care provision for people with learning disabilities. *Health and Social Care* **2:** 11–7

Singh P (1997) *Prescriptions for Change: A Mencap Report on the Role of GPs and Carers in the Provision of Primary Care for People with Learning Disabilities*. Mencap, London

Stein K (2000) Caring for people with a learning disability: A survey of general practitioner's attitudes in Southampton and South-West Hampshire. *British Journal of Learning Disabilities* **28:** 9–15

Thornton C (1997) Meeting the needs of people with learning disabilities. *Nursing Times* **93**(20): 52–4

Weiss CH (1998) *Evaluation: Methods for Studying Programs and Policies* (2nd edn.) Prentice Hall, Upper Saddle River, NJ

CHAPTER 8

Epilepsy and specialist learning disability practice

Fiona Rich and Catherine Doherty

Introduction

The development of the learning disability nurse as an epilepsy specialist practitioner is long and convoluted, largely due to the fact that the role of the learning disability nurse has been in contention for decades. Uncertainty over this role is something that these nurses have encountered frequently: from the emphasis in the 1970s on meeting the social care needs as proposed in the Briggs Report (1972) and the Jay Report (1979) going full circle back to the emphasis in the 1990s on meeting the health needs as proposed in the Department of Health's *Continuing the Commitment Report* (1996)

Alongside this was the UKCC's (now the NMC), Post-Registration Education and Practice (PREP) Project in 1993 which proposed a new post-registration education framework based on three distinct areas of nursing practice: the primary practitioner, the clinical nurse specialist and the advanced nurse practitioner. The learning disability nurse, as a result of these initiatives, is finally able to exercise higher levels of judgement and discretion in clinical care to meet the demands of specialist care as well as providing leadership, teaching and support to others. One particular area in learning disability nursing requiring this area of expertise is in the care of people who have the dual diagnosis of learning disability and epilepsy. The uniqueness of the learning disability nurse in developing this role is the experience and expertise gained through supporting people with learning disabilities who are up to 40 times more likely to have epilepsy than the general population (Department of Health, 2001). It is this uniqueness of the learning disability nurse that prompted the Clinical Standards Advisory Group (1999) report to recommend that those with learning disability nursing experience would be best placed to carry out this role.

This chapter aims to introduce the incidence, severity, patterns and causes of epilepsy and consider the problems and consequences associated with a misdiagnosis of epilepsy in relation to the challenges of the learning disability nurse. It also considers the role of the learning disability nurse as an epilepsy specialist practitioner using a case study to illustrate the domains of the role. Finally, there is a consideration of the impact of the epilepsy specialist practitioner on meeting the needs of individuals with a dual diagnosis of learning disability and epilepsy.

Introduction

According to Sander and Shorvon (2001), epilepsy is the most common serious neurological condition and the Department of Health (2001) suggests a prevalence rate of 1 in 130. Epilepsy is a condition that does not hold any barriers to class, race or gender; however it is often misinterpreted and misunderstood, largely because of the social stigma attached to it. Today, although attitudes have changed somewhat, and despite greater knowledge among the general population, there are still misconceptions and stigmas associated with epilepsy. One of the many challenges of the learning disability nurse is supporting those who have epilepsy in coping with the stigma attached to the condition in every sphere of life.

What is epilepsy?

When we think of seizures, many people tend to think of the classic grand mal seizure with visions of thrashing limbs and frothing at the mouth. There are however, many different types of seizure and not all of them involve convulsions. For example, some seizures involve changes in the level of consciousness or unexpected movements, strange feelings, fluctuating emotions or altered behaviour such as appearing to 'loiter with intent' or stripping off clothes, all of which cause problems with diagnosis when supporting a person who has the dual diagnosis of epilepsy and a learning disability.

Jackson (1873) defined epilepsy as 'an episodic disorder of the nervous system arising from the excessively synchronous and sustained charges of a group of nerve cells'. Over the following 130 years, there was little change in the definition. Epilepsy is now defined as 'the transient clinical manifestations that result from an episode of epileptic neuronal activity' (Shorvon, 2005).

Epilepsy is a characteristic sudden, brief change in the function of the brain cells. In an epileptic seizure, excessive electrical activity builds up causing uncontrolled stimulation of the brain. Excitatory cells fire in rhythmic, uncontrolled bursts which can spread from a localised area of the brain to a generalised area, eventually involving the whole brain. The seizure activity can affect muscle groups, sensations, behaviour, emotions, consciousness, or a combination of these.

Classification of seizures

As Panayiotopoulos (2002) notes, the epilepsies and epilepsy syndromes are now classified under the auspices of the International League Against Epilepsy (ILAE). In 1981, the ILAE divided seizures into two categories and then re-defined them in 1989 (Panayiotopoulos, 2002). The two categories are partial (or focal) seizures, affecting only a part of the brain where the seizure activity starts and remains, and generalised seizures affecting the whole or most of the brain.

Table 8.1 summarises the seizure types found in these categories; however there are numerous texts and websites which explore these in more detail (for example, see Shorvon, 2005; the Joint Epilepsy Council website, http://www.jointepilepsycouncil.org.uk/; the National Society for Epilepsy website, http://www.epilepsynse.org.uk; or the Epilepsy Action website, http://www.epilepsy.org.uk/).

Unclassifiable seizures

Despite the fact that the clinical features of seizures can lead to a classification, no two individuals have exactly the same seizures – each person is unique and may present with very idiosyncratic seizures. For example, for some individuals their seizures may be shorter in duration than

Table 8.1. Seizure types

Partial or focal	Only part of the brain affected by seizure activity
Simple	Seizure activity with no loss of consciousness
Complex	Seizure activity with impairment of consciouness
With secondary generalisation	Seizure activity begins as a partial seizure and spreads to involve the whole of the brain
Generalised	The whole of the brain is affected by seizure activity and there is loss of consciousness
Tonic–clonic	The body stiffens, the person falls followed by involuntary jerking
Tonic	Sudden increase in muscle tone and the person falls backwards like a board
Atonic	Sudden loss of muscle tone and the person falls like a puppet wih its strings cut
Absence	Abrupt, fleeting moment of loss of consciousness

typically found or a tonic-clonic seizure may appear more like a tonic or atonic seizure. Electroencephalograph (EEG) patterns can help to support the diagnosis of the seizure type. Nevertheless, according to Shorvon (2005), up to one-third of seizures are considered unclassifiable using the current ILAE system, taking forms that do not conform to typical clinical features and EEG patterns.

Diagnostic techniques

The invention of the EEG, to measure minute electrical discharges within the brain, was the impetus to advances with regards to diagnostic measures including neuro-imaging and neuro-physiology techniques. *Table 8.2* illustrates techniques used to assess and identify lesions within the brain. EEGs proved to be the initial breakthrough in measuring brain function and an individual's seizure activity. As well as aiding diagnosis, current use of EEG has enabled specific epilepsy syndromes to be identified due to the EEG manifestations (Panayiotopoulas, 2002).

EEG readings have aided the diagnosis of non-convulsive status, a manifestation in the past that has been misdiagnosed by some as behavioural difficulties, particularly in the field of learning disabilities. This may result in individuals being treated with drugs such as chlorpromazine, a phenothiazine which has a sedating effect and is used for difficult behaviour, but can cause EEG changes and convulsions (Shorvon, 2000). The strategy of prescribing individuals with drugs for problem behaviour when in fact they are experiencing seizures would obviously make the apparent problem behaviour worse. The difficulties lie in distinguishing what is true challenging behaviour and what is non-convulsive status, as this type of non-convulsive status does not resemble 'typical seizures', i.e. there is no thrashing of the limbs or frothing at the mouth, etc. Communication problems in people with learning disabilities may make diagnosing this type of seizure more difficult as they may be unable to describe what is happening to them

However, the EEG still continues to offer support in the diagnosis of epilepsy where clinical recordings or descriptions of the seizure can be sketchy. Nevertheless, the standardised 10:20 electrode positions on the scalp are not able to give the advanced readings now obtainable through magnetoecephalography (MEG). This is supported by the work of Lewine et al (1999) who demonstrated linkage between children with Landau-Kleffner syndrome (LKS) and autism spectrum conditions (ASC) and epileptiform activity. The results indicated that 'MEG showed significantly greater sensitivity to this epileptiform activity than simultaneous EEG'. Due to evolving technological advances clinical practice is constantly taking on new dimensions, as for example the use of MEG, which enables brain

Table 8.2. Investigations to aid diagnosis of epilepsy: Neurophysiological and neuro-imaging techniques

Technique	Function	Diagnosis	Date utilised
Electroencephalogram (EEG)	Evaluates the paroxysmal discharges of cerebral neurones causing seizures	Can support diagnosis of epilepsy	1929
Ambulatory EEG	Helpful where clinical information inadequate		
Video-telemetry and EEG	Aided by visual images during EEG recording		
Magnetoencephalography (MEG)	Non-invasive neurophysiological technique, measures magnetic fields generated by neuronal activity in the brain	Direct measurement of brain function Diagnostic brain function	1994 First used in epilepsy surgery (4-D neuro-imaging 2004)
Magnetic resonance imaging (MRI)	Identification of small lesions and abnormalities of the cerebral cortex Defines structural abnormalities that underlie seizure disorders	Diagnosis of epilepsy Aids surgical planning Functional measure	1997
Computed tomography (CT)	Less sensitive than MRI, results can be masked by bone artefact. Useful in detection of cortical calcifications	Can support and aid diagnosis Cannot be relied on	1973
Positron emission tomography (PET)	Assesses cerebral metabolism. Used only when data are not good between MRI, EEG. Would utilise fluorodeoxyglucose (FDU) PET for temporal lobe epilepsy	Functional measure inadequate for assessment of brain structure	1970s
Single photon emission computed tomography (SPECT)	Useful scan for ictal or early post-ictal examination when compared with an inter-ictal scan	Functional measure Inadequate for assessment of brain structure	1970s

function to be measured within millimetre precision. The readings can then be superimposed onto a magnetic resonance imaging (MRI) illustration of the individual's brain, giving the clinician/surgeon details of the structure and function of the brain (FourD/Neuro-imaging, 2004). With this calculated information, neurosurgery for the individual with a diagnosis of learning disability and partial (focal) seizures should be more readily available. In the past this client group, even if they met the clinical criteria for brain surgery, were frequently denied this opportunity and management option as the verbal and intellectual skills of the individual would not be sustainable to undertake the psychological assessment required for neurosurgery. Although psychological assessment is still a prerequisite for neurosurgery, people with this diagnosis may benefit from the technological advances that MEG and MRI can offer.

Koppel (2002) notes that seizures are always a symptom of brain dysfunction, and advises that although a single seizure may not be epilepsy, it may indicate a susceptibility to seizures or a low seizure threshold and, as such, an accurate diagnosis is critical.

The signs and symptoms for an individual's diagnosis and aetiology must be carefully examined so as to ensure misdiagnosis does not occur. The lay person presenting such signs and symptoms and other critical information to a neurologist or health professional must recall information accurately as this could have life saving implications for the individual if, for example, the epilepsy is related to a tumour or other underlying condition or disease.

Incidence and prevalence of epilepsy

A change of basic physiology for any reason may invoke a seizure and about one in 20 people will have a major seizure at some time in their lives. Reuber et al (2002) state that 20% of people have minor, irrelevant EEG abnormalities which are frequently misinterpreted as confirming a diagnosis of epilepsy. However a single seizure does not indicate that a person has epilepsy and the person may need to undergo medical investigations to discover the cause. Causes for a one-off seizure could include binge drinking, alcohol withdrawal, hyper-pyrexia, chronic stress or recreational drugs to name but a few.

Shorvon (2005) suggests that the incidence of epilepsy is approximately 80 new cases per 100000 persons per year, but depending on the source examined, this varies between 50 and 120 per year. The cumulative incidence of epilepsy, i.e. the risk of an individual developing epilepsy in his or her lifetime, is between 3% and 5%. The highest rates of epilepsy occur in neonates and young children (congenital and genetic conditions being the most common cause). In older children and young adults, inherited predisposition, hippocampal sclerosis, alcohol or drug abuse and trauma are known causes. In the elderly, there is a second peak of prevalence with vascular disease being a common cause. (Taylor, 1996; Shorvon, 2000)

Shorvon (2005) however notes that more recently, the rate of epilepsy in children seems to be falling and the rate in the elderly is rising. The suggestion is that this is due to better public health and perinatal care in respect of children and higher incidence of degenerative cerebrovascular disease and demographic changes in respect of older adults.

Epilepsy is however more common in developing countries, largely as a result of the poorer standards of nutrition (Hackett and Iype, 2001), the prevalence of infectious diseases and the higher proportion of children in a population. Most, but not all, studies found slightly more males than females have epilepsy.

Epilepsy is also much more prevalent in the learning disabled population – 30% of people with learning disabilities will have epilepsy compared with 0.7% of the general population. The greater the severity of the learning disability however, the more likely the person is to have epilepsy (National Society for Epilepsy, 2006a). In people with profound, multiple learning disabilities, the incidence is 1 in 50 and for those with severe learning disability it is 1 in 30 (Webb et al, 1991).

In addition, approximately 50% of people with autistic spectrum conditions have abnormal EEGs. The National Society for Epilepsy (2006b) suggests that epilepsy occurs in between 25 and 35% of people with autistic spectrum conditions. It should be pointed out though that people with autistic spectrum conditions do not necessarily have a learning disability.

Severity of epilepsy

According to Shorvon (2005), of those who have active epilepsy, i.e. those who have had at least one seizure in the preceding 2–5 years and are not in remission, only 5–10% have more than one seizure a week and require intensive regular medical attention. Sander and Shorvon (2001) estimate that in the UK there are about 160000 people with epilepsy who require continuing hospital-based medical treatment. However, over 60% of people have between one seizure a month and one a year: the majority of people who have a current diagnosis of epilepsy therefore have well-controlled epilepsy (Shorvon, 2005).

Causes of epilepsy

There are numerous causes of epilepsy, and it is human nature to search for reasons for someone's epilepsy. When making a diagnosis, the terms idiopathic, cryptogenic or symptomatic may be used. This provides us with an indication as to the cause of the epilepsy.

- Idiopathic: meaning that the epilepsy is part of a genetic syndrome (such as benign childhood epilepsy). In this case, the epilepsy is not precipitated by an underlying condition such as a tumour.
- Cryptogenic: meaning that the cause is unknown (consider the analogy of the cause being hidden in a crypt). However, Shorvon (2005) notes that as technology advances and more sophisticated neuro-imaging techniques become available, the number of cases in this category is reducing.
- Symptomatic: meaning that a cause can be identified for the seizures, e.g. as a result of a tumour or vascular disease.

Table 8.3 illustrates the wide range of causes of epilepsy.

Seizure patterns

Some people with epilepsy develop a regular pattern of seizures. When this is recognised it can help in everyday life, because the seizures are no longer unpredictable. The more common patterns are during sleep, on waking or whilst going to sleep.

It is common for seizures to occur during these times as, when people pass through the normal stages of wakefulness to drowsiness to sleep, there is a change in the electrical activity of the brain. It is thought that these changes may allow uncontrolled electrical discharges. Most people have experienced electrical changes within the brain when drifting off to sleep and are then unexpectedly disturbed by a sudden bodily jerk. This is referred to as 'motor sleep start' (Betts, 1998) and, although not epilepsy, occurs because of changing electrical activity in the brain.

Other patterns of seizure activity occur during the menstrual cycle, such as catamenial epilepsy (Duncan et al, 2004). Catamenial epilepsy is the term used for epilepsy that is triggered by hormonal changes of the menstrual cycle. Progesterone (the hormone that occurs in the last two weeks of the menstrual cycle) has some protective effects against seizures. Prior to the onset of the woman's period, progesterone levels drop and the protective effect is lost. Equally, oestrogen is known to be mildly epileptogenic and therefore without the protective effect of progesterone, seizures may occur in the first few days of the menstrual period. In addition, as oestrogen is at its highest level at the point of ovulation, many women have seizures at this time in their cycle.

Menopausal women also have a reduction in progesterone, therefore

Table 8.3. Causes of epilepsy

Cause	Condition	Risk of epilepsy	Reference
Prenatal disorder of brain development	Lissencephaly	High	
	Tuberous sclerosis	High	Soryal (2005)
	Sturge-Weber Syndrome	High	
	Polymicrogyria	High	
	Schizencephaly	High	Sisodiya (2004, 267)
	Porencephalic cysts	High	
Vascular occlusion			Soryal (2005)
In-utero infection	Rubella	High	
	Toxoplasmosis Æ	High	
	Hydrocephalus	High	
Drug ingestion			
Metabolic errors	Pyridoxine dependent	High	
	Amino acid	No increased	Beghi (2004, 55)
	Endocrine	risk	Beghi (2004, 55)
Intrapartum obstetric complications	Pre-eclampsia/eclampsia	Slight increase	Beghi (2004, 59)
	Intracranial haemorrhage	High	
	Birth trauma	High	
	Anaesthetic intoxication	High	Soryal (2005)
Post-natal metabolic causes	Hypoglycaemia	High	
	Hypocalcaemia	High	
	Hypomagnesaemia	High	
	Infantile seizures	High	Beghi (2004, 59)
	Febrile convulsion	High	Dodson (2004, 16)
	Angelman's syndrome	High	
Syndromes	Prader-Willi syndrome	Slight increase	Beghi (2004, 55)
Gene disorders	Fragile X syndrome	High	
Chromosome disorders	Trisomy 13 syndrome	High	
	Trisomy 21 syndrome	Slight increase	Beghi (2004, 55)
Neurocutaneous disorders	Neurofibromatosis type 1	Slight increase	
	Neurofibromatosis type 2	No increase	Beghi (2004, 55)
Central nervous system	Location in brain	High	
	Centrotemporoparietal region	High	
Brain tumours	Cortical tumour	Low	Beghi (2004, 62)
	Non-cortical tumour	High	
	Meningioma	No risk	
	Astrocytoma	High	
	Glioma	Increase	
	Intracranial metastasis	High	
Head trauma	Missile wounds	High	
Penetrating injury	Brain contusion	Slight increase	
	Subdural haematoma	Slight increase	Beghi (2004, 61)
	Linear fracture	High	
	Depressed fracture	High	

Table 8.3 continues/

Table 8.3 cont/

Cause	Condition	Risk of epilepsy	Reference
Infections	Encephalitis	High	
	Bacterial meningitis	High	
	Aseptic meningitis	Slight increase	
Brain abscess	Supratentorial lesion	High	
Infectious agents	Herpes simplex virus I	High	
Viruses	Cytomegalovirus	Slight increase	
	Epstein-Barr virus	Low	
	HIV	High	
	Arboviruses	High	Goldstein &
	CJD	Low	Harden (2002,
	Syphilis	Slight increase	102, 111, 113)
Cerebrovascular disease			
Ischaemia	Transient ischaemic attack	Slight increase	
	CVA/stroke	High	
Arteriovenous	Subarachnoid haemorrhage	High	Bromfield and
Malformations	Aneurysm	High	Henderson
			(2002, 269, 276)
Other	Eclampsia	Symptomatic seizures high Slight increase for long-term epilepsy	
	Hypertension	Slight increase	Beghi (2004, 61)
Degenerative	Alzheimer	High	
disease	Multi-infarct dementia	High	
Dementia			Beghi (2004, 61)
Demyelination	Multiple sclerosis	Low	
Inheritance	Mendelian inheritance simple complex inheritance	Unknown	
Unknown	60% of population have unknown cause of epilepsy	Unknown	
Systemic causes 'Seizures are manifestation of the underlying disease process and not of epilepsy'	Metabolic		
	Hypoglycaemia	Increase	
	Hypoatraemia	Increase	
	Hypocalcaemia	Increase	
	Hyperosmolar	Increase	
	Hyperthyroidism	Increase	
	Thyrotoxicosis	Increase	Rowan (2002, 434)
	Porphyria	Increase	

Table 8.3 continues/

Table 8.3 cont/

Cause	Condition	Risk of epilepsy	Reference
Toxic cause	Withdrawal of:		
Drugs	Benzodiazepines (sudden)	High	
	Barbiturates (sudden)	High	
	Opiates	Slight increase	
	Sedatives/hypnotics	Increase depends on drug	
	Theophylline	High	
	Overdose of:		
	Cyclic antidepressants	High	
	Opoid analgesics	Slight increase	
	B Blocker	Low	
	Increase risk if prescribed: antipsychotic drugs:		
	Aliphatic phenothiazines	High	
	Piperazine phenothiazines	Slight increase	
	Antidepressants:		
	Clomipramine	High	
	SSRIs	Low	
	(This list is not exhaustive)		
Alcohol	Alcoholism (chronic)	High	
	Alcohol abstinence syndrome	Slight increase	Beghi (2004, 54)
Carbon monoxide	Carboxyhaemoglobin Levels over 50%	Increased risk	
Solvents	Organic solvent exposure	Increased risk	
Heavy metals	Exposure to lead, mercury, tin	Unknown	

women who previously had 'cluster seizures' around the time of their period may find seizures are less predictable and occur at any time of the month because of the reduction in progesterone.

The challenge to the learning disability nurse is to accurately record or support the person with a learning disability in identifying any patterns of seizures which may indicate catamenial epilepsy or sleep-related seizures.

Precipitating factors

Some individuals with epilepsy often have firm ideas about factors that precipitate seizures and there are a number of factors which are said to trigger them. One of the most common triggers is thought to be emotional stress. Although stress is difficult to define or pin down, it is commonly thought to provoke seizures in many individuals. It is unclear however whether stress results as a primary or secondary cause of epilepsy: people who are in stressful situations may well have poor sleeping patterns, may drink more alcohol to relax and generally have poorer health which may lower the seizure threshold and make a seizure more likely to happen. We would refer to this as a secondary cause of epilepsy. Stress as a primary cause is where the actual stress itself causes the seizures.

In the UK, research by Betts (1996) has suggested that aromatherapy can help to control epilepsy in some individuals by reducing stress. The use of various oils, such as ylang ylang, camomile and lavender appear to act on parts of the brain and help relaxation. However, some oils can trigger seizures, therefore should be avoided by people with epilepsy. These include rosemary, sage, hyssop, fennel, and wormwood, although when used in food and drinks they are perfectly safe, with the exception of wormwood which should be avoided (Epilepsy Action, 2006)

Sleep deprivation and fatigue is another common trigger of epilepsy and a few people only have seizures following sleep deprivation. Young adults with idiopathic epilepsy are more prone to having seizures triggered by sleep deprivation (Shorvon, 2005)

Excitement, whether emotional or sexual, leads to the brain becoming more active and may lead to excessive electrical discharge, triggering a seizure. Pain, as with excitement, can increase electrical activity within the brain and may also trigger a seizure. Conversely low levels of activity and boredom can sometimes trigger seizures. This is particularly relevant for people with profound and multiple learning disabilities, where stimulating activities that they are cognitively able to participate in are limited. The challenge for the learning disability nurse is to ensure that activities for all levels of ability are available and that peaks and troughs of engagement levels are avoided.

Another common trigger is thought to be constipation and although there is a paucity of literature on the subject, there is a great deal of anecdotal evidence. It is believed that there are direct sensory pathways from the bowel to the brain via the vagus nerve and that abdominal pressure from the colon as a result of chronic constipation is transferred to the brain resulting in seizure discharges (Meridian Institute, 1999). A combination of a history of over-use of laxatives in institutional care and the side effect of constipation in many of the drugs used in caring for people with learning disabilities means that the learning disability nurse must be vigilant in monitoring for signs of constipation, especially in the case of older adults with learning disabilities and those with profound, multiple learning disabilities who are more likely to have sluggish peristaltic movement of the bowel.

Alcohol can make anti-epileptic drugs (AEDs) less effective and cause seizures if too much is drunk at one time. Seizures are also known to increase by 20 times in people consuming large quantities of alcohol. Research suggests that drinking more than two units of alcohol increases the risk of seizures in people with epilepsy. Seizures are also common in the 24 hours after alcohol withdrawal.

Hypoglycaemia from missed meals is also a common trigger of epilepsy and those with epilepsy are advised to maintain healthy low fat, high fibre diets; 'crash dieting' is not advised. Hackett and Iype (2001) suggest that malnutrition leads to a low dietary intake of the amino acids from protein which affects levels of inhibitory amino acid neurotransmitters (which 'switch off' electrical discharges). Vegetarians and more especially vegans therefore need to ensure they maintain adequate protein levels from other sources such as nuts, grains and pulses. People who have learning and physical disabilities and associated feeding difficulties may require additional protein supplements in order to maintain an adequate intake of protein.

If triggers of epilepsy can be identified, then they can be avoided as far as possible. This means that seizures will be less unpredictable and the person will be more in control of his or her life.

Non-epileptic attack disorder (NEAD)

Various studies have estimated the misdiagnosis rate of epilepsy to be very high and, alarmingly, between 20% and 45% of people who have been diagnosed with epilepsy do not have the condition. More worryingly, between 10% and 30% of patients referred to a specialist epilepsy centre by their GP do not have epilepsy. The National Institute of Clinical Excellence (2004a) indicate a misdiagnosis of up to 31%. These people may have been treated as having epilepsy for years by their GP, and may have been prescribed numerous drugs needlessly.

According to Taylor (1996) the major difficulty lies in distinguishing epilepsy from other causes of disturbed consciousness or 'black-outs'. Betts (1998) suggests that epilepsy is frequently over-diagnosed because the initial diagnosis is often made by primary care doctors whose knowledge of the wide differential diagnosis of the disorders is insufficient.

It is very important to rule out any other form of 'black-out' before deciding that the person has epilepsy. As learning disability nurses can be involved in witnessing seizures or reporting seizures, it is important to have an awareness of conditions that can be mistaken for epilepsy. If a person is misdiagnosed with epilepsy, then there will be a neglect of the real cause of the 'black-out' and the incorrect treatment will be given. It is critical that a correct diagnosis is made, not only to reassure individuals and their families but to ensure the appropriate treatment is initiated to manage a condition that causes 1000 known deaths per year, 500 of which are classified as sudden unexpected death in epilepsy (SUDEP) (Hanna et al, 2002). The incidence of mortality for those with convulsive seizures is two to four times greater than that of the general population (Taylor, 1996; Sander, 2001).

In addition, many people with NEAD are receiving expensive treatments for seemingly intractable epilepsy which in times of massive overspending within NHS Trusts should be avoided.

Conditions that may be mistaken for epilepsy

There are a number of conditions that may be mistaken for epilepsy including syncope, transient ischaemic attack, migraine, hyperventilation, narcolepsy and cataplexy. These are summarised in *Table 8.4*.

In order to diagnose NEAD, true epilepsy must first be ruled out. The diagnosis of epilepsy depends on the clinical description, supported by investigative procedures. Unfortunately everything that happens in epilepsy can also be a feature of non-epileptic attacks and vice versa, making diagnosis extremely difficult. As we know, a diagnosis of epilepsy is supported by investigations such as EEGs which record abnormal electrical discharges. If the clinical description points to a specific seizure type and an EEG is found to be abnormal, then epilepsy cannot be ruled out.

Definition of NEAD

NEAD is described as recurring paroxysmal episodes that resemble epileptic attacks but lack characteristic clinical and electrographic features. When diagnosing NEAD, there needs to be evidence of sudden, recurring attacks (paroxysmal episodes) which may look like epilepsy but which do not have any clinical or electrographic features. In other words the person may have a normal EEG and the witness accounts may differ from specific seizure types (Betts, 2003).

According to Shorvon (2000) NEAD broadly speaking falls into two main categories.

- Attacks of motionless collapse: These attacks are often prolonged, continuing for minutes or even hours. This may also occur in true epilepsy, but it is very rare. Often the person is able to demonstrate partial awareness in NEAD, e.g. resistance to eye opening. Tone is usually flaccid and attacks are sometimes triggered by external events
- Attacks with motor phenomena: These also differ from epileptic seizures in that they often have a slow build-up. There are periods of motor activity but this is not constant. There may be resistance to eye opening and signs of volition or semi-purposeful movement on

Table 8.4. Conditions that may be mistaken for epilepsy

Condition	Description	Rationale for mistaken diagnosis
Syncope: Vasovagal or provoked cardiac	Caused by pain, emotion, hot surroundings, prolonged standing or may be post-traumatic Ischaemic heart disease or cardiac arrhythmia leading to fainting	Syncopal episodes can look very neurological and can occur when individuals are sitting or even lying, particularly in the elderly. Tonic spasms, twitching and incontinence can all occur as part of syncope
Postural Vascular Respiratory	Caused by alcohol and drugs, old age, diabetes Caused by embolism or thrombosis Resulting from coughing	
Transient ischaemic	A brief transient stroke lasting only a few minutes	Symptoms include numbness or weakness in the face, arm or leg, visual problems, dizziness, loss of balance and coordination, shaking and involuntary movements which may mimic symptoms of epilepsy
Migraine	Often accompanied by flashing lights	May be mistaken for complex partial epilepsy or a prodromal symptom
Psychiatric conditions	Panic attacks and night terrors	Features of panic attacks include twitching of peripheries and blurred vision which may be mistaken for partial temporal lobe epilepsy
Hyperventilation	Classical history of rising panic, feeling that not enough air can get into the lungs	Symptoms usually accompanied by peripheral tingling, dizziness, weakness, fatigue, and loss of consciousness. Additionally severe hyperventilation can be accompanied by apparent foaming of the mouth all of which may be mistaken for epilepsy

Table 8.4 continues/

257

Table 8. 4 Contl

Condition	Description	Rationale for mistaken diagnosis
Fictitious disorder	Individuals who simulate seizures	May superficially resemble epilepsy
Narcolepsy	Episodes of suddenly falling asleep	May superficially resemble epilepsy
Cataplexy	Sudden loss of postural tone precipitated by strong emotions such as anger	May superficially resemble epilepsy
Paroxysmal dystonias	Sudden loss of tone or sudden movements such as athetoid movements in those with cerebral palsy	May superficially resemble epilepsy

examination, and urinary incontinence, although uncommon, may occur, as can self-injury.

The incidence of NEAD is 100 000 persons per year. According to Betts (2003), up to 20% of people with a confident diagnosis of epilepsy turn out later to have some other disorder which has been misdiagnosed, and nearly 50% of patients admitted to casualty in 'status epilepticus' turn out not to have epilepsy. NEAD is also common in people who have a learning disability – unfortunately, this client group, who are most in need of accurate investigation and assessment are least likely to receive it.

In cases of NEAD, there is often an association with epilepsy; the person may actually have true epilepsy. There may also be a history of neurological or physical disease, however, this is often found in true epilepsy as well. The condition is much more common in females than males, and usually commences in adolescence or early adulthood, before the age of 40. A history of childhood abuse is common

In cases of NEAD, there is an associated occurrence with genuine past or current epilepsy – the individual may have both epileptic and non-epileptic attacks, but usually one type predominates. In those who present with NEAD, there are often problems in diagnosis; there may be difficulty in getting a true diagnosis of epilepsy as there will be problems in identifying specific true seizure types.

Compared to people with epilepsy, people with NEAD are more likely to have family histories of psychiatric disorder; the parents may have had psychiatric treatment which should be examined. They themselves are more likely to have past personal history of psychiatric disorder and to have attempted suicide. Eighty five per cent of individuals with NEAD also have current affective syndromes (affecting mental health). Paroxysmal changes in feeling or internal awareness resembling those of epilepsy are commonly found in people who are stressed, highly aroused, anxious or depressed, e.g. déja vu, derealisation, depersonalisation, or changes in the perception of taste or smell, which can be mistaken for temporal lobe epilepsy. Conversely, people with complex partial status may present with behaviours over a prolonged period of time which closely mimic the symptoms of mental illness (Betts, 1998).

In addition, compared to people with epilepsy, people with NEAD are more likely to have a current diagnosis of post-traumatic stress disorder, family and marital problems, conversion reactions (where feelings of fear/trauma are converted into physical symptoms), hysterical personality and disassociative disorders (disruption in the integrated function of consciousness, memory and perception). These are traditionally associated with NEAD and it is likely that previous sexual abuse is a cause.

What presents may not always be epilepsy but what would be termed as a differential diagnosis. Diagnosis should never be hurried and should never be an unconsidered reaction to one particular feature of the seizure. The diagnosis depends on rational consideration of a full medical, neurological and psychiatric history and examination and there should be a careful appraisal of the seizure history.

As already stated, in order to diagnose NEAD, epilepsy itself must be excluded as the cause of the 'blackouts'. Investigation must establish whether there is evidence of:

- Anticonvulsants being ineffective. If there has been little or no change in the number of episodes despite high doses of anticonvulsants, this might lead to the belief that something other than epilepsy is the cause.
- Descriptions of ictal behaviour being inconsistent with that of epilepsy. Eye-witness reports are vital for this to happen. If the descriptions do not indicate a seizure type, the 'blackout' may be something else. However, the seizures may well be true epilepsy, but idiosyncratic.
- Normal EEGs during and after seizures. There is a possibility of a normal EEG during seizures if the activity occurs deep within the brain. However a normal EEG might lead to the belief that this is something other than epilepsy. If epilepsy is still suspected, there may be a call for more invasive EEGs such as MEG or the use of sphenoidal electrodes (electrodes, which are fine wires inserted under the cheekbone).
- Video-EEG telemetry yielding normal EEG recordings during the clinical episode. If the videotape shows an episode but it is not recording on the EEG, this might indicate something other than epilepsy.
- A rise in serum prolactin levels immediately after a person has a seizure. However, if the test is taken 20 minutes after the seizure or following a second seizure, the prolactin levels will return to normal. In people who have NEAD, there will be no rise in the prolactin levels. There needs to have been a baseline recording of prolactin levels in order to identify any raise following a seizure.

Table 8.5 summarises the differences between NEAD and true epilepsy.

In assessing people with newly presenting seizures and those whose intractable epilepsy is being reviewed, the possibility that it is not epilepsy should always be considered. The consequences of not diagnosing NEAD include the inappropriate use of anti-epileptic drugs with their associated risks of toxicity and polypharmacy, and use of other hazardous and inappropriate

Table 8.5. Differences between NEAD and true epilepsy

Feature	NEAD	Epilepsy
Precipitated by trauma	Many	Some
Onset	May be gradual	Sudden
Duration	Many minutes	Seconds or minutes[1]
Retained consciousness	Common	Rare
Clonic movements	Out of phase	In phase[2]
Side-to-side movement/pelvic thrusting	Present	Absent
Cyanosis	Unusual	Common
Weeping	Present	Absent
Tongue biting and other injuries	Less common[3]	Common
Post-ictal drowsiness and confusion	Often absent	Usual

[1] True epilepsy tends to be stereotyped and brief, while non-epileptic attacks are prolonged, relatively non-stereotyped (although they can look stereotyped) and behaviour may be modified by the observer.

[2] Conversely, frontal lobe epilepsy is often accompanied by bizarre movements such as bicycling movements of the legs therefore can be mistaken for non-epileptic episodes.

[3] Usually only the tip of the tongue.

interventions, e.g. surgery, etc. There are additional consequences related to the demands on health and social services by spending time and resources in trying to reach a diagnosis or treating an incorrect diagnosis. Finally, there is the consequence of neglecting the psychological disorder or underlying behaviour or encouraging secondary gain if the behaviour is aimed at achieving input from health professionals.

Once epilepsy has been excluded, investigations need to take place in order to diagnose NEAD. This will include a complete medical and psychosocial history including investigation of any history of child abuse, family psychiatric conditions, previous/current psychiatric conditions or post-traumatic stress disorder. A behavioural analysis will help to look for unintentional or intentional reinforcement of the behaviour during each episode. Investigations should also include consideration of the circumstances of the first episode and any association with epilepsy, whether experienced personally or by witnessing another's seizures.

Betts (1998) notes that if a diagnosis of NEAD has been made, it is important to prepare the individual for the change in diagnosis. It is possible that the individual is reliant on these episodes to convey some meaningful message and therefore should have a full mental health assessment. The episodes should be ignored to avoid rewarding the behaviour – this may result in an initial increase in frequency, but it will reduce eventually. Praise and positive reinforcement should be given to episode-free periods and medication should be slowly withdrawn or, if the non-epileptic episodes are combined with epilepsy, medication review, with a view to monotherapy. The individual's dignity and self-respect must be maintained or the episodes will continue. The whole family should be involved in counselling to prevent reinforcement of seizures. This is also particularly important if abuse counselling is needed.

If there is no evidence of epilepsy, ensure the diagnosis of NEAD is correct and treat the underlying cause so that there is no neglect of any underlying psychological disorder. As Betts (1998) states: 'It is possible to be 100% certain that a seizure is an epileptic one; it is rarely possible to be completely sure that it is not'.

Treatment of epilepsy

The last century has witnessed a revolution in relation to the development of anti-epileptic drug treatments. Leach and Mohanraj (2004) identify anti-epileptic drugs (AED) since the launch of phenobarbitone in 1912, classifying their modes of action (*Table 8.6*). Understanding this information will enable a greater chance for the individual to be rendered seizure free. However it has to be noted there is no conclusive evidence that newer drugs are more efficacious than older drugs (National Institute for Clinical Excellence, 2004b: 12). However it should be noted the evidence and publication of the SANAD study (SANAD Study Group 2007), has prompted NICE to review the pharmacological management of the epilepsies in adults and children in primary and secondary care. The update relating to pharmacological management of the epilepsies is due to be published in 2010.

Crawford (1996) advises that 60–70% of people will become seizure free on monotherapy (i.e. a single anti-epileptic drug). For the remaining 30–40% of the population, seizure freedom does not exist (Sander, 1993).

Monotherapy is always the first choice of drug therapy for an individual; if the first drug is unsuccessful, other drug therapies should be attempted sequentially. Monotherapy which is the preferred management plan and recommended by the National Institute for Clinical Excellence (2004a, b) does not always prevail, thus the rationale for polytherapy must then be considered. The practice of polytherapy may support an individual to become seizure free or at least result in a reduction in their seizure activity and/or severity.

The advantages and disadvantages of polytherapy need to be discussed in order for a physician and an individual to decide if polytherapy has a place in that individual's life. Addressing the issues of anti-epileptic drugs and the use of polytherapy, the medical fraternity and in particular the prescribing doctor or nurse, must consider all the advantages and disadvantages of this practice. The prescribing of polytherapy does not always mean success and a seizure-free life for the individual. The treatment regime must be specific for the individual, taking into account numerous variables. The following issues will influence the practitioner's clinical decision.

Epilepsy issues

- Seizure type
- Epilepsy syndrome
- Co-morbidity
- Co-medication.

Table 8.6. Molecular targets of AEDs and year launched/UK licence

Drug	Sodium channels	Calcium channels	GABA system	Glutamate receptors	Year
Predominant ion channel activity					
Phenytoin	√				1938
Carbamazepine	√				1965
Oxcarbazepine	√				2000
Lamotrigine	√	√			1991
Zonisamide	√	√			2005
Rufinamide	√				2007
Lacosamide	√				2008
Mixed actions or uncertain mechanisms					
Valproate	√	√	√		1973
Topiramate	√	√	√	√	1995
Ethosuximide	√	√			1955
Gabapentin		√	√		1993
Levetiracetam		√			2000
Phenobarbital		√	√	√	1912
Pregabalin		√	?		2004
Felbamate	√	√	√	√	1993
GABA-mediated mechanisms					
Benzodiazepines			√		1960's
Vigabatrin			√		1989
Tiagabine			√		1998

(Adapted from Leach and Mohanraj 2004). GABA = gamma-aminobutyric acid

Drug-related issues

- Pharmacodynamics
- Pharmacokinetics
- Tolerability
- Efficacy
- First line drugs monotherapy
- Second line drugs polytherapy
- Drug serum levels
- Side effects.

Lifestyle Issues

- Age
- Quality of life including:
  - Driving
  - Sexual health
  - Gender issues including pregnancy and childbearing
  - Mental health
  - Social isolation
  - Stigma
  - Concordance
  - Compliance
  - Employment/unemployment
  - Education
  - Dependence
  - Morbidity
  - Mortality.

For those labelled with 'drug resistant', 'therapy resistant' or 'refractory' epilepsy, the question should be asked: is polytherapy the answer? To render individuals seizure-free on polytherapy but disabling them and reducing their quality of life would not be viewed as a positive outcome. Using a polytherapy drug regime will require a greater commitment by the clinician to reduce side effects, ensure efficacy, reduce interactions and combine desirable drugs of choice (all of which could be difficult to manage). However, this could have a positive outcome for the individual including reduced seizure activity or severity of seizures and a reduction in morbidity.

The treatment and management of epilepsy will only be further improved for the individual if medical professionals not only collaboratively support the individual but also are pioneering in their clinical decisions, assessing the risk of drug treatments and lifestyle issues. The development of novel treatment plans and pathways arc required in order to impact positively on the individual thereby improving quality of life, reducing morbidity and mortality risks for the individual. Treatment plans do not solely relate to drugs but also to surgery, vagal nerve stimulation, complementary therapy and other therapies such as neuromodulation therapy as described by Cuellar-Herara et al (2004).

Epilepsy and learning disability

Besag (2004) identified that a dual diagnosis of epilepsy and learning disability and/or psychiatry require careful consideration. Thus management of this group of people at times needs to be multidisciplinary in nature. Kerr (2005: 416) reports a community prevalence rate of epilepsy of 32.2% for people with a learning disability and psychiatric and emotional disturbance which can affect diagnosis, assessment and treatment. Not only are people with epilepsy predisposed to psychiatric symptoms, many people with epilepsy present with behavioural or emotional difficulties. This is also reported by Piazzini and Canger (2001), Kaye et al (2000) and Devinsky (2003) in their work on depression, anxiety and psychiatric illness among those with epilepsy. However, research indicates that little has changed in the management and treatment of this particular group of people. This is corroborated by the work of Starr and Sporty (1994) and Kanner (2003). Research has indicated that people with this dual diagnosis need to be appropriately managed as failure to do so can have devastating effects on the individuals, their lives and their families. Although the science of epilepsy has indicated a link between the co-morbidity of epilepsy and psychiatric illness in some individuals, the management of this group poses yet another question. Professionals cannot separate the mind and the physical brain; they must be managed and treated simultaneously. This may require tertiary and primary or secondary care, working collaboratively on treatment plans. The stigma associated with these conditions and the psychosocial effect is the impetus for the scientific research to continue. The unknown entities in this area need further work in order to support the families more fully, because, as noted by Starr and Sporty (1994), 'the family found the seizures to be more socially acceptable than the psychiatric disorder', the psychiatric disorder being psychosis. In other words, the seizures becomes controlled with anticonvulsant therapy, however ensuing psychosis occurs (a phenomenon known as 'forced normalisation'). The science of epilepsy, with the utilisation of EEG, has been able to portray and illustrate the experience of anti-epileptic medication suppressing seizures but which promotes the development of a psychosis. In all populations, but particularly among people with a learning disability, this occurrence can be misdiagnosed and therefore mismanaged.

The role of the learning disability nurse as an epilepsy specialist practitioner

There is no one definition of the job title, epilepsy specialist nurse, and what is expected from him or her is dependent on where the individual is employed. Specialist nursing was born out of restructuring based on the Salmon career structure, with the first specialist nurse taking up post in the 1970s. Doncaster was revolutionary in appointing the first epilepsy specialist nurse in 1973. The 1990s witnessed the small explosion of epilepsy specialist nurses working in adult care, paediatrics and learning disabilities. Many of these posts were initially supported by Epilepsy Action, one of the national charities for epilepsy in the UK.

Kelly (1996) advises the 'reality of the specialist practitioner is directed towards prevention, restoration and amelioration'. The role of the specialist epilepsy nurse is supported by evidence-based practice; authors include Wallace et al (1997), the Clinical Standards Advisory Group (1999), Meads et al (2001), Hanna et al (2002) and the Department of Health (2002). Within learning disability practice this health professional has also been identified as a key player in the management of an individual with the dual diagnosis of epilepsy and learning disability (Zaagman, 1998; Graydon, 2000). *The National Service Framework for Long-Term Conditions* (Department of Health, 2005) failed to identify the specific need for epilepsy specialist nurses within learning disabilities but this does not mean there is not a recognised role for this professional. The Clinical Standards Advisory Group (1999) report, however, recommended the appointment of nurses with learning disability experience when appointing epilepsy specialist nurses. The employment of such practitioners is dependent on local Primary Care Trusts and health and social care trusts. To engage the services of this professional will enhance the multidisciplinary team and enable collaborative working across the domains of primary and secondary care, thus supporting improved outcomes for individuals and their families/carers.

The National Service Framework for Long-Term Conditions refers to people with long-term neurological conditions having support in the community from specialist nurses and practitioners, it is no more specific in its definition of specialist nurse support than this. Unlike the Scottish Intercollegiate Guidelines Network (SIGN) document (2003) *Diagnosis and Management of Epilepsy in Adults*, it advises on the role of the epilepsy nurse specialist although not specifically in learning disability. The same document advocates specialist epilepsy clinics for people with a learning disability. The National Institute for Clinical Excellence (2004a 18) document states:

People with a learning disability should receive the same support and care as the general population of people with epilepsy. They also need the care of the learning disabilities team. The management and treatment of epilepsy in a person who has learning disabilities should be undertaken by a specialist, working within a multidisciplinary team.

In order to achieve the status of specialist practitioner, the Nursing and Midwifery Council (2001) requires the successful completion of specialist practitioner outcomes which must be attained in order to be granted the Specialist Practitioner Award. *Table 8.7* illustrates the clinical competencies required in order to meet these specialist practitioner outcomes.

The learning disability nurse practising as an epilepsy specialist nurse is supported and recognised by Greenhill et al (2001). This specialist practitioner will have the knowledge, skills and attributes as identified within the epilepsy nurse specialist competencies (*Table 8.7*). These skills and modern approaches to epilepsy care will enable the nurse to support and manage the individual who presents with the complex health needs of a dual diagnosis of epilepsy and learning disability.

The Chief Nursing Officer, who identified the 10 Key Roles for Nursing in the NHS Plan (Department of Health 1999), defined the clinical tasks to be undertaken by a practitioner working at a specialist level. Miller (1995) identified the clinical nurse specialist as having five main sub-roles:

- Clinical expert
- Researcher
- Consultant
- Teacher
- Change agent.

These sub-roles inter-link with the 10 key roles identified in the NHS Plan (Department of Health, 1999)

- Ordering diagnostic investigations
- Triaging of patients
- Making and receiving direct referrals
- Managing patient caseload
- Nurse-led clinics
- Prescribing medication and treatment
- Admitting and discharging patients
- Taking the lead in organising local health services
- Extending the role of resuscitation procedures
- Performing minor surgery.

Table 8.7: Clinical competencies

Specialist practitioner outcomes (NMC, 2001)	Suggested competencies for epilepsy specialist practitioner (UCE, 2005)
Specialist clinical practice	
1. Assess health, health-related and nursing needs of service users, their families and other carers by identifying and initiating appropriate steps for effective care for individuals and groups	• Demonstrate and critically apply a good knowledge of normal and abnormal neurophysiological functioning related to diagnosing seizure types • Demonstrate good knowledge of the characteristics of epileptic seizures and critically apply knowledge to history taking/interviews with patients/clients/carers during the diagnosis process • Demonstrate and critically apply good knowledge of seizure types and identify with justification seizure types in patients/clients
2. Set, implement and evaluate standards and criteria of nursing intervention by planning, providing and evaluating specialist clinical nursing care across a range of care provision to meet the health needs of individual and groups requiring specialist nursing	• Describe, justify and critically evaluate the management and nursing care required for a specific group of people with epilepsy, e.g. women, elderly, learning disability, children
3. Assess and manage critical and clinical events to ensure safe and effective care	• Respond efficiently and effectively to a person presenting with a major generalised epileptic seizure • Respond efficiently and effectively to a person presenting with prolonged seizures or convulsive/non-convulsive status epilepticus

NMC = Nursing and Midwifery Council
UCE = University of Central England (now Birmingham City University)

Table 8.7: cont/

Specialist practitioner outcomes	Suggested competencies for epilepsy specialist practitioner
4. Support and empower service users, their families and other carers to influence and participate in decisions concerning their care by providing information on a range of specialist nursing care and services	• Critically discuss the information that service-users/carers may need regarding lifestyle implications of epilepsy • Critically discuss the information that service-users/carers may need regarding treatment options for epilepsy
5. Facilitate learning in relation to identified health need for service users and carers	• Demonstrate an ability to effectively teach carers to administer rectal diazepam in situations of status epilepticus • Demonstrate an ability to effectively teach service-users/carers to understand the action and side effects of anti-epilepsy drugs and the implications of polypharmacy
6. Provide counselling and psychological support for individuals and their carers	• Demonstrate an ability to provide appropriate support and counselling to service users and carers during the diagnosis process • Demonstrate an ability to provide appropriate support and counselling to service users and carers in addressing the needs of specific groups of people with epilepsy, e.g. women, elderly, learning disability, children • Demonstrate an ability to provide appropriate support and counselling to service users and carers when considering treatment options

Table 8.7 continues/

Table 8.7: cont/

Specialist practitioner outcomes	Suggested competencies for epilepsy specialist practitioner
7. Act independently within a multi-disciplinary/multi-agency context	• Perform efficiently, and contribute with justifiable arguments to multidisciplinary team meetings regarding consent to treatment • Perform efficiently and contribute with justifiable arguments to discussions regarding treatment options
8. Support and empower patients clients and their carers to influence and use available services, information and skills to the full and to participate in decisions concerning their care	• Critically discuss with service users and carers the role of anti-epileptic drugs in the treatment of epilepsy to encourage full compliance of medication

Care and programme management

9. Supervise and manage clinical practice to ensure safe and effective holistic research-based care	• Critically evaluate the care of specific groups of people with epilepsy, e.g. women, elderly, learning disability, children
10. Initiate and contribute to strategies designed to promote and improve health and prevent disease in individuals and groups by identifying and selecting from a wide range of health and social agencies, those that will assist and improve care	• Identify with justification measures which may be taken to avoid precipitating factors of seizures

Table 8.3 continues/

Table 8.7: cont/

Specialist practitioner outcomes	Suggested competencies for epilepsy specialist practitioner
Leadership	
11. Recognise ethical and legal issues which have implications for nursing practice and take appropriate action	• Critically discuss with service-users and carers the role of anti-epileptic drugs in the treatment of epilepsy to encourage full compliance of medication
12. Lead and clinically direct the professional team to ensure the implementation and monitoring of quality assured standards of care by effective and efficient management of finite resources	• Participate efficiently and effectively in the operational/strategic management of the service
13. Identify individual potential in registered nurses and specialist practitioners, through effective appraisal systems. As a clinical expert advise on educational opportunities that will facilitate the development and support of their specialist knowledge and skills to ensure they develop their clinical practice	• Actively participate in the educational and professional development of the nursing team and positively contribute to the dynamic learning culture
14. Ensure effective learning experiences and opportunity to achieve learning outcomes for students through preceptorship; mentorship, counselling, clinical supervision of an educational environment	• Actively participate in the educational and professional development of the nursing team and positively contribute to the dynamic learning culture

Table 8.3 continues/

Table 8.7: cont/

Specialist practitioner outcomes	Suggested competencies for epilepsy specialist practitioner
Clinical practice development	
15. Create an environment in which clinical practice development is fostered, evaluated and disseminated	• Develop and critically evaluate specialist clinical teaching packages used for the development of practice
16. Identify specialist learning activities in a clinical setting that contribute to clinical teaching and assessment of learning in a multi-disciplinary environment within scope of expertise and knowledge	• Develop and critically evaluate specialist clinical teaching packages used for the development of practice
17. Initiate and lead practice developments to enhance the nursing contribution and quality of care	• Demonstrate active engagement in setting standards, developing quality initiatives, monitoring and quality assurance strategies within the framework of clinical effectiveness
18. Identify; apply and disseminate research findings relating to specialist nursing practice	• Identify, evaluate, critically apply and disseminate research findings relating to specialist needs of specific groups of people with epilepsy, e.g. women, elderly, learning disability, children • Identify, evaluate, critically apply and disseminate research findings relating to the use of AEDs
19. Explore and implement strategies for quality assurance and quality audit. Determine criteria against which they should be judged, how success might be measured and who should measure success	• Demonstrate active engagement in setting standards, developing quality initiatives, monitoring and quality assurance strategies within the framework of clinical effectiveness

Thus the role of specialist epilepsy nurse is to improve care and enhance quality of life through rehabilitation for people who have a diagnosis of epilepsy. These nurses, working in the specialist field of learning disabilities, will adapt these key roles to the environment in which they are employed. The organisation will have job role expectations and practitioners will be expected to work at an advanced level and function intuitively within their job role. Higgins (2003) advised 'the epilepsy specialist nurse role is extremely varied, often dependent on organisational, individual and client-based boundaries'.

The epilepsy specialist nurse working in learning disability practice will identify key domains of the job role. These need to be considered by the nurse in order to provide a first class service to the individual. These domains, based on Doherty's (2003: 247) contemporary issues, highlight some new challenges for the epilepsy nurse specialist, e.g. nurse prescribing (either independent or supplementary) and telemedicine.

The domains of the epilepsy specialist nurse's role are as follows:

- Age-related needs
- Assessment
- Audit
- Communication
- Education and training
- Fast track treatment
- Gender-specific issues
- Medication
- Mortality
- Morbidity
- Multi-disciplinary working
- Nurse-led clinics
- Nurse prescribing (independent and supplementary prescribing)
- Review and evaluation of care
- Sudden unexpected death in epilepsy
- Support for surgery candidates
- Telemedicine
- Treatment options.

The epilepsy specialist nurse in learning disabilities will in particular have to recognise the following domains:

- Cognition
- Consent
- Risk assessment linked to quality of life
- Status epilepticus – rescue medication issues.

The following case study illustrates the domains of the epilepsy nurse specialist role:

Case study

Connie is a 30-year-old lady with a diagnosis of cerebral palsy, moderate learning disabilities and epilepsy. She currently lives at home with her parents and sister. Her health needs, including epilepsy, are currently monitored by a consultant psychiatrist (learning disabilities) and epilepsy specialist nurse (learning disabilities). Connie has had previous admissions and out-patient monitoring at epilepsy tertiary centres and several admissions at her local hospital. Her diagnosis is that of tonic-clonic seizures, absence seizures and status epilepticus. Her current medication is lamotrigene, sodium valproate, clobazam and rectal diazepam. However the seizures remain poorly controlled at times.

The family are now seeking a short break service (respite care) for their daughter on a regular basis due to the deteriorating health needs of Connie's mother. The day service is currently reviewing Connie's placement due to prolonged seizures, which culminate in admissions to hospital from their unit, as being an invasive procedure. Their medication policy does not allow staff to administer rectal diazepam as a rescue medication. In the past, changes to Connie's lifestyle have affected her seizure activity thus the current situation needs to be managed with sensitivity and understanding.

Immediate points to consider by the epilepsy specialist nurse

- Appropriate respite unit that can manage epilepsy, including nocturnal seizures.
- Consider current rescue medication in consultation with the consultant psychiatrist and Connie and her family as this could have implications on both the day placement and the respite service (an alternative buccal preparation may be a more appropriate rescue medication).
- Health facilitation plan to be updated in conjunction with Connie's community learning disability nurse and circulated to the multidisciplinary team.
- Training and education for family, day service and respite service staff if rescue medication is changed.
- Rescue medication protocol to be established.
- Ongoing monitoring of Connie's epilepsy via the nurse-led clinic to include patterns and triggers of seizures and the updating of assessment information as required.

- Ongoing monitoring of Connie's anti-epileptic medication via the nurse-led clinic.
- Ongoing monitoring of Connie's mental well-being utilising, for example, the Glasgow Epilepsy Outcome Scale (Watkins et al, 2006)
- Appropriate risk assessment including the issue of sudden unexpected death in epilepsy, and nocturnal seizures which needs to be circulated to all involved in Connie's care, to ensure understanding by the staff team.
- Gender-specific issues, including catamenial epilepsy and the use of clobazam, confirming with staff how it is prescribed.
- Communication between all involved in Connie's care through collaborative working.
- Ensure Connie's quality of life is maintained and not marginalised due to her diagnosis of epilepsy.

The epilepsy specialist nurse in learning disabilities will be required to identify the needs and concerns not only of the carer but, most importantly, the needs and concerns of the individual; this is supported by Watkins et al (2006).

Epilepsy nurse-led clinics are commonplace within secondary and tertiary care centres and learning disabilities services where an epilepsy specialist nurse is employed. The role within the clinic will vary depending on the qualifications of the nurse practitioner, for example whether the nurse prescribes medication or not. Fast track service and triage could be options for the nurse within a clinic setting (Greenhill et al, 2001). The epilepsy specialist nurse, via the clinics, is a link to many services with which a person with this dual diagnosis may come into contact, including general practitioners, practice nurses, midwives, health visitors and social care and health staff.

The epilepsy specialist nurse within learning disabilities will play a key role in gathering and collating basic information to commence the assessment process. The initial assessment may occur within the individual's home or via the nurse-led clinic prior to the first hospital/out-patient appointment with the consultant psychiatrist. Each individual healthcare trust will have policies and procedures as to the information required and how to document such data, for example, it could be recorded through a care pathway document or the current epilepsy health record (Doherty, 2003). It is paramount at this point of contact that the facts are determined in relation to what either the individual or his/her carer thinks/knows what happened in relation to the episode. The nurse will discuss basic information in relation to epilepsy with the individual, carer and family including what to do should the person have another seizure; a recording sheet/diary would be left with the family for this purpose.

The seizure diary is an on-going recording tool that would be brought to the nurse-led epilepsy clinic for continued monitoring of the individual's epilepsy. The seizure diary is an important document when trying to diagnose epilepsy and to evaluate if there are any precipitating factors/ triggers. The diary should be completed every time the individual has a seizure. This is helpful for the management and treatment plan and it will support rationalisation of the medication regime. Information to be recorded includes:

- Date
- Day
- Time of seizure
- Precipitating factors (if any)
- What actually happened during the seizure
- Duration of the seizure
- What the individual did after coming out of the seizure
- Any post-ictal signs
- Whether paramedics where called.

Some of the precipitating factors/triggers that would be discussed with the individual/family/carer are listed below:

- Sleep pattern
- Use of alcohol
- Use of recreational drugs
- Changes to prescribed medication
- Excitement
- Boredom
- Change in body temperature
- Illness
- Skipping of meals
- Constipation
- Menstruation
- Changes in lifestyle
- Stress
- Photosensitivity (this is only present in a small proportion of people with a diagnosis of epilepsy)
- Pain
- Medical procedures, e.g. anaesthetic

It must be remembered that, at this stage, a diagnosis has not been confirmed and the nurse is not in a position to make such a diagnosis no matter what information has been given. The issue of epilepsy specialist nurses diagnosing is currently being debated. Although there is no evidence to date with regards to nurses diagnosing epilepsy, it may be incorporated into job descriptions of nurse consultants in epilepsy in the future as the profession awaits the outcome of a recent research study in the UK in relation to this subject.

The clinical role of the epilepsy specialist nurse is ever changing, from merely managing nurse-led clinics a few years ago, to now offering independent and supplementary prescribing within the clinics. The Department of Health (2005: 25) advocates 'using medicines effectively to manage long-term conditions'. The nurse's primary role in relation to medication is to monitor epilepsy drug treatment, to ensure efficacy and establish side effect profiles of the treatment for the individual. Nurses who do not prescribe would discuss this clinical information with the doctor who would rationalise the prescription if necessary. However, as from May 2006 independent prescribing for registered nurses that have successfully completed the extended prescribing course can now prescribe independently of a doctor. However, some nurses may chose to continue to prescribe through supplementary prescribing following the clinical management plan agreed with the medical practitioner.

The epilepsy specialist nurse has a responsibility to ensure carers of the individual are familiar with the individual's epilepsy drug regime including any rescue medication that they may be prescribed. The consequences of the individual not taking their medication as directed by the prescriber needs to be established with both the person with epilepsy and the carer.

Nurse-led clinics, although now frequent within epilepsy services, do not detract from domiciliary visits when these are deemed to be more appropriate. Follow up appointments from the nurse-led clinic could be at the individual's home in order to advise on detailed information, for example a complex treatment/care plan which has been formulated by the epilepsy specialist nurse for learning disabilities and agreed by the consultant psychiatrist. Although the nurse-led clinic allows greater numbers of people to be monitored, there remain certain tasks expected of the epilepsy specialist nurse that cannot be performed within such an environment, e.g. education and training to a care team or environmental risk assessment of a short-break service.

Research and audit of this population is limited due to reasons of consent. Therefore, as professional nurses involved in the treatment of people with this dual diagnosis, the evaluation of services and treatment plans (an essential role of the epilepsy specialist nurse) may be problematic. Some NHS trusts may audit carers and family members to establish if they are satisfied with current care, however this does not necessarily give an accurate conclusion.

Understanding of whether an individual's quality of life has improved is not just a number crunching exercise to establish if the number of seizures the person has had in the last month has reduced, although these domains could form part of the audit. Audit should take into account thoughts and feelings of the individual, and utilising the Glasgow Epilepsy Outcome Scale (Watkins et al, 2006) could be a start. The outcome of such an audit using this tool would enable greater understanding of the way people with this dual diagnosis feel about their epilepsy.

Gold standard research is not available in the learning disability arena in relation to the benefits of the epilepsy specialist nurse to patients. However, anecdotal evidence within learning disabilities indicates that it is comparable to that of adult population studies. The British Epilepsy Association, now known as Epilepsy Action, presented such findings in their document *Making It Happen*. They concluded the following:

- Improved medication compliance and reduced side effects.
- Improved seizure control.
- Improved safety during seizures (less incidence of recorded injuries: audit of accident and emergency).
- Improved knowledge of condition.
- Improved quality of life.
- Improved care for women during pregnancy, labour and postpartum.

If epilepsy specialist nurses within learning disabilities can facilitate the above findings within their job role for the individual with a dual diagnosis of learning disability and epilepsy, they will be able to support individuals in a unique way.

Conclusion

The Department of Health (2005: 9) categorises epilepsy as an intermittent and unpredictable condition where relapses and remissions lead to a marked variation in the care needed. The challenge to epilepsy specialist nurses in learning disability is to ensure that appropriate care is provided for individuals with a whole spectrum of needs. This includes an ability to reduce anxiety and the psychological and psychosocial effects that the impact of a diagnosis of epilepsy may have on an individual by examining all causes of epilepsy and its various differential diagnoses. People with epilepsy can sometimes feel marginalised within society, causing social isolation and feelings of stigmatisation, consequences which could affect their prospects in society, e.g. education, employment and dependence on others. In achieving appropriate care the quality of life of individuals will be enhanced and new opportunities may be open to them, e.g. employment, sports, relationships, social functioning, elimination of dependence on others, removal of labels and social isolation, reduced hospitalisation, improved mental well-being and mood, reduction in morbidity events, e.g. fractures, and reduced risk of sudden unexpected death in epilepsy.

Treatment and management plans, whatever the diagnosis, need to be established to address morbidity and mortality of the condition and improve the individual's quality of life. History taking and investigations (e.g. videotelementry/EEG), although often viewed as time consuming and costly, could resolve the diagnosis. Merely changing medication is not always the answer if seizures persist, but ensuring a prompt and correct diagnosis as recommended by the Department of Health (2005) is a critical factor in the treatment profile.

There is now greater understanding through scientific research of the causes of epilepsy, identifying chromosomal linkage to some seizure types, new and improved neurophysiological and neuro-imaging techniques, aiding diagnosis and surgery work up. Sophisticated, efficacious drug therapies with a reduced side effect profile are now increasingly available. This in turn has contributed to the change in clinical practice for both medical and nursing professionals. The epilepsy specialist nurse, working in the field of learning disabilities, has a defined role within the multidisciplinary team offering a service not only to the individual diagnosed with epilepsy but also to families and carers. The role as educator and trainer of staff within the private, voluntary and health and social care sectors, confirms the cross boundary working of this professional, contributing to the care of the individual to reduce risks, increase life expectancy and enhance quality of life.

References

Beghi E (2004) Aetiology of epilepsy. In: Shorvon SD, Fish DR, Perucca E, Dodson WE (eds.) *The Treatment of Epilepsy* 2nd edn. Blackwell Science, 50–63

Besag FMC (2004) The Department of Health Action Plan "Improving services for people with epilepsy": A significant advance or only a first step? *Seizure* **13:** 553–64

Betts T (1996) Further experience of the Smell Memory Technique in the behavioural treatment of epilepsy. *Epilepsia* **37**(Suppl 4): 60

Betts T (1998) *Epilepsy, Psychiatry and Learning Difficulty*. Martin Dunitz, London

Betts T (2003) *Non-Epileptic Attack Disorder*. Available from: http://www. e-epilepsy.org.uk

Briggs A (1972) *Report of the Committee on Nursing.* HMSO, London

Bromfield EB; Henderson GV (2002) Seizures and cerebrovascular disease. In: Ettinger AB, Devinsky O (eds.) *Managing Epilepsy and Co-Existing Disorders.* Butterworth-Heinemann, Woburn, pp 269–89

Clinical Standards Advisory Group (CSAG) (1999) *Services for Patients with Epilepsy.* Department of Health, London

Crawford P (1996) Adult drug treatment - The best way forward in an even more complex maze. *Everyday Neurology.* (Supp 1A): 2–5 Neuroeducation, York

Cuéllar-Herraera M, Velasco M, Velascol F, Velasco AL, Jimenez F, Orozco S, Briones M, Rocha L (2004) Evaluation of GABA system and cell damage in parahippocampus of individuals with temporal lobe epilepsy showing anti-epileptic effects after subacute electrical stimulation. *Epilepsia* **45**(5): 459–66

Department of Health (1996) *Continuing the Commitment: The Report of the Learning Disability Nursing Project.* HMSO, London

Department of Health (1999) *The Chief Nursing Officer's 10 Key Roles for Nursing.* HMSO, London

Department of Health (2001) *Annual Report of the Chief Medical Officer.* Available from: www.doh.gov.uk/cmo [last accessed 14 April 2002]

Department of Health (2002) *Improving Services for People with Epilepsy: Department of Health Action Plan in Response to the National Clinical Audit of Epilepsy Related to Death.* HMSO, London

Department of Health (2005) *The National Service Framework for Long-Term Conditions.* HMSO, London

Devinsky O (2003) A 48-year-old man with temporal lobe epilepsy and psychiatric illness. *Journal American Medical Association* **290**(3): 381–92

Dodson WE (2004) Definitions and classifications of epilepsy and its treatment. In: Shorvon SD, Fish DR, Perucca E, Dodson WE (eds.) *The Treatment of Epilepsy* 2nd edn. Blackwell Science, Oxford, pp 3–20

Doherty CC (2003) Epilepsy and learning disability. In: Jukes M, Bollard M (eds.) *Contemporary Learning Disability Practice.* Quay Books Division, Wiltshire, pp 244–59

Duncan S, Fairey A, Gomersall S, Kerr M, March A, Morrow J, Sander L, Simons S (2004) *Primary Care Guidelines for the Management of Females with Epilepsy.* Epilepsy Guidelines Group, The Royal Society of Medicine Press Ltd, London

Epilepsy Action (2006) Epilepsy Information. Living with Epilepsy:

Complementary Treatments. Available from: http://www.epilepsy.org. uk/info/complementary.html [last accessed 13 July 2006]

Four-D/Neuroimaging (2004) Magnetoencephalography. Available from: www.4dneuroimagining.com/whatisMEG/what % 201s%20MEG.html [last accessed 25 February 2005]

Goldstein MA, Harden CL (2002) Infectious States. In: Ettinger AB, Devinsky O (eds.) *Managing Epilepsy and Co-existing Disorders.* Butterworth-Heinemann, Wofura, pp 83–133

Graydon M (2000) Do learning disability services need epilepsy specialist nurses? *Seizure* **9:** 294–6

Greenhill L, Betts T, Pickard N (2001) The epilepsy nurse specialist – expendable handmaiden or essential colleague? *Seizure* **10:** 615–24

Hackett R, Iype T (2001) Malnutrition and childhood epilepsy in developing countries. *Seizure* **10**(8): 554–8

Hanna NJ, Black M, Sander JWS, Smithson WH, Appleton T, Brown S, Fish DR (2002) *The National Sentinel Clinical Audit of Epilepsy-Related Death: Epilepsy – Death in the Shadows.* The Stationary Office, London

Higgins S (2003) Meeting the challenge. *Epilepsy Care* **1**(3): 6–8

Jackson (1873) In lecture notes from Carey (2004) University of Birmingham, umpublished

Jay P (1979) *Report of the Committee of Enquiry into Mental Handicap Nursing and Care.* Department of Health and Social Security, London

Kaye J, Morton J, Bowcutt M, Maupin D (2000) Depression: The forgotten diagnosis among hospitalised Adults. *Journal of Neuroscience Nursing* **32**(1): 7–16

Kanner AM (2003) When did neurologists and psychiatrists stop talking to each other? *Epilepsy and Behaviour* **4:** 597–601

Kelly A (1996) The concept of the specialist community nurse. *Journal of Advanced Nursing* **24:** 42–52

Kerr M (2005) Epilepsy and learning disability. In: Sander JW, Walker MC, Smalls JE (eds.) *Epilepsy 2005 From Neurone to NICE – A Practical Guide.* Oration Group Ltd, West Sussex: 415–26

Koppell BS (2002) Contribution of drugs and drug interactions (prescribed, over the counter, and illicit) to seizures and epilepsy. In: Ettinger AB, Devinsky O (eds.) *Managing Epilepsy and Co-Existing Disorders.* Butterworth-Heineman, Woburn, pp 155–73

Leach JP, Mohanraj R (2004) The reality of rational polytherapy. *Mims Advances* **Nov:** 6–9

Lewine JD, Andrews R, Chez M, Patil AA, Devinsky O, Smith M, Kanner A, Davis JT, Funke M, Jones G, Chong B, Provencal S, Weisend M, Lee RR, Orrison WW, Jr MD (1999) Magnetoencephlographic patterns of epileptiform activity in children with regressive autism spectrum disorders. *Pediatrics* **104**(3): 405–18

Meads C, Bradley P, Burls A (2001) *The Effectiveness of Specific Epilepsy Services*. West Midlands Health Technology Assessment Course, Birmingham

Meridian Institute (1999) A complementary medicine approach to abdominal epilepsy. Available from: http://www.meridianinstitude.com/epilepsy.htm [accessed 13 July 2006]

Miller L (1995) The clinical nurse specialist: A way forward. *Journal of Advanced Nursing* **22**: 494–501

National Institute for Clinical Excellence (2004a) *The Epilepsies: Diagnosis and Management of the Epilepsies in Adults in Primary and Secondary Care*. National Collaborating Centre for Primary Care, London

National Institute for Clinical Excellence (2004b) *Newer Drugs for Epilepsy in Adults*. Technology Appraisal 76. NICE. (www.nice.org.uk/TA076 guidance)

National Society for Epilepsy (2006a) Information on epilepsy: Epilepsy and learning disability. Available from: http://www.epilepsynse.org.uk/pages/info/leaflets/learning.ifm [accessed 13 July 2006]

National Society for Epilepsy (2006b) Epilepsy Review Extracts: Epilepsy and Autistic Spectrum Disorders. Available from: http://www.epilepsynse.org.uk/pages/whatsnew/review/autumn04_1.cfm [accessed 13 July 2006]

Nursing and Midwifery Council (2001) *Standards for Specialist Education and Practice*. NMC, London

Panayiotopoulos CP (2002) *A Clinical Guide to Epileptic Syndromes and their Treatment*. Bladon Medical Publishing, Oxfordshire

Piazzini A, Canger R (2001) Depression and anxiety in individuals with epilepsy. *Epilepsia* **42**(supp 1): 29–31

Reuber M, Fernandez G, Bauer J, Singh DD, Elger CE (2002) Interictal EEG abnormalities in individuals with psychogenic nonepileptic seizures. *Epilepsia* **43**: 1013–20

Rowan AJ (2000) Epilepsy and seizures in the aged. In: Ettinger AB, Devinsky O (eds.) *Managing Epilepsy and Co-existing Disorders*. Butterworth-HJeinemann, Woburn, pp 433–44

SANAD Study Group (2007) The SANAD study of effectiveness of carbamazepine, gabapentin, lamotrigine, oxcarbazepine or topiramate for treatment of partial epilepsy: an unblinded randomised controlled trial. *Lancet* **369:** 1000–15

Sander JW (1993) Some aspects of prognosis in the epilepsies: A review. *Epilepsia* **34:** 1007–16

Sander JW (2001) The mortality of epilepsy. In: Duncan JS, Sisodiya SM, Smalls JE (eds.) *Epilepsy 2001. From Science to Individual. 8th Epilepsy Teaching Weekend.* Burleigh Press Ltd, Bristol: 153–6

Sander JW, Shorvon S (2001) The incidence and prevalence of epilepsy. In Duncan JS, Sisodiya SM, Smalls JE (eds.) *Epilepsy 2001 From Science to Patient.* International League Against Epilepsy 8th Epilepsy Teaching Weekend, September 28–30, St Anne's College, Oxford, pp 1–12

Scottish Intercollegiate Guidelines Network (SIGN) (2003) *Diagnosis and Management of Epilepsy in Adults. A National Clinical Guideline.* Royal College of Physicians, Edinburgh

Shorvon S (2000) *Handbook of Epilepsy Treatment.* Blackwell Science, Oxford

Shorvon S (2005) *Handbook of Epilepsy Treatment* 2nd edn. Blackwell Science, Oxford

Sisodiya SM (2004) Treatment of epilepsy in general medical conditions. In: Shorvon SD, Fish DR, Perucca E, Dodson WE (eds.) *The Treatment of Epilepsy* 2nd edn. Blackwell Science, London, pp 763–74

Soryal I (2005) Causes of epilepsy. Lecture Notes. University of Birmingham, Unpublished.

Starr A, Sporty LD (1994) Similar disorders fiewed with different perspectives. A challenge for neurology and psychiatry. *Archives of Neurology* **51:** 997–80

Taylor M (1996) *Managing Epilepsy in Primary Care.* Blackwell Science Ltd, Oxford

UKCC (1993) *The Council's Proposed Standards for Post-Registration Education.* Annex Two to Registrar's Letter, 8/1993, London, UKCC

Wallace H, Shorvon S, Hopkins, Donohoghue M (1997) *Adults with Poorly Controlled Epilepsy.* Royal College of Physicians, London

Watkins J, Espie CA, Curtice L. Mantala K, Corp A, Foley J (2006) Development of a measure to assess the impact of epilepsy on people with an intellectual disability: The Glasgow Epilepsy Outcome Scale-Client version (GEOS-C). *Journal of Intellectual Disability Research*

50(3): 161–71

Webb DW; Fryer AE, Osborne JP (1991) On the incidence of fits and mental retardation in tuberous sclerosis. *Journal Medical Genetics* **28**(6): 395–7

Zaagman P (1998) Epilepsy and learning disability nursing – The case of expert knowledge. *Journal of Association of Practitioners in Learning Disability* **15**(1): 4–9

CHAPTER 9

Nursing people with profound and multiple learning disabilities

Colin Griffiths and Carmel Doyle

Introduction

> *I hear footsteps coming down the hall. I've been lying awake for the last hour trying to figure out which day it is. I would have moved but my legs won't do that for me. I would have asked but my tongue won't do that for me so I'll have to wait... I think it's my turn now, and the door is opened up... 'Good morning Patrick... Oh, you've messed your bed again...' I know, it's not my fault and anyway I had to lie in it for the last hour. (Anon, 1990).*

The history of the care of people such as Patrick; that is people with profound and multiple learning disabilities (PMLD) is one of a slow emergence from the shadows. The shadows were generally construed as being the mental handicap hospital that was the main form of provision for persons with PMLD up until the 1970s. A typical staff attitude from those days was reported by Oswin (1978) who interviewed a charge nurse in a unit for multiply handicapped children. This nurse said, 'I am a realistic man. I have no sentimental ideas about the children; we keep them clean, feed them, give them medication, that's all we can do for them' (1978: 90).

Since that time people with learning disabilities have mostly gradually, but in some cases very quickly, been discharged from large long-stay hospitals and institutions. The last group to leave has consisted of those with the most severe disabilities of all; those with PMLD (Lacey, 2000). The trend for deinstitutionalisation has been driven largely by the abandonment of the medical model that informed care up until this period. In 1971, in the UK, the White Paper *Better Services for the Mentally Handicapped* (Department of Health and Social Security, 1971) opened up the idea that the provision of day and residential services for people with learning disability might be better provided in local small-scale services. This trend has been supported by various reports and legislative measures that culminated in England in the White Paper *Valuing People* (Department of Health, 2001), in Scotland by the Scottish Executive's policy *The Same as You* (Scottish Executive, 2000), in Wales by *Fulfilling the Promises* (National Assembly for Wales, 2002), in Northern Ireland by the policy review *Equal Lives* (Department of Health, Social Services and Public Safety, 2004) and in the Republic of Ireland by the Disability Act (Government of Ireland, 2005).

These policy and legal changes mark significant milestones in the change of residential provision from large-scale institutions to smaller community-based support facilities and also in the attitudinal changes that drive such developments. The spirit behind such developments may best be summed up by the Scottish document which states: 'At the centre of this is a major shift to person-centred and needs-led approaches, which put the individual at the heart of any decisions made' (Scottish Executive, 2000: 94). This 30-year paradigm change owes its genesis to concepts such as normalisation (Wolfensberger, 1972) that emerged from Scandinavia in the 1960s, subsequently crossed the Atlantic and returned in the guise of Social Role Valorisation which has been given most meaningful expression in O'Brien's five valued experiences: community presence, choice, competence, respect and community participation. (O'Brien and Tyne, 1981). These were seen as providing a meaningful template to inform the development of person-centred services. However, while trends in person-centred support have been universal not all countries took such a radical approach to deinstitutionalisation. Some countries, such as The Netherlands and Ireland, have retained some large institutions. These tend to be modelled on campus-based communities in which residents live in houses that accommodate between four and 10 people. While most people with less severe degrees of disability live in the community, those with PMLD largely remain in such cloistered settings. Thus, there are a variety of residential and day service places where people with profound and multiple disabilities spend their lives. They may be community-based houses where people live ordinary lives or, by contrast, secluded residential facilities that are set apart. It is in these varied contexts that the nurse is to be found.

Care models for people with profound and multiple learning disabilities

In the UK, there are between 250000 and 350000 persons with a profound disability (Foundation for People with Learning Disabilities, 2005). Approximately 160000 adults with PMLD live in the family home initially and then subsequently enter residential care (Department of Health,

2002a). In Ireland, records illustrate that 25 613 people with intellectual disability are in receipt of services and 1028 of these have PMLD (Kelly et al, 2007). As people with PMLD age, care needs increase and alter family circumstances which result in a move to some form of residential care. In the UK, residential care for people with PMLD centres on supported living, with care workers and nurses being the main providers of care. With a move from a medical model of care to a social model of care some houses are staffed solely by care workers. Respite facilities in the UK are an important part of the service provided to people with PMLD. The desire for the availability of more respite care has led, in many parts of the country, to the development of citywide respite strategies with the goal of providing a specialist respite service to those with profound intellectual and multiple disabilities.

Nursing practice

The nurse in learning disability practice is a key figure in the multi-professional team caring for the person with PMLD. Nurses have many roles which include: clinician, educator, therapist, supporter and advocate (Lacey and Ouvry, 2001). Nurses also possess vital skills that are required in order to meet the holistic needs of the person with PMLD. The nurse's role may be very different depending on the context in which he or she is working, it may include organising co-ordinated support for an individual in the community or home environment, or alternatively it may involve the provision of direct care in a residential setting. In particular, the role involves the deployment of specific skills and abilities that are detailed in the next part of this chapter. Based upon a health action plan type format the following case study illustrates some of the key areas for inclusion in the assessment and planning of care for a person with a profound learning disability.

Case study

Jack is a 23-year-old man who lives at home with his parents, two brothers and a sister. Jack has a profound learning disability; he has been diagnosed as having cerebral palsy. He is unable to mobilise without the use of a wheelchair. He requires support in order to sit and has little mobility of his limbs. He is reliant on his carers to tend to his personal hygiene needs and for feeding. He displays signs of intermittent diarrhoea and constipation on a daily basis and is incontinent. His communication is limited to vocalisations and facial expressions. He is known to cry at intervals throughout the day. Jack attends a day centre for work, leisure and recreational pursuits and also attends a respite care centre for two nights per month.

Assessment

A nursing assessment of the individual is generally undertaken as part of a wider assessment by the multidisciplinary team. Jack's assessment may cover areas such as his health needs, living skills, mobility, activity programmes, mental health needs, social issues, support requirements, finance, respite requirements, spiritual needs and any accommodation issues (Sox, 2004). Assessment is frequently carried out in order to provide an input to the person-centred planning process. Jack will have a thorough assessment carried out as part of his health action plan and the key areas will be discussed further in this chapter.

The assessment will involve the nurse deploying skills of acute observation and precise recording of what the person with PMLD does, how he or she lives life and what influences pertain to that life. Physical assessment will be coordinated with the doctor, physiotherapist and occupational therapist. Assessment of challenging behaviour and any mental health difficulties will require specific assistance from the psychiatrist and the relevant clinical nurse specialist. Lifestyle assessment demands a concerted input from Jack, his relatives and friends and lastly from other nurses and care staff who know him.

The nurse often takes the role of key worker which means that the coordination and integration of information is a central part of what the nurse has to do. It should be noted that recent approaches to meeting people's needs in a comprehensive manner include care mapping. This involves trained mappers observing behaviours and getting the views of the service user. Care mapping is grounded in the philosophy of person-centred care and takes a holistic approach to formalised care (Leyshon et al, 2004). Its value in meeting the multiple and complex needs of individuals with PMLD is increasingly emphasised (Leyshon et al, 2004). Health action plans, which detail the actions that are required to maintain and improve the health of an individual and outline any help needed to accomplish these (Department of Health, 2002b), are being developed and used by nurses, and this approach will be adopted with Jack. In addition, the OK Health check assessment is being widely used by nurses and interdisciplinary teams and is not only valued in the identification of physical difficulties for the person with intellectual difficulties but also in identifying staff training needs and areas in need of development (Matthews, 2004; Gates, 2006).

Physical care

One of the most important aspects of the role of the nurse working with people with PMLD is the organisation and delivery of specialist physical care on a 24-hour basis (Gravelle, 1997). This specialist care is generally deployed in three areas: eating and drinking, promotion of continence and the establishment of good posture and seating. Good nursing practice is based on the premise that support in these key areas is provided by the nurse only in so far as the service user cannot manage the activity him/herself. Therefore a central part of the nurse's role is to involve Jack in his self-management of personal activities of living as much as possible.

Eating and drinking

As Tait and Genders (2002) note, eating and drinking constitute two of the many physical difficulties that persons with PMLD must contend with. Poor muscle tone and body posture alongside difficulties in chewing and swallowing (Gates, 2003) may make eating and drinking difficult. Many people with PMLD are unable to feed themselves and are dependent upon the nurse for this task. Jack is dependent upon the nurse and carers to tend to his feeding requirements. The nurse must ensure he is comfortable and in an upright sitting position to enhance digestion and prevent aspiration. Food should be offered at the right consistency and temperature and should be what he actually likes to eat. Dysphagia is a common condition in persons with a profound learning disability and cerebral palsy (Gates, 2006), and it must be considered in this case. As Jack needs to be fed, the nurse must closely observe the way in which Jack swallows his food and tailor her approach to feeding him so that food is swallowed comfortably by him and not inhaled. Following meals, close observation by the nurse can detect reflux problems which, if undetected, may lead to aspiration and respiratory difficulties. As management of eating and drinking skills is a primary role of the nurse in learning disability (Gates, 2007) it is essential that the nurse has access to a speech and language therapist with specific training in feeding difficulties and their management to advise on this. If Jack was at high risk of aspiration on a continuous basis, a gastrostomy feeding tube may be recommended (Todd et al, 2005). However, this method of non-oral feeding requires much consideration and the decision should not be taken lightly.

Diet

A well-balanced diet is of utmost importance for persons with PMLD as constipation is a common problem associated with lack of mobilisation (Boyd-Carson, 2003). Jack displays signs of intermittent diarrhoea and constipation on a daily basis. The diarrhoea may be overflow as a direct result of the constipation. A successful management approach to dealing with constipation needs to be considered. Therefore Jack's diet will require increased fibre and adequate fluid intake, in general this will be of the order of 2–3 litres per day. In the interim, medication may be used but prevention of the condition is the preferred method of management. An increase in exercise may also assist in the prevention and management of constipation. Additionally, in order to decrease the risk of developing pressure sores, correct nutritional and fluid intake is required and is essential for wound healing (Russell, 2001). To maintain skin integrity and prevent pressure sores, correct amounts of protein, energy, vitamins and minerals are required and, therefore, are an important part of Jack's daily dietary requirements.

Oral hygiene

Physical abnormalities associated with feeding emphasise the need for regular administration of oral hygiene (Gates, 2007). Jack should have an oral hygiene assessment and plan for the daily management of his oral hygiene. The nurse should attend to this as part of the daily care and can adopt a range of techniques such as use of an electric toothbrush, desensitisation for the face and mouth and relaxation techniques prior to brushing the teeth (Fenton et al, 2003). The nurse also has a responsibility to observe for dental problems such as plaque build up or decay and report these to ensure management is instigated before they become major problems for Jack. Were Jack to be fed non-orally, the nurse must consider the potential risks for oral mucous membrane breakdown.

Continence

Both urinary and faecal incontinence are a primary problem for persons with PMLD (Stanley, 1997). The nurse must ensure that suitable continence aids are used that meet the individual needs of the person, that they fit comfortably, do not leak and that an appropriate changing regime is instituted. Jack will require consideration of all of these issues. The impact of wearing such continence aids needs to be addressed by the nurse and they should not be visible beneath clothing. The nurse must also ensure suitable skincare regimes are adopted along with the use of barrier creams and repositioning if the person is immobile (Lacey and Ouvry, 2001).

Mobility

Many persons with PMLD are unable to mobilise and are dependent on the nurse for movement (Gates, 2003). Jack is dependent upon his carers to mobilise him within his wheelchair. He also needs to be moved into and out of other seating and his bed. Therefore, the nurse must be aware of the impact of Jack's dependency. A suitable functional assessment needs to be undertaken to ensure that active measures can be implemented to prevent potential mobility problems (Gates, 2007). This will be done in conjunction with other multi-disciplinary team members including the physiotherapist and occupational therapist. The aim of any intervention is to enhance comfort and positioning for Jack as well as preventing the development of such problems as kyphosis, scoliosis and muscle wasting. A variety of suitable seating systems exist that may be combined with the use of appropriate frames and supports. With the use of supportive strapping, improved neck · control, the prevention of further physical deformities and optimal mobility can be achieved. Additionally, the observation and prevention of pressure sores using a suitable risk assessment tool such as that recommended by Waterlow (1992) should be an integral part of Jack's nursing care.

Mental health

With recognition of the higher incidence of mental health problems in persons with learning disability (Priest and Gibbs, 2004), continuous observation is required to ensure that their mental health needs are met and deviations diagnosed and managed. Approximately 40% of the population of persons accessing learning disability services have additional mental health needs (Emerson et al, 2001) and there is evidence to suggest that the percentage increases with the degree of disability (Tonge et al, 1996; Stromme and Diseth, 2000). Mental health difficulties are more likely to go unnoticed in persons with PMLD than in the general population due to the difficulties in communication and diagnostic overshadowing (Marston et al, 1997; Priest and Gibbs, 2004). Jack cries at intervals throughout the day and no explanation has been offered for this. According to his parents and carers there does not seem to be a physical explanation. Therefore, a mental health assessment would need to be carried out. The skills of staff that care for persons with PMLD are crucial in this process (Markwick and Parrish, 2003). Quigley et al (2001) report that nurses, when educated in mental health issues, are able to recognise and describe symptoms of anxiety, depression and psychosis. Raghavan and Patel (2005) are of the view that for persons in this group third party information is important for nurses to obtain but so are 'direct observations of the person's behaviour and functioning in different settings' (2005: 80).

Although little is documented about the role of the nurse in caring for persons with PMLD and mental health difficulties the nurse is often the first person to suspect an individual has mental health difficulties and therefore plays an essential role in the assessment of the individual. Matthews (1996) encourages the direct assessment of the individual through identifying key symptoms such as frequent emotional distress, irrational mood swings, obsessions and altered perceptions. Jack displays signs of emotional distress on a daily basis and this will be considered in his assessment. The nurse should document his mental health symptoms including a clear description of each symptom, the duration of the symptom and the possible circumstances surrounding the display of such a symptom (Gates, 2007). The effect of the mental health difficulty upon the individual is also important. Effective management and intervention for individuals with PMLD and mental health difficulties warrants an appropriate assessment to ensure that mental health issues are not missed and that distressing experiences are limited. The development of appropriate assessment tools for persons with a learning disability and mental health problem is in its infancy (Deb et al, 2001; Bush and Beail, 2004; Dagnan and Lindsay, 2004; Novaco and Taylor, 2004). Appropriate management of Jack's mental health difficulties will involve the deployment of supportive therapies, behaviour therapies and pharmacological treatments.

Leisure

According to Lacey and Ouvry (2001) there are several barriers to persons with PMLD taking part in leisure activities. As this client group tends to be confined to wheelchairs with multiple physical and sensory deficits, dependency upon the nurse or carer for leisure activities is common. Leisure activities have both physical and psychological benefits for the individual (Gates, 2003). The nurse working with Jack has a challenging role in ensuring that his leisure activities are fun and enjoyable and that participation, no matter how minimal, is achieved (Lacey and Ouvry, 2001). Choosing a leisure activity may appear difficult but is facilitated by careful assessment of his likes and dislikes. There are several activities that the nurse can introduce that may provide pleasure and enjoyment as well as exercise for the individual with PMLD.

Multi-sensory activities including exposure to Snoezelen and massage therapy are recommended (Gates, 2007). Other activities that may be of use include cookery, horticulture, motor movement games in the local gym, and swimming. All of these activities are available to Jack. Of particular importance is the person's participation in the local community. The nurse can enhance the person's exposure to a variety of environments. These may include obtaining suitable transport so that access can be gained to local leisure pursuits which may include being wheeled along a pier at the beach, spending time in the countryside, attending local clubs and visiting parks, cinemas and shopping centres. Lastly, Jack's nurse will be able to assist him to participate in community life to the maximum by utilising the principles of partial participation (Ferguson and Baumgart, 1991) which suggest that Jack and his nurse should work together to accomplish tasks in his life. Partial participation indicates that Jack should be supported to carry out as much of a task as he is able to accomplish and his nurse should support him by doing any elements of the task that he is unable to do.

Family support

The nurse plays a supportive role with families from birth to end of life care spanning from diagnosis of the learning disability to actual provision of care and support as the person grows and develops. In partnership with families, nurses not only provide physical management and psychological support but advice on the holistic needs and care of the individual with PMLD and support for the family in meeting their individual needs (Gates, 2003). Each family is unique and, therefore, the nurse must adapt to the individual needs of each family member. Individual needs can be determined by assessing the family, which will provide a baseline for the care and support that may be required (Gates, 2007).

Jack's family have the support of the local service for persons with a disability. The nurse must communicate in an open manner with family members and demonstrate commitment to collaborate on care issues whether the nurse is the primary carer or working in a supportive role (Hastings and Taunt, 2003). The nurse must be willing to recognise the contribution the family makes in the life of the person with PMLD. Patterson (1995) identified principles that are useful in supporting families. These include focusing on the family's strengths, acknowledging the emotional issues that arise and working with the family to devise solutions. Jack also attends respite care which plays a key role in the supportive process for both Jack and his family (Lindgren, 1990; Neufeld et al, 2001).

Finally the support and care that Jack requires from his keyworker and other staff is best delivered in a coordinated holistic manner. In view of the fact that the nurse is generally the healthcare professional who spends most time with the person with PMLD, he or she is the person with both the responsibility and the opportunity to ensure that the supports that Jack requires fit seamlessly with his needs.

New developments in nursing care

Percutaneous endoscopic gastrostomy

The nurse's role in supporting people with PMLD has changed over recent years, partially as a result of developments and trends in the general bio-medical field. None has had more impact on the lives of service users than percutaneous endoscopic gastrostomy (PEG) feeding. This is a method of artificial feeding whereby an incision is made in the abdominal wall and a permanent gastrostomy tube is fed into the stomach and pulled through the abdominal wall so that an artificial tract leads directly into the stomach. All nutritional requirements can then be delivered by means of a pump connected by a tube to the plug in the person's abdominal wall. In this way the need for the individual to drink, masticate food and swallow is removed.

The main reasons for carrying out this procedure and instituting PEG feeding are due to the service user's inability to swallow (Ponsky and Gauderer, 1989). Although widespread use of PEG feeds is a relatively recent development in Ireland and the UK, in the USA such approaches are more common. Kobe et al (1994) reported that 25% of a sample of 203 non-ambulatory children and adults with PMLD required gastro-intestinal feeding. Decisions regarding whether a service user should be offered a PEG and then exactly how the autonomy of the service user is respected within the decision making process are difficult, most particularly when the benefits to the service user are unclear (Todd et al, 2005). A full multi-dimensional assessment of the benefits and disadvantages of PEG for the service user should be undertaken. Special attention should be paid to the value to the service user of the eating process, questions should be asked such as: Does he/she savour food? Is the sensory process of eating something important to the person? Furthermore, the effects of losing an interaction process which occurs three times daily needs to be very carefully considered. On the other hand if a service user has difficulty swallowing or has a tendency to aspirate food and consequently cannot obtain sufficient nutrition or gets frequent chest infections, then the procedure should be considered.

These authors suggest that the nurse's role is pivotal in the decision making process and also that consultation with an independent advocate may be of help in order to ensure that the procedure is being undertaken transparently to promote the quality of life of the service user. Further consideration of the necessity for a service user to have a PEG feed inserted may be assisted by consulting documents that have been published by the Clinical Resource Efficiency Support Team which is based in Northern Ireland. These documents offer a model for managing enteral tube feeding as well as guidelines for the process (Crest 2004a, b).

Complementary therapies and the nurse

Another development in interventions for people with PMLD is the utilisation of various complementary therapies, primarily aromatherapy and massage. Aromatherapy oils placed in a diffuser or as an adjunct to a massage session can be used to provide multi-sensory stimulation or simply as a tool for relaxation. The aim of the session will determine the particular oil that is used and the massage approach. In general the nurse's role is to assist and complement the role of the therapist. However, some nurses take up such training as an addition to their nursing practice. Sanderson et al (1991) note that massage can be used as a tool to promote interaction and participation for service users with multiple disabilities. By way of contrast drama therapy has been used as participative entertainment for this group. The best known approach is termed 'Odyssey Now' (Grove and Park, 1996). Developed by speech and language therapists who thought that well-known stories and poems could be dramatised in a way that would make them accessible to all, this approach has had some success as a way of drawing people with PMLD into both the acting out of stories and the co-creation of new ones. Some limited empirical evidence exists to suggest that this approach is effective in facilitating increased interaction levels (Mitchell and Van der Gaag, 2002).

In some circumstances new developments in related fields can be of benefit to people with PMLD, such as art therapy and music therapy. Interestingly, Jackson (2004) reports that music therapy can be a useful mechanism to assist in achieving care planning outcomes. The authors suggest close collaboration between the nurse and the relevant therapist in order to make use of these powerful therapeutic approaches in a way that most suits the service user. If this happens, the authors are of the view that these multi-disciplinary approaches may be of help in promoting therapeutic nursing outcomes for people with PMLD.

Advanced nursing practice

Several key areas of nursing practice have been highlighted so far in this chapter. It should be noted that insofar as new therapeutic approaches that enhance life for people with profound multiple disabilities are being developed, new areas of learning disability nursing practice have also emerged in the last decade (Barr, 2004). Of greatest importance is the need for specialist practice in learning disability nursing (Government of Ireland, 1998, Bollard and Jukes, 1999). Specialist roles have been developed for nurses working in specific areas of care. These include supporting persons with PMLD when they display challenging behaviours and mental health problems (Priest and Gibbs, 2004) and community nursing in learning disability services. The development of advanced nursing practice roles in learning disability is something that is currently evolving. Crouch (2002) suggests there are minimal nurse consultant posts in the UK while in Ireland there are no advanced nurse practitioners in this discipline. According to Jukes (1996) the difficulties surrounding the development of advanced nurse practice posts result from traditional perceptions of nursing and the lack of awareness regarding the role of the learning disability nurse. However in July 2006 the UK Learning Disability Consultant Nurse Network published its vision for learning disability nursing (Northway et al, 2006) which detailed that the field of nursing people with PMLD is an area where nurses have developed in depth knowledge. Such specialist nurses possess a myriad of skills required to care for persons with PMLD, as the vision document notes. Changing methods of service provision implies that nurses must have a commitment to lifelong learning. This will mean that nurses acquire research skills and skills of analysis that will enable them to expand the knowledge base of nursing of people with profound intellectual and multiple disability. Specialist nurses will find that their role within the multi-disciplinary team becomes one where they posses a deep theoretical knowledge of the field which, combined with a commitment to being present with service user's implies an unprecedented combination of competencies being available to support individuals with PMLD.

Communication

Every person, regardless of the severity of their disabilities, has the right and the ability to communicate with others, express everyday preferences and exercise at least some control over his or her daily life
(Williams, 1989: 1).

Williams's assertion, which was written in the context of an article that examined the communication possibilities for people with severe intellectual disability, still holds true some 20 years later. The statement makes some challenging points; not only does everyone have the right to communicate; everyone has the ability to do so.

However, difficulties arise, as highlighted by Roy McConkey, who noted at the IASSID Europe conference in Dublin in 2002 that:

We used to think that it was the person with the intellectual disability who had the communication problem, now we realise it is we who are unable to understand ... we need to find ways to unravel the communications of people with intellectual disability.

If one believes, as these authors do, that the essence of the role of the nurse occurs at the interface with the service user and that that interface is expressed in the communication that takes place between the person with the disability and the nurse then the primary role of the nurse consists of trying to understand the person with the disability and his/her communications.

Interpreting communication

How then can the nurse start to unravel and interpret the communications of people with PMLD? Members of this client group have great difficulty communicating and when they do communicate their interactions manifest in various different ways; the most salient being: unformed vocalisations, gestures, and variations in their posture, gaze and alertness. These difficulties mean that they have, according to Grove et al (1999: 190–1):

- A high dependence on the interpretation of others to make themselves understood.
- A level of awareness of their own intentions that is low, or difficult to determine.
- A level of comprehension that is low, or difficult to determine.
- Limited independent ability to use a formal linguistic code.
- Inconsistent ways of communication leading to ambiguity of meaning.
- A tendency to acquiesce with the suggestions of others.
- Inability to contradict an interpretation.

Information regarding the communications of others can be obtained through observation or by proxy reports. In the latter situation, the views of staff or others who spend time with the service user are correlated with the aim of producing an overview of what the service user does to communicate. The difficulties with this approach are that each person's judgement of the meaning of a communication relies on their understanding of the communication, the context, and his/her prior knowledge. This may mean that nurses project their hopes, fears or own issues onto the service user and misinterpret the communications (Grove et al, 2001) a situation that arose in the 1990s with facilitated communication (Crossley, 1997).

In order to elude the subjective difficulty of interpretation of the meaning of communications it is necessary to carry out systematic observations of people with PMLD in the context of their ordinary lives. This can be done in different ways. Particular behaviours can be targeted as part of the observation strategy. Some behaviours will be clearly indicative of communicative intent, such as when the service user orients to another person and displays direct eye contact, a gaze that observes a partner's response or repetition of behaviour where the object of the behaviour is clear. Some communicative behaviour may be less clear, thus changes of gaze direction, posture, hand or arm movements may be indicative of communicative intent or may not. Intent in itself can be said to be present when a communication is 'goal directed, purposeful behaviour whose origin is within the self' (Grove et al, 1999: 92). Some behaviour may be apparently lacking in communicative intent. This category refers to such micro-communications as small facial gestures, small changes of posture, certain arm, hand and finger gestures, eye gaze and eye blink. These communications may vary with the context in which they occur and may be quite subtle (Porter and Ouvry, 2001).

It is the contention of the authors that the capacity to observe, note and contextualise these behaviours and discriminate which are communicative and which are not is one of the skills that the nurse who works with this group of people needs to set out to acquire. As yet little research has been carried out systematically to analyse the importance of the micro-communications of people with PMLD. However, this may be a fruitful field for future research (Timmins et al, 2005). In terms of the nurse's practice the observation of micro-communications is a skill that nurses largely acquire through watching service users and seeing what they do and how they react in different situations and subsequently incorporating this information into their personal practice knowledge. Where formal research has been carried out, these observations have largely been made through the use of video which, as Grove et al (2001) note, is the most powerful tool available for the observation of communications.

A related approach to the ascertaining of how a person with PMLD communicates that may be helpful to the nurse is the use of 'zoning theory' (Gray, 2006) which proposes that people with sensory disabilities, and particularly people with intellectual disability and accompanying sensory disability, can be classified into different communication zones through ascending levels of sensory ability. The initial level, zone 1, is where the person responds through touch to sensory stimuli and also by varying muscle tone and breathing patterns. Zone 2 implies that the person also responds to basic auditory and visual stimuli. Zoning theory proposes six levels at the highest of which the person communicates normally with no assistance. Through being with the person the nurse establishes in which zone the person is communicating and modifies the nursing interactions accordingly. The general approach is that nursing communications are tailored to the service user's level and are based very much on the behaviours that the service user displays. This approach has some similarities with that of intensive interaction (Nind and Hewitt, 2001).

Facilitating meaningful self-determination

Although the primary aim of the nurse's understanding of the communications of people with PMLD is to establish a better comprehension of who the person is and what his or her inner world is like, a secondary aim is to establish what are the person's needs, wants, likes and dislikes. The purpose of this is to enable people to express themselves and as a result to take greater control of their life and facilitate greater self-determination and an enhanced quality of life.

Currently the main vehicle for planning and implementing individualised care is person-centred planning (PCP). Having been developed over the last 30 years PCP has become important in the UK and Ireland and is a component of the 2001 White Paper *Valuing People* (Department of Health 2001). The elements of PCP that distinguish it from previous approaches to multi-disciplinary care planning approaches are as follows.

Firstly, rather than just considering the needs of the service user emphasis is placed on individuals' abilities and their wishes for their life. Secondly, the support group for the service user is not simply based on the service but mobilises the person's family and friends. Furthermore people with profound multiple disabilities should take a far more central role in the planning and delivery of the plan than that of the service personnel. Lastly, and most crucially, the plan emphasises the provision of support to achieve the service user's goals rather than the goals that the service deems it can achieve (Mansell and Beadle-Brown, 2004a). Therefore, ideally, PCPs expand the possibilities that life offers for the service user.

The nurse is crucial to this process in that he or she will often spend the most time with the service user, know them best and have the most valuable information to feed into the process. The difficulty that nurses need to acknowledge is that because the process shifts the decision making power away from the service provider, nurses may find themselves caught between two conflicting requirements; that of the service provider and that of the service user. There remains the danger that disparate assessments that are contributed to a PCP may not reflect the whole of the person with PMLD's life. These problems can be resolved to some extent if an appropriate multi-disciplinary assessment of the person takes place in advance of the PCP and if the evidence of the service user's needs is presented clearly in the outcome of the assessment as it feeds in to the PCP process. The assessment should be truly collaborative so that each professional's expertise is brought to the support of the individual in a coordinated manner (Vlaskampf, 2005). If the nurse is the keyworker for the service user he or she will be in position to assess the validity of the inputs into the PCP process because he or she will know the service user better than any of the other members of the team. By deploying some of the strategies outlined in the section on communication above, the nurse may be in a position to cross-check these inputs. This exercise may improve both the holistic nature of the eventual plan that emerges from the process and also the chances of the PCP process tackling the service user's needs as he or she perceives them. In England personalised care is regarded as the lynchpin upon which good care planning and delivery hinge for people with complex needs (Department of Health, 2009); it is the nurse's challenge to realise this aim.

In the totality of the PCP process the nurse's role can be said to be primarily one of skilled advocate whereby nurses advocate for the service users on the basis that they have listened and achieved a thorough understanding of the service users' needs, wishes, preferences and the conditions that constitute a high quality of life. The nurse should then translate these understandings into concrete inputs in the PCP process and subsequently facilitate the carrying out of the plan. This is important in that so many plans are 'notional or aspirational' (Mansell and Beadle-Brown, 2004b: 32) and become paper exercises. This delicate role has to be carried out by balancing nurses' obligations towards the service provider and their duty of care to act as an advocate for the service user. Kendrick (2004: 9) illustrates this point when he notes that professionals 'may recognise that their presence and possible dominance of the PCP process can be an issue if not properly subordinated to the higher goal and responsibility of keeping the person's needs and interests central'.

Quality of life

The aim of self-determination should be to establish the best possible quality of life for the person. According to Schalock (2004), current thinking on quality of life situates the debate in three areas: Firstly, economic rationalism and the allocation of resources to people with PMLD. Secondly, the disability reform movement, which emphasises the rapid emergence of the self-advocacy movement. The final aim is concerned with ascertaining which outcomes best provide evidence that services and supports for people with PMLD have really enhanced personal well-being.

Quality of life for people with PMLD has been shown to be a multi-dimensional construct that has five domains: physical well-being, material well-being, social well-being, development and activity, and emotional well-being (Felce and Perry, 1995: 53). These domains have been examined for their relevance to people with PMLD by Petry et al (2005). They interviewed 76 parents and direct support staff who validated the application of these domains to this group. However, the researchers also found that the sub-domains differed somewhat. For instance, emphasis was placed on hygiene, nourishment, rest, technical aids, communication, basic security and individual attention. Less important were some of the sub-domains that applied to the homogeneous population with learning disability, these included 'fitness, personal safety, finance and income, stress, mental health, sexuality and faith' (Petry et al, 2005: 44). Petry et al (2005) also note that they are developing a procedure for evaluating the quality of life of people with PMLD and this is a development that nurses should await with interest.

Conclusion

This chapter has examined nursing care for persons with PMLD and given an overview of the key areas to be considered in the assessment and planning of care for persons with PMLD. The nursing practice involved in caring for this client group has been discussed. It is suggested that the skills nurses possess are deeply rooted in nurses' humanity. How nurses exercise their practice flows from the way that they conceive the personhood of the other. The validity of this assertion can be judged by some of the more troubling actions or inactions that nurses have engaged in during the 20th century and indeed the quote at the start of this chapter which reflects this point of view.

In the light of the subjects that have been discussed in this chapter the following recommendations are made:

- Good nursing practice should be based on a holistic nursing assessment of the person with PMLD.
- Assessment should provide the basis for development of care plans that support the highest quality of life for the person with PMLD.
- Communication will always be a central issue of consideration for persons with PMLD as it lies at the heart of nursing people with intellectual disabilities. It is therefore important that the nurse should make understanding of the service user's communication a priority.
- New developments in supporting people with PMLD occur constantly, nurses should be aware of these and incorporate those that are supported by the evidence into their practice. Furthermore, as highly skilled practitioners, nurses have a responsibility to share this learning with others with whom they work.

In conclusion, the nurse's role is to facilitate a life for the person with a disability that is fulfilling and to support people with PMLD to envision and to realise the same possibilities in their life as everyone else (Department of Health, 2009). This chapter has pointed in various ways to different aspects of what can be broadly classed as good nursing practice which has that aim. The authors have also attempted to offer certain incitements in this chapter that may collectively act as a catalyst for thought and reflection by nurses who work with this inspiring client group and that enable nurses to support service users in achieving the life they wish for.

References

Anonymous (1990) *The Frontline of Learning Disability* **4:** 16–7

Barr O (2004) Nurses for people with learning disabilities within the

United Kingdom: An overview and some challenges for the future. *International Journal of Nursing in Intellectual and Developmental Disabilities* **1**(1): 5–10

Bollard M, Jukes M (1999) Specialist practitioner within community learning disability and the primary healthcare team. *Journal of Learning Disabilities for Nursing, Health and Social Care* **3**(1): 11–9

Boyd-Carson W (2003) Faecal incontinence in adults. *Nursing Standard* **18**(8): 45–51

Bush A, Beail N (2004) Risk factors for dementia in people with Down syndrome: Issues in assessment and diagnosis. *American Journal of Mental Retardation* **109**(2): 83–97

Crest (2004a). *A Model for Managing Enteral Tube Feeding*. Stormont. Crest Secretariat.

Crest (2004b). *Guidelines for the Management of Enteral Tube Feeding in Adults*. Stormont. Crest Secretariat.

Crossley R (1997). Remediation of communication problems through facilitated communication training: A case study. *European Journal of Disorders of Communication* **32:** 61–9

Crouch D (2002) What Valuing People really means. *Nursing Times* **99**(18): 38–9

Dagnan D, Lindsay WR (2004) Research issues in cognitive therapy. In: Emerson E, Hatton C, Thompson T, Parmenter TR (eds.) *The International Handbook of Applied Research in Intellectual Disabilities*. Wiley, Chichester

Deb S, Thomas M, Bright C (2001) Mental disorder in adults with intellectual disability: Prevalence of functional psychiatric illness among a community-based population aged between 16 and 64 years. *Journal of Intellectual Disability Research* **45:** 495–505

Department of Health (2001) *Valuing People: A New Strategy for Learning Disability for the 21st Century: Implementation*. HMSO, London

Department of Health (2002a) *Policy and Guidance: Learning Disability*. Available from http://www.dh.gov.uk/PolicyAndGuidance/ HealthAndSocialCareTopics/LearningDisabilities/FactsAndFigures/ fs/en?CONTENT_ID=4001882&chk=MFHYV8 [accessed on 2 November 2006]

Department of Health (2002b) *Action for Health – Health Action Plans and Health Facilitation. Detailed Good Practice Guidance on Implementation for Learning Disability Partnership Boards*. Stationary Office, London

Department of Health (2009). Valuing People Now: a new three-year strategy for people with learning disabilities. HMSO, London

Department of Health and Social Security (1971) *Better Services for the Mentally Handicapped*. HMSO, London

Department of Health, Social Services and Public Safety (2004) *Equal Lives: Review of Policy and Services for People With Learning Disabilities in Northern Ireland*. Stormont, Belfast

Emerson E, Hatton C, Felce D (2001) *Learning Disabilities: The Fundamental Facts*. Mental Health Foundation, London

Felce D, Perry J (1995) Quality of life: Its definition and measurement. *Research in Developmental Disabilities* **16:** 51–74

Fenton SJ, Perlman S, Turner H (2003) *Oral Health Care for People with Special Needs: Guidelines for Comprehensive Care*. River Edge, New Jersey

Ferguson DL, Baumgart D (1991) Partial participation revisited. *Journal of the Association for Persons with Severe Handicaps* **16:** 218–27

Foundation for People with Learning Disabilities (2005) Available rom: http://www.learningdisabilities.org.uk/page.cfm. [accessed 28 June 2005]

Gates B (2003) *Learning Disabilities: Toward Inclusion*. 4th Edn. London. Churchill Livingstone.

Gates B (2006) *Care Planning and Delivery in Intellectual Disability Nursing*. Blackwell Publishing, Oxford

Gates B (2007) *Learning Disabilities: Toward Inclusion*. 5th Edn. London. Churchill Livingstone.

Government of Ireland (1998) *Report of the Commission on Nursing – A Blueprint for the Future*. Stationary Office, Dublin

Government of Ireland (2005) *The Disability Act*. Stationary Office, Dublin

Gravelle A (1997) Caring for a child with a progressive illness during the complex, chronic phase. *Journal of Advanced Nursing* **25:** 738–45

Gray M (2006) Practical ways of involving users in everyday planning. In: Jukes M, Aldridge J (eds.) *Person-Centred Practices. A Therapeutic Perspective*. Quay books, London

Grove N, Bunning K, Porter J (2001) Interpreting the meaning of behaviour by people with intellectual disabilities. Theoretical and methodological issues. In: Columbus F (ed.) *Advances in Psychology Research* Vol 7. Nova Science, New York

Grove N, Bunning K, Porter J, Olsson C (1999) See what I mean:

Interpreting the meaning of communication by people with severe and profound intellectual disabilities. *Journal of Applied Research in Intellectual Disabilities* **12:** 18–27

Grove N, Park K (1996) *Odyssey Now*. Jessica Kingsley, London

Hastings RP, Taunt HM (2003) Positive Perceptions in Families of Children with Developmental Disabilities. *American Journal on Mental Retardation* **107**(2): 116–27

Jackson R (2004) Music: Fun, Relaxation, training or Therapy? *The Frontline of Learning Disability* **60:** 26–8

Jukes M (1996) Advanced practice within learning disability nursing. *British Journal of Nursing* **5**(5): 293–8

Kelly F, Kelly C, Craig S (2007). *Annual Report of the National Intellectual Disability Database Committee 2007*. Dublin. Health Research Board.

Kendrick M (2004) Some predictable cautions concerning the over-emphasis and over-reliance on person-centred planning. *The Frontline of Learning Disability* **58:** 8–9

Kobe FH, Mulick JA, Rash TA, Martin J (1994) Nonambulatory persons with profound mental retardation: Physical, developmental and behavioural characteristics. *Research in Developmental Disabilities* **15**(6): 413–23

Lacey P (2000) Meeting complex needs through collaborative multidisciplinary teamwork. In: Lacey P, Ouvry C (eds.) *People With Profound and Multiple Learning Disabilities. A Collaborative Approach to Meeting Complex Needs*. David Fulton, London

Lacey P, Ouvry C (2001) *People with Profound and Multiple Learning Disabilities. A Collaborative Approach to Meeting Complex Needs*. David Fulton, London

Leyshon S, Clark L, Epstein L, Higgins S (2004) Caring for people with learning disability using care management. *British Journal of Nursing* **13**(14): 845–7

Lindgren CL (1990) Burnout and social support in family caregivers. *Western Journal of Nursing Research* **12**(4): 469–87

Mansell J, Beadle-Brown J (2004a) Person-centred planning or person centred action? Policy and practice in intellectual disability services. *Journal of Applied Research in Intellectual Disabilities* **17:** 31–5

Mansell J, Beadle-Brown J (2004b) Person-centred planning or person centred action? A response to the commentaries. *Journal of Applied Research in Intellectual Disabilities* **17:** 1–9

Markwick A, Parrish A (2003) *Learning Disabilities Themes and Perspectives*. Elsevier, UK

Marston GM, Perry DW, Roy A (1997) Manifestations of depression in people with intellectual disability. *Journal of Intellectual Disability Research* **41**(6): 476–80

Matthews D (1996) *The OK Health Check*. Fairfield, Preston

Matthews D (2004) *The 'OK' Health Check: Health Facilitation and Health Action Planning*. 3rd Edn. Fairfield Publications, Preston

Mitchell JR, Van der Gaag A (2002) Through the eye of the cyclops: Evaluating a multi-sensory programme for people with complex disabilities. *British Journal of Learning Disabilities* **30**: 159–65

National Assembly for Wales (2002a) *Fulfilling the Promises: Proposals for Services for People with Learning Disabilities. Consultation Documents*. National Assembly for Wales, Cardiff

Neufeld SM, Query B, Drummond JE (2001) Respite care users who have children with chronic conditions: Are they getting a break? *Journal of Pediatric Nursing* **16**(4): 234–44

Nind M, Hewett D (2001) *A Practical Guide to Intensive Interaction*. British Institute of Learning Disabilities, Kidderminster

Northway R, Hutchinson C, Kingdon A (2006) *Shaping the Future: A Vision for Learning Disability Nursing*. UK Learning Disability Consultant Nurse Network, United Kingdom

Novaco RW, Taylor JL (2004) Assessment of anger and aggression in male offenders with developmental disabilities. *Psychological Assessment* **16**: 42–50

O'Brien J, Tyne A (1981) *The Principle of Normalisation: A Foundation for Effective Services*. CMH, London

Oswin M (1978) *Children Living in Long-Stay Hospitals*. Heinemann, London

Patterson J (1995) Promoting resilience in families experiencing stress. *Pediatric Clinics of North America* **42**(1): 47–63

Petry K, Maes B, Vlaskamp C (2005) Domains of quality of life of people with profound multiple disabilities: The perspective of parents and direct support staff. *Journal of Applied Research in Intellectual Disabilities* **18**: 35–46

Ponsky JL, Gauderer M (1989) Percutaneous endoscopic gastrostomy: Indication, limitations, techniques and results. *World Journal of Surgery* **13**: 165–70

Porter J, Ouvry C (2001) Interpreting the communication of people with profound and multiple learning difficulties. *British Journal of Learning Disabilities* **29:** 12–6

Priest H, Gibbs M (2004) *Mental Health Care for People with Learning Disabilities*. Churchill Livingstone, London

Quigley A, Murray G, McKenzie K, Elliot G (2001) Staff knowledge about symptoms of mental health problems in people with learning disabilities. *Journal of Learning Disabilities* **5**(3): 235–44

Raghavan R, Patel P (2005) *Learning Disabilities and Mental Health. A Nursing Perspective*. Blackwell Publishing Ltd, Oxford

Russell L (2001) The importance of patients' nutritional status in wound healing. *British Journal of Nursing* **10**(6): 42–7

Sanderson H, Harrison J, Price S (1991) *Aromatherapy and Massage for People with Learning Difficulties*. Hands On Publishing, Birmingham

Schalock RL (2004) The concept of quality of life: What we know and do not know. *Journal of Intellectual Disability Research* **48**(3): 203–16

Scottish Executive (2000) *The Same As You? A Review Of Services for People sith Learning Disabilities*. The Stationary Office, Edinburgh

Sox HF (2004) *Care Plans: Comprehensive Care Planning for Long Term Care Facilities: A Guide to Resident Assessment Protocols (RAPS) and Interdisciplinary Care Plans*. Vol 1. Robin Technologies, Ohio

Stanley R (1997) Treatment of continence in people with learning disabilities: 3. *British Journal of Nursing* **6**(1): 12, 14, 16

Stromme P, Diseth TH (2000) Prevalence of psychiatric diagnoses in children with mental retardation: Data from a population based study. *Developmental Medicine and Child Neurology* **42:** 266–70

Tait T, Genders N (2002) *Caring for People With Learning Disability*. Hodder Arnold, London

Timmins F, McCabe C, Griffiths C, Gleeson M, O'Shea J (2005) Lessons from practice – reflecting on communication across the nursing disciplines. The 2005 International Nursing Research Conference of the RCN. Belfast 8–11 March

Todd V, Van Rosendaal G, Duregen K, Verhoef M (2005) Percutaneous endoscopic gastrostomy: The role and perspective of nurses. *Journal of Clinical Nursing* **14**(2): 187–94

Tonge B, Einfeld S, Krupinski J, Mackenzie A, McLaughlin M, Florio T (1996) The use of factor analysis for ascertaining patterns of psychopathology in children with intellectual disability. *Journal of Intellectual Disability Research* **40:** 198–207

Vlaskampf C (2005) Interdisciplinary assessment of people with profound intellectual and multiple disabilities. In: Hogg J, Langa A (eds.) *Assessing Adults with Intellectual Disabilities: A Service Provider's Guide*. Blackwell, Oxford

Waterlow J (1992) *The Waterlow Scale*. Newlands, Taunton

Williams B (1989) Communication, Control and Choice. Available from: http://www.nrec.org/synapse32/williams.html [accessed 3 June 2005]

Wolfensberger W (1972) *The Principle of Normalisation in Human Management Services*. National Institute of Mental Retardation, Toronto

CHAPTER 10

Mental health and learning disability

Dave Ferguson

Introduction

Mainstream, as well as specialist health and social care services, have undergone significant changes in the UK over recent decades (Gravestock, 1999). Learning disability hospitals are more or less closed, the use of mainstream services is the goal of inclusion strategies (Department of Health, 2001), and the development of a range of specialist services models, working alongside mainstream services, are promoted (and sometimes contested) as an appropriate service response to people who have a learning disability and mental health need (Piachaud, 1999).

Priest and Gibbs (2004) suggest that an effective service can only be successful if it is founded on nationally agreed policies. A contemporary mental health service for people who have a learning disability should have its roots in mainstream services but we must also recognise the important role that specialist learning disability services play and indeed the role of the learning disability nurse, not only in providing care for these individuals but also in educating mainstream providers and family or paid carers.

However, with the merger of some NHS trusts, the challenges facing learning disability services are both similar to and different from general adult mental health services. A similar challenge that faces both services is the modernisation of the NHS, which aims to improve the quality of life for people with a learning disability and for people who have mental health needs. A different challenge for learning disability services however, is that organisational boundaries do not hinder access to essential expertise and support (Hollins and Courtenay, 2000).

The focus of this chapter is twofold – to discuss service model responses to governmental policy concerning the mental health needs of people with a learning disability and, secondly, to discuss the role of the learning disability nurse as mental health specialist.

Service model responses

In some areas of England, service responses to people who have a learning disability and mental health need have underdeveloped partnerships and joint approaches. A systematic approach to developing services is required (Simpson, 1997) and a general consensus must emerge to determine the necessary service model responses, components and responsibilities of mainstream adult mental health and specialist learning disability services when responding to this significant group of individuals.

Perceptions concerning the difficulties people who have a learning disability and mental health need have affected the delivery of services required to meet individual need (Reiss, 2001) and today it would still seem that mental illness is overshadowed by the primary diagnosis of learning disability.

In my experience, when service users have needs that require the input of more than one service, they are often at risk of being excluded by most of the services that they require. People with learning disabilities and additional mental illness are known to be excluded, in many instances, from accessing mainstream services because they may not meet the eligibility criteria of having a severe and enduring mental illness.

Xenitidis et al (2004) consider the implications of meeting the needs of this specific client group in their research into generic and specialist (learning disability) units. They sampled service users across three London boroughs that used either generic psychiatric in-patient services or specialist learning disability in-patient services. The research study followed a comparative descriptive study of all patients admitted to a specialist unit and those admitted into general psychiatric wards and an evaluative study of immediate outcome of in-patient treatment in the specialist unit.

The conclusion from this research was that where there was a need to admit a service user into an in-patient facility, those who were admitted into a specialist learning disability facility showed significant improvements on a number of outcomes such as psychopathology, global level of functioning, behavioural distress and severity of mental illness.

Similarly, Alexander et al (2001) compared two models of in-patient services for people who have a learning disability and mental illness – the specialist learning disability in-patient service model and the mainstream mental health model. Their preliminary findings have suggested that there were differences in the profiles of those who used the services; the specialist learning disability provision attracted more people with severe learning disabilities and pervasive developmental disorders whereas the mainstream provision attracted more individuals with mild learning disability.

So one could assume from this study that not one service can meet the needs of this client group. Perhaps, then, both approaches to service delivery will be necessary.

Although staff training and experience in the mental health needs of people who have a learning disability are not identified specifically in the paper by Xenitidis et al (2004), the reason for the significant improvements in those people admitted into a specialist in-patient facility would appear to suggest a workforce with specialist skills and knowledge when working with this specific client group, therefore making the patient experience a more positive one for all concerned.

The knowledge and skills of staff in the assessment and treatment of mental health in learning disability would appear to be a crucial consideration in whether a service model is successful or not in meeting the specific mental health needs of this client group. Kwok (2001) suggests that in general psychiatric wards there are inadequate opportunities for staff to gain experience of working with this specific client group and yet on the other hand it could be suggested that it is vital that staff have the expertise to accurately diagnose mental illness in people who have a learning disability and are able to provide the (often) adapted therapeutic interventions required in treating their illness.

So how does this apparent deficit meet the access and inclusion agendas about which the present Government are resolute?

Recently, a number of reports and Government policies have had a significant effect on the development of the service models used (Bouras et al, 2003). The present position is that people who have a learning disability should have access to mainstream health services but with additional support from specialist learning disability services when this is needed.

This has been recognised in the *Valuing People* (Department of Health, 2001) White Paper which states: 'Generic mental health services need to become more responsive, with specialist learning disability services providing facilitation and support.'

However, like Kwok (2001), Bouras and Holt (2001) also express concerns in relation to admitting adults with learning disabilities into general adult mental health wards. They suggest that staff often lack training and experience in the assessment and treatment of this client group and Kwok (2001) suggests that in some cases people who have a learning disability are often vulnerable to exploitation and abuse by more intellectually able and, at times, disturbed patients.

Moss et al (2000) claim that in the UK generic mental health services have often been unable to meet the mental health needs of people with learning disabilities and other authors suggest that, as a result, specialist psychiatric services are becoming an increasingly preferred option in many countries (Moloney, 1993; Day, 1994; Doyle, 2000).

It would appear from the literature that there are two specific service model responses that are captured in the national and international research, but these are at various stages of development:

- To develop specialist provision (in-patient and community).
- To secure generic services with the knowledge, skills and resources necessary to provide an effective service to those people with a learning disability and mental illness who are able to use them.

Learning disability specialist services are usually delivered in multi-disciplinary community teams. Introduced in the late 1970s they have survived a number of organisational changes and provide a comprehensive range of skills involving both health and social care workers (Hollins and Courtenay, 2000).

However, there is tension between the development and provision of specialist mental health services for the needs of what could be constituted as a minority, while not providing for the needs of the majority. Often, a final course of action is to admit the client into a generic mental health in-patient provision where their needs and difficulties can be misunderstood (Chaplin and Flynn, 2000).

Barlow (1999) claims that service delivery for this client group is often hampered with wrangling over responsibility for management and resource allocation and suggests that the solution to this lies in effective multi-agency collaboration. He argues that multi-disciplinary team working is the only way forward because the needs of this client group are too complex for one service provider to respond to effectively. In support of this, Gravestock (1999) suggests that local services should have agreed inter-agency and inter-professional service coverage when meeting the needs of this client group.

The key issue within the *Valuing People* White Paper would appear to concur with this and it suggests that the key to meeting the mental health needs of people who have a learning disability lies in the close collaboration required between adult mental health and learning disability services, with the provision of clear local protocols outlining joint working as well as the importance of care co-ordinators having expertise of both mental health and learning disabilities. *Valuing People* also comments that each local service should have access to an acute assessment and treatment resource for those people who have a significant learning disability (severe or profound) and mental health need who could not be admitted into general psychiatric in-patient areas, even without specialist learning disability support, due to the nature of their level of cognitive impairment.

Priest and Gibbs (2004) discuss policy and guidance documents that address the specific needs of this client group. These consist of psychiatric services for children and adolescents with learning disabilities (Royal College of Psychiatrists, 1998) and the *Count Us In* report (Foundation for People with Learning Disabilities, 2002). In addition the inclusion agenda promoted by *Valuing People* and the report by the Valuing People Support

Team (2002) means the needs of people with learning disabilities should be included in all relevant policies that guide service development.

From an ideological and philosophical perspective the literature reviewed would suggest that the service model delivered will reflect the way in which mental health needs for people who have a learning disability are conceptualised (Lindsey, 2000). Indeed, there has been a historical shift from institutionalised care to community services, and the changing of public opinion and attitudes has been a key player in accepting people with learning disabilities into the mainstream of local communities; but this acceptance is variable across Europe (Day, 1995; Holt et al, 2000).

The basis for the argument for generic service provision lies in the philosophy of normalisation which promotes the view that all people who have a learning disability should be exposed to the culturally normative experiences of the society in which they live (Priest and Gibbs, 2004: 170), this includes receiving generic services available to the rest of the population and there is increasing support for this.

However, there is also a considerable counter-argument that, whether through default or design (Priest and Gibbs, 2004), mainstream mental health services cannot totally meet the needs of this client group (Day, 1995).

Chaplin (2004) suggests that while *Valuing People* spells changes in patterns of service delivery with a greater emphasis on the use of mainstream services whenever possible, increased staff training and support are required as well as the involvement of mainstream mental health services in the planning process to avoid negative attitudes and a perception of being deskilled.

Mental health service evaluation

The Green Light Toolkit for Mental Health (Department of Health, 2004) is a joint initiative by the National Institute for Mental Health in England (NIMHE) and the Valuing People Support Team (VPST).

The toolkit has been designed as a multi-service self-assessment for improving mental health support services for people with learning disabilities. It makes suggestions, based upon evidence in practice, of what good mental health support services for people with learning disabilities look like, and suggests ways of assessing how well local services measure up to it.

Within the document the term 'mental health support services' is used as it claims that support for people with learning disabilities with their mental health is not the exclusive responsibility of just one service. People may get support from primary care services, mental health services, learning disability services, public and voluntary sector services, and others. This document is therefore concerned with what all of those services can do to improve mental health support for people with learning disabilities.

If implemented locally, the Green Light Toolkit will go a long way, I believe, in addressing some of the concerns already expressed in some of the literature examined. It will also be an essential resource for commissioners, service providers, service users and their carers and other stakeholders to work in partnership to deliver a high quality service to this client group.

Person-centred approaches

Person-centred approaches will ensure individualised quality of care is at the very heart of mental health in learning disability services. People with mental health problems who have learning disabilities, whose support is co-ordinated through the care programme approach (CPA), must also be offered the opportunity to develop a person-centred plan (PCP). In essence the CPA should come from the PCP.

Both mental health and learning disability policy highlight the importance of good individual planning and coordination so that people receive services and support to match their needs. The CPA is the framework for co-ordinating support and treatment for people receiving secondary mental health services. CPA encompasses care management, i.e. there is a single assessment process that provides access to both health and social services support. People with learning disabilities who are receiving support from specialist mental health services, are required to be on the CPA, and it applies to people regardless of setting (Kingdon, 2004).

Therefore, the challenge that faces both mental health and learning disability services is to develop a person-centred care plan with an individual that also meets the requirements of the CPA. To be effective, person-centred planning approaches require a transfer of power from services to client. It is not the same as assessment and care planning, but it can add to its quality and effectiveness. It can help get the plans right for people and is now seen as a central characteristic of quality service provision.

One of the challenges of the modernisation, inclusion and access agendas is working out how best to use all the resources, human, environmental and financial, within the specialist learning disability and generic mental health services, to provide services that 'fit' with the principles of the *National Service Framework for Mental Health* (Department of Health, 1999) and *Valuing People* (Department of Health, 2001).

Based upon the two service model options (mentioned earlier in this chapter) that are consistently discussed in the literature, it would seem logical to not only consider these two evidence-focused models as service model responses in more detail, but to also be much more radical and create a service model that is not only responsive to the dual diagnoses of learning disability and mental illness but also to the modernisation, access and inclusion agendas which underpin the *National Service Framework for Mental Health* and *Valuing People*.

There is an exciting opportunity to develop a service model that delivers a person-centred, high quality mental health service to people who have a learning disability. A model that recognises that some people may need to access specialist learning disability services and, for others, mainstream services, or both.

Indeed from the literature reviewed so far, it would appear that from an ideological perspective, responding to individual need is more important than having one prescribed service model response. However, the agenda for service provision is clear:

- Include and address the needs of people with learning disabilities within mainstream mental health provision.
- Deliver integrated mental health support services to people with learning disabilities.

Specialist role of the learning disability nurse

A significant number of people with learning disabilities are likely to experience mental health problems at some time in their lives. As a result they and their families will require accurate assessment, diagnosis, treatment and care. However, apart from psychiatry, there are not a vast number of skilled professionals in the field of learning disability who can carry out detailed mental health assessments and implement mental health care to this client group. Although there is increasing interest from the range of professionals working in the field, nursing would appear to be leading these developments.

The breadth and depth of nursing practice is varied and, as a body, learning disability nurses have all the core skills that are used in the day-to-day work of meeting the healthcare needs of users. However, some will acquire further knowledge and skills in specific areas of practice, such as mental health, and as a result will apply knowledge and skills in a unique way in the areas in which they work.

Evolution of the role

Learning disability nursing has undergone significant changes over many years and has evolved into a health-focused role.

Norman (1998) suggests that the role of psychiatric and learning disability nurses has been under scrutiny since the closure of long-stay institutionalised care. This has perhaps occurred over the last decade in a way that did not occur when most nursing care was hospital based. Specific policy directions have certainly had an influence on the role direction of these two disciplines (Department of Health, 1993, 2004, 2006; Kay et al, 1995).

Across the four countries of the UK, policies describe a holistic approach for supporting people with learning disabilities to reach their potential (Royal College of Nursing, 2006). These policies (Scottish Executive, 2000; National Assembly for Wales, 2001; Department of Health, 2001, 2005) focus upon similar concerns, including joint working between mainstream health services and specialist learning disability services particularly to improve access for people who have a learning disability, as well as mainstream staff receiving training in the needs of people with learning disabilities.

Moulster and Turnbull (2004) suggest that changes in governmental policy have had a major impact upon the role of the learning disability nurse and there are a number of descriptors of the profession which have changed over time. They suggest the purpose of learning disability nursing is to work in partnership with the individual to improve his or her personal autonomy. With the policy challenge of users and their carers having access to and effectively using mainstream service provision, learning disability nurses must continue to develop their specialist skills and knowledge, to use effectively the evidence base as well as consider their contribution to the evidence base through research activity.

Aldridge (2004) suggests that there are a range of practices used by learning disability nurses to promote the (mental) health, autonomy and social inclusion of people who have a learning disability. He adds that although learning disability nursing is a dynamic and varied professional activity, there is still the need to provide a clearly articulated and coherent framework for practice.

Interestingly, in relation to mental health practice, Gilbert et al (1998) and Raghavan and Patel (2005) suggest that learning disability nursing does not 'presently operate within a clear model of mental health'. Although that may, in some quarters, be true it could be argued that there are a number of models learning disability nurses can utilise within a multi-disciplinary context. Some are specifically developed for use with this client group (e.g. DASH-II: Matson, 1995; Mini PAS-ADD: Moss, 2002; LCDNS: Raghavan et al 2004; Aldridge and Ferguson, 2007) and in many areas nursing models are used within mental health practice (e.g. Peplau, 1991; Orem, 1995). It is how these models are applied by learning disability nurses to assess and respond to the mental health needs of individuals that highlights the specialist contribution they make.

Table 10.1 details with some nursing models and frameworks, assessments and classification systems learning disability nurses can access and use for mental health work.

Table 10.1. Nursing models and frameworks, assessments and classification systems

Nursing Models/frameworks	Assessments	Classification systems
Aldridge (2007)	CANDID (2003)	DC-LD (2001)
King (1981)	DASH-II (1995)	ICD-10 (1992)
Sands (1993)	LCDNS (2004)	
Orem (1995)	Mini PAS-ADD (2002)	
Peplau (1991)		

Towards the application of person-centred contemporary specialist learning disability nursing

Valuing People (Department of Health, 2001) and *Valuing People Now* (Department of Health, 2009) promote the principles of person-centred approaches when working with people with learning disabilities and supporting them in the planning of their care.

Ferguson et al (2006), cited in Blair et al (2008: 25), have defined learning disability nursing, they suggest

'It is the application of specialist knowledge of the causation and development of learning disability and its impact on the person's enjoyment of good health. Through the informed integration of professional and clinical judgement the nurse enables people who have learning disabilities to improve, maintain or recover health, to cope with health problems and to achieve the best quality of life.'

This definition clearly underlines the learning disability nurse as a specialist in learning disability and the importance of having a specialist professional qualification that centres on the principles of enabling an individual to lead an independent healthy life (Raghavan and Patel, 2005). This definition can be applied to all areas of clinical practice including mental health.

Gilbert et al (1998: 1155) suggest 'the skills and attitudes of the learning disability nurse make a considerable contribution to the mental health of people with learning disabilities'. Utilising the specialist knowledge and skills learning disability nurses possess enables them to identify, articulate and distinguish the underlying cause of specific conditions and the impact this will have upon an individual's mental health and vice versa. This will support the formulation of hypotheses to make specific diagnoses and ultimately improve the mental health status of individuals as key members of the multi-disciplinary team.

Gilbert et al (1998) also claim that mental health service practitioners do not have the necessary skills to meet the mental health needs of people who have a learning disability. There is therefore an opportunity for learning disability nurses to develop their knowledge and skills in this clinical area, as well as facilitate mental health practitioners to acquire the necessary knowledge and skills in this discrete area of practice. They suggest potential could be realised to establish a common ground between the discourses of learning disability nursing and those of psychiatric nursing, which could be related to the needs of this specific client group. However, the learning disability nurse should not replace the mental health practitioner and therefore deny individuals access to mainstream services if they are able to use them effectively.

Clearly learning disability nurses need to have good working knowledge and application of national and local policy and the impact this has upon their specific area of clinical practice. In the past few years policy developments have been more prescriptive:

- Scotland: *The Same as You: A Review of Services for People with Learning Disability* (Scottish Executive, 2000).
- England: *Valuing People: A New Strategy for Learning Disability in the 21st Century* (Department of Health, 2001), and *Valuing People Now: A New Three year Strategy for People with Learning Disabilities* (Department of Health, 2009).
- Wales: *Fulfilling the Promises: Report of the Learning Disability Advisory Group* (National Assembly for Wales, 2001).
- Northern Ireland: *Equal Lives: Review of Policy and Services for People with a Learning Disability* (Department of Health and Social Security, 2005).

These policies were briefly cited earlier in this chapter. However, learning disability nurses must consider the influence they have upon their roles and how they can influence the roles of others in maximising the mental health outcomes for this client group.

Nationally, learning disability nurses make a significant contribution to the assessment, formulation, diagnostic, therapeutic and evaluative processes. Learning disability nurses work with individuals with mental health needs in a variety of settings (e.g. primary care, mainstream mental health in-patient provision, specialist learning disability in-patient provision, assertive outreach teams, home treatment teams and community learning disability teams).

It is often the learning disability nurse who is at the forefront in detecting an individual who may have a mental health problem and will provide an extensive collection of evidence through nursing assessment to ascertain a person's mental health status. The learning disability nurse will need to understand and consider the evidence base (the reliability and validity) for the use of any assessment tool, and especially if they have been adapted, as some have been, from those used with the general population.

As the purpose of the assessment is to identify, articulate and discriminate specific difficulties in a person's life that may be causing physical or mental imbalance or indeed harm, the knowledge and skill of the learning disability nurse in the assessment process is paramount. Specific knowledge and skills would include:

- Articulating a holistic approach to assessment.
- Understanding the aetiology of the person's learning disability.
- Understanding the factors that may have contributed to the person's mental health status.
- Understanding how the person's learning disability has an impact upon his or her mental health and vice versa.
- Understanding and effectively applying standardised and adapted assessment tools.

From formulation through to diagnosis the learning disability nurse will be actively involved as a member of the multi-disciplinary team. The input learning disability nurses will contribute to the diagnostic process will require them to make clinical judgements derived from a systematic assessment process. Within this process, learning disability nurses will:

- Undertake mental health assessments including a detailed history.
- Assist in determining formulation, hypothesis(es) and diagnosis.
- Identify health need.
- Plan and deliver therapeutic interventions.
- Deliver mental health promotion/education to users and carers.
- Educate other professionals.
- Evaluate care.

The learning disability nurse as mental health promoter

As mentioned previously, the promotion of health is a key role for the learning disability nurse, and this includes mental health promotion. Learning disability nurses will work to promote, improve and protect the mental well-being of individuals. Indeed Raghavan and Patel (2005) suggest that 'in learning disability nursing the development of personal competence through teaching and empowerment is seen as an integral part of nursing practice'.

Mental health promotion is the first standard in the Department of Health's *National Service Framework for Mental Health* (1999). The standard states: 'Health and social services should promote mental health for all, working with individuals and communities, combating discrimination against people with mental health problems and promoting their social inclusion.' Therefore the present Government wants to ensure that mental health promotion materials and information about services are provided in accessible formats for people with learning disabilities, including those from minority ethnic communities (Department of Health, 2001).

Priest and Gibbs (2004) rightfully claim that there are many professional barriers which prevent effective mental health promotion for people with learning disabilities and there is evidence which indicates that, as their health needs are not adequately met by primary care services, this results in poor uptake of health promotion.

Mental health promotion is therefore an even more important role for the learning disability nurse as promoting and educating about mental health issues does place significant value for individuals and for their networks of support (Moss and Lee, 2001). Learning disability nurses are regularly involved in promoting mental health within primary and specialist services and there are a number of national initiatives wherein this is undertaken in partnership with primary care colleagues (Department of Health, 2004).

Nurse education (mental health in learning disability)

It is strongly suggested that there is a need for trained nurses specialising in learning disabilities who can work with users and carers in fighting health inequalities (Raghavan and Patel, 2005) and this is evident within mental health practice.

In their research concerning educational preparation, Alaszewski et al (2001) examined the role of learning disability nurses within multi-professional and multi-agency teams. Although they found that there were overlaps in role with other members of the multi-disciplinary team, they also found that major changes in the role of learning disability nurses had occurred from the provision of support and care within hospital settings to the provision of diverse roles and activities.

A large number of learning disability nurses have received very little formal mental health training in pre-registration education (Haut et al, 2000). Wallace (2002) queries the ability of learning disability nurses to identify signs indicative of mental illness which are derived through the pre-registration curricula.

The aim of any pre-registration curricula must be to prepare students to meet Nursing and Midwifery Council (2004) requirements for registration to a standard that makes them suitable for employment. Therefore education programmes must continue to be health focused. Gibbs and Priest (1999) suggest that within common foundation programmes, the bio-psycho-social needs of people with mental health and learning disability need to be addressed within the social context of where they live. However, although learning disability nurses have a key role in the care of people with mental health needs, the time allocated to explore the impact of one condition on another is limited.

Although some learning disability pre-registration nurse programmes include some mental health-related issues, on the whole these would appear to be marginalised to a limited number of sessions. It is therefore often the role of the mentor in practice to facilitate insights for the student into the mental health needs of people with a learning disability with opportunities to experience and undertake supervised practice.

It would appear that the majority of learning disability nurses gain further knowledge and skills acquisition through attendance at further education sessions (Priest and Gibbs, 2004). Nationally there are only a small number of higher education institutions offering academic qualifications in mental health in learning disability, e.g. MSc and Post-Graduate Diploma in Mental Health Studies (Learning Disabilities) Kings College, London.

Conclusion

This chapter began by describing the current policy concerning service model responses to people who have a learning disability and who experience mental health problems. The debate concerning how or why individuals should access either mainstream mental health services or learning disability services, or a mixture of both, will continue as further research and service evaluation demonstrate the health outcome for the user.

The challenge for learning disability nurses within contemporary services is to continue to develop, articulate and apply their specialist skills and knowledge when working with the mental health needs of individual service users.

Learning disability nurses are not only the largest professional group working within learning disability services but the only professional group who are trained exclusively to work with this client group. As members of the multi-disciplinary team, they are pivotal in identifying, articulating and responding to the mental health needs of this specific client group.

References

Alaszewski A, Gates B, Motherby E, Manthorpe J, Ayer S (2001) *Educational Preparation for Learning Disability Nursing: Outcomes Evaluation of the Contribution of Learning Disability Nurses Within the Multi-Professional, Multi-Agency Team*. English National Board, London

Aldridge J. (2004). Learning disability nursing: A model for practice. In Turnbull J (cd.) *Learning Disability Nursing*, Chapter 13. Blackwell Publishing: 169

Aldridge J, Ferguson D (2007). The ecology of mental health framework. In Jukes M, Aldridge J (eds.). *Person-centred practices: a holistic and integrated approach*, London, Quay Books, pp 91–123

Alexander RT, Piachaud J, Singh I (2001) Two districts, two models: In-patient care in the psychiatry of learning disabilities. *British Journal of Developmental Disabilities* **47**(2): 105–10

Barlow C (1999) Issues in the management of clients with the dual diagnosis of learning disability and mental illness. *Journal of Learning Disabilities for Nursing, Health and Social Care* **3**(3): 159–62

Belfast: DHSSPS IN Royal College of Nursing. (2006). Meeting the health needs of people with learning disabilities: guidance for nursing staff, p. 8, Royal College of Nursing, London.

Bouras N, Holt G (2001) Community mental health services for adults with learning disabilities. In: Thornicroft G, Szmukler G eds. *Textbook of Common Psychiatry*. Oxford University Press, London: 397–407

Bouras N, Holt G, Jones M, Ditchfield H, Spiller MJ (2003) *Services for people with learning disabilities and mental disorders: working paper 1*. Estia Centre: 4

Chaplin R (2004) General psychiatric services for adults with intellectual disability and mental illness. *Journal of Intellectual Disability Research* **48**(1) 1–10

Chaplin R, Flynn A (2000) Adults with learning disability admitted to psychiatric wards. *Advances in Psychiatric Treatment* **6**: 128–34

Day K (1995) Psychiatric services in mental retardation: generic or specialised provision? In: Bouras N ed. *Mental Health in Mental Retardation*. Cambridge University Press: 275–92

Department of Health (1999) *National Service Framework for Mental Health*. DoH, London

Department of Health (2001) *Valuing People: a new strategy for learning disability for the 21st century*. DoH, London

Department of Health (1993) *Challenging Behaviours and/or Mental Health Needs of People with Learning Disabilities.* HMSO, London

Department of Health (2004) *Green light for mental health: how good are your mental health services for people with learning disabilities? A service improvement toolkit.* HMSO, London

Department of Health (2006) *From values to action: the chief nursing officer's review of mental health nursing.* DoH, London: 1–78

Department of Health. (2007). Good practice in learning disability nursing, Department of Health, London.

Department of Health (2009) Valuing People Now: a new three year strategy for people with learning disabilities, Department of Health, London.

Department of Health and Social Security (2005) Equal lives: review of policy and services for people with a learning disability in Northern Ireland, Belfast: DHSSPS IN Royal College of Nursing. (2006). Meeting the health needs of people with learning disabilities: guidance for nursing staff, p. 8, Royal College of Nursing, London.

Doyle J (2000) The dual diagnosis facility: a renewed engagement with the psychiatry of intellectual disability? *Contemporary Nurse* **9**(1): 62–70

Ferguson D, Howard F, Trenowden N (2006) Directory of learning disability nursing. Cited in Blair J, Bollard M, Ferguson D, Trenowden, N. (2008) Health for all? *Learning Disability Today*, **September**: 25

Foundation for People with Learning Disabilities. (2002). Count Us In: the Report of the Committee of Inquiry into Meeting the Mental Health Needs of Young People with Learning Disabilities. Mental Health Foundation, London. Cited in Priest H, Gibbs M. (2004) *Mental Health Care for People with Learning Disabilities.* Churchill Livingstone, Edinburgh, 151

Gibbs M, Priest HM (1999) Designing and implementing a "dual diagnosis" module: A review of the literature and some preliminary findings. *Nurse Education Today* **19**: 357–63

Gilbert T, Todd M, Jackson N (1998) People with learning disabilities who also have mental health problems: practice issues and directions for learning disability nursing. *Journal of Advanced Nursing* **27**: 1151–7

Gravestock S (1999) Adults with learning disabilities and mental health needs: conceptual and service issues. *Tizard Learning Disability Review* **4**(2): 6–13

Haut F, Hull A, Irons A (2000) Learning disability nursing staff: a response to psychiatric teaching. *British Journal of Learning Disabilities* **28**: 154–6

Hollins S, Courtenay K (2000) Issues and dilemmas for learning disability community psychiatric services. *The Mental Health Review* **5**(2): 26–9

Holt G, Costello H, Bouras N, Diareme S, Hillery J, Moss S, Rodriguez-Blazquez C, Salvador L, Tsiantis J, Weber G, Dimitrakaki C (2000) BIOMED-MEROPE* project: service provision for adults with intellectual disability: a European comparison. *Journal of Intellectual Disability Research* **44**(6): 685–96

Howard F, Trenowden N (2003) *Competencies for learning disability nursing*. Surrey and Hampshire Borders NHS Trust, Unpublished

Kay B, Rose S, Turnbull J (1995) *Continuing the Commitment: The report of the learning disability nursing project*. Department of Health, London

King, I.M. (1981). The theory of nursing: systems, concepts and process, New York: John Wiley Kingdon A (2004) Person centred planning and the care programme approach. *Learning Disability Practice* **7**(7): 14–5

Kwok HWM (2001) Development of a specialised psychiatric service for people with learning disabilities and mental health problems: report of a project from Kwai Chung Hospital, Hong Kong. *British Journal of Learning Disabilities* **29**: 22–5

National Assembly for Wales (2001) *Fulfilling the Promises: Report of the Learning Disability Advisory Group*. Cardiff: National Assembly for Wales.

Lindsey M (2000) Services for people with learning disabilities and mental health problems. *Mental Health Review* **5**(2): 5–14

Matson JL (1995) *The Diagnostic Assessment for the Severely Handicapped 11*. Scientific Publishers, Baton Rouge

Moloney H (1993) Mental health services for people with intellectual disability: Current developments. *Australian Journal of Public Health* **18**: 169–76

Moss S (2002) *The Mini PAS-ADD Interview Pack*. Estia Centre/Pavilion

Moss S, Bouras N, Holt G (2000) Mental health services for people with intellectual disability: A conceptual framework. *Journal of Intellectual Disability Research* **44**: 97–107

Moss S, Lee P (2001) Mental health. In: Thompson J, Pickering S (eds.) *Meeting the Health Needs of People who Have a Learning Disability*. Chapter 13, 235–63

Moulster G, Turnbull J (2004) The purpose and practice of learning disability nursing. In Turnbull J (ed.) *Learning Disability Nursing*. Chapter 5, Blackwell Publishing, 57–63

Norman IJ (1998) Priorities for mental health and learning disability nurse education in the UK: A case study. *Journal of Clinical Nursing* **7**: 433–41

Nursing and Midwifery Council (2004) *Standards of Proficiency for Pre-Registration Nursing Education.* Nursing and Midwifery Council, London

Orem DE (1995) *Nursing: Concepts of Practice,* 5th edn. Mosby, St. Louis

Peplau H (1991) *Interpersonal Relationships in Nursing: A Conceptual Frame of Reference.* Springer, New York

Piachaud J (1999) Issues for mental health in learning disability services. *Tizard Learning Disability Review* **4**(2): 47–8

Priest H, Gibbs M (2004) *Mental Health Care for People with Learning Disabilities.* Churchill Livingstone, Edinburgh

Raghavan R, Marshall M, Lockwood A, Duggan L (2004) Assessing the needs of people with learning disabilities and mental illness: Development of the learning disability version of the Cardinal Needs schedule. *Journal of Intellectual Disability Research* **48**: 25–37

Raghavan R, Patel P (2005) Learning disability nursing. In Raghavan R, Patel P (eds.) *Learning Disabilities and Mental Health: A Nursing Perspective.* Chapter 6. Blackwell Publishing, 116–27

Reiss S (2001) Available from http://thearc.org/faqs/mimrqa.html [accessed 21 April 2006]

Royal College of Nursing (2003) *Defining Nursing.* Royal College of Nursing, London

Royal College of Nursing (2006) *Meeting the Health Needs of People with Learning Disabilities: Guidance for Nursing Staff.* Royal College of Nursing, London

Royal College of Psychiatrists (1998) *Psychiatric services for children and adolescents with learning disabilities. Council Report CR70.* Royal College of Psychiatrists, London

Royal College of Psychiatrists (2001) *DC-LD: Diagnostic Criteria for Psychiatric Disorders for Use with Adults with Learning Disabilities/ Mental Retardation,* Gaskell, London

Sands KS (1993) *Betty Neuman: The Neuman Systems Model.* Sage Publications.

Scottish Executive (2000) *The Same As You: A Review of Services for People with Learning Disability,* Edinburgh: Scottish Executive

Simpson N (1997). Developing mental health services for people with learning disabilities in England. *Tizard Learning Disability Review* **2**(2): 35–42

Valuing People Support Team (2002) *Improvement, Expansion and Reform – Ensuring that All Means All, Handy Hints for Primary Care Trusts and Strategic Health Authorities.* Department of Health, London

Wallace B (2002) Boxed in: The challenge of "dual diagnosis". *Learning Disability Practice* 5(4): 24–6

World Health Organisation (1992) *The ICD-10 Classification of Mental and Behavioural Disorders*, WHO, Geneva

Xenitidis K, Gratsa A, Bouras N, Hammond, Ditchfield H, Holt G, Martin J, Brooks D (2004) Psychiatric inpatient care for adults with intellectual disabilities: Generic or specialist units? *Journal of Intellectual Disability Research* 48(1): 11–8

Xenitidis K, Slade M, Thornicroft G, Bouras N (2003) *CANDID: Camberwell Assessment of Need for Adults with Developmental and Intellectual Disabilities.* Gaskell, London

CHAPTER 11

Challenging behaviour: The contribution of nurse specialists

Tony Osgood

Introduction

Modern behavioural approaches can result in significant short and medium term reductions in the severity of the behaviour. Learning Disability Partnership Boards should ensure that local services develop the competencies needed to provide treatment and support within the local area.

Valuing People (Department of Health, 2001:8.44)

The front line

When I was asked to write this chapter I spoke with a number of nurse colleagues. How does being a learning disability nurse (LDN) impact on what you might be expected to provide in regard to people with intellectual or developmental disabilities (IDD) who challenge the system (Lehr and Brown, 1996)? Fortunately, working in the NHS, there were plenty of nurses to question about their experiences.

One of the concerns many LDNs voiced was the issue of time constraints when dealing with challenging behaviour. Many examples of challenging behaviour occur in people with complex needs, and thorough assessment and understanding of all the influences on people can be very time-consuming. Behavioural interventions that are fit for purpose (effective, reliable, valid, and long-lasting) tend not to follow from hit-and-run consultations (British Psychological Society, 2004). Behavioural assessments are not simply a matter of ticking boxes, looking at contingency records and implementing off-the-shelf interventions. The specialist worker in behavioural issues requires more time to undertake this invariably complex work. Why? Because there are few quick and yet clinically effective and socially valid interventions for complex behaviours. Intervention tends to need to last for some time (Emerson, 2001).

One of the fundamental benefits nurse training offers is its emphasis upon reflection. What this chapter aims to do is reflect a little on current issues for nurses in regard to people with IDD who have a reputation for challenging behaviours; nurses who, in many cases, are at the frontline of implementing interventions in families, schools and services. The chapter provides a brief overview of some issues associated with the challenging behaviour LDNs might encounter. Behavioural issues are part of the LDNs professional life: between 5% and 15% of people with IDD may present with behaviour that is challenging (Emerson et al, 2001), and these behaviours tend to persist (Murphy et al, 1993). Challenging behaviours (for example, aggression, self-harm and self-injurious behaviour, damage to property and environment) are a major cause of stress to families and service staff (Rose, 1995) and have a high cost for funding agencies. People whose behaviour challenges others are often themselves neglected (Department of Health, 1993) and are one of the 'at risk' groups for experiencing restrictive or dangerous treatments and of being abused (Rusch et al, 1986).

Influences on practice

LDN practice is determined not just by education and skills, but also by the personal and professional values and service architecture (structure, culture, expectations, policy) surrounding them. LDN functions in the UK today are multi-faceted, despite the future of the profession having been under almost continual examination for some time (e.g. Kay et al, 1995; Mitchell, 2004). In response to an uncertain environment the LDN role has evolved specialisms, and practitioners have become assertive in their vision of themselves as a profession (e.g. Jukes and Bollard, 2003; Turnbull, 2004). A number of ecological niches have been filled by dedicated varieties although all have fundamentally developed from the principles of health enablement for vulnerable people (Chief Nursing Officers of the UK, 1991; Mobbs et al, 2002). One of the domains the LDN has often been considered to have experience and knowledge of is challenging behaviour (Stewart and Todd, 2001). With regard to challenging behaviour, LDN Diploma training should be considered an introduction to the topic only: specialist longitudinal training is required.

In England, perhaps the most influential recent document on LDN was *Valuing People* (Department of Health, 2001). This White Paper's guidance and aspirations have been generally welcomed, and its implementation-in-part has coincided with the move to more joined-up provision. *Valuing People* has many implications for the nursing role: there is a clear move toward facilitation, and today health promotion, education and collaboration with those providing support are at the heart of the LDN function. The LDN will continue to contribute to the development of a skilled social workforce as well as directly enabling individual's health support. *Valuing People* notes those people supporting individuals whose behaviour is challenging must not lose sight of the guiding principles of independence, choice, rights and inclusion.

Many LDNs work in residential provision, including assessment and treatment units, traditionally the bastion of the NHS but increasingly provided by private organisations. Assessment and treatment units have been criticised on a number of counts but their benefits have also been highlighted (Blunden and Allen, 1987; Newman and Emerson, 1991). Many LDNs also work within community teams, and historically, these have often not had the resources to commit to the prolonged periods of intensive support required when working with people whose behaviour challenges. Over the last two decades specialised peripatetic support teams have been established to provide support to people with IDD and those living or working with them in their home, learning or working environments. Many nurse specialists will find themselves either working within or closely alongside such peripatetic teams. A good deal of research into the effectiveness of challenging behaviour provision has been accumulated (Allen and Felce, 1999; Emerson et al, 1993, 1996) and a 'bed free' service option has been found to work well in some situations (McBrien, 1994), but it is likely such an approach does function best when other elements of a comprehensive service perform well. Peripatetic teams alone are not sufficient to ameliorate the impact of challenging behaviour in the longer term for all people, and comprehensive commissioning of an integrated model (outreach, 'in-patient') is clearly still required (Mansell, 2005).

Having noted that, peripatetic teams can bring about significant changes in severe challenging behaviour within natural settings (McGill, 2000), cost less than residential units (Magiure and Piersel, 1992; Allen and Lowe, 1995), improve the quality of life of service users (Toogood et al, 1994), and improve carer's skills and capacity (Davidson et al, 1995; Kushlick et al, 1997). However, peripatetic teams alone may not be able to prevent placement breakdowns and cannot compensate for fundamental deficiencies in IDD services or commissioning generally (Department of Health, 2007). LDNs who take on a specialist function require an array of clinical and personal skills. According to Allen and Felce (1999: 288):

Being a member of a specialist support team is a complex job, and one that requires staff to be good at hands-on work, to be able to remain calm under fire, to possess didactic/participative teaching skills, to be effective role models, to be experienced in group work, and to be effective behaviour analysts. This is not a readily occurring combination, and a considerable investment in training team members will therefore be required. Credibility, confidence and competence in high stress situations are generally of more value than academic qualifications.

Challenging behaviour

People with the catch-all label 'challenging behaviour' are as diverse as any randomly selected group: if we were to ask everyone with blonde hair to leave the Royal College of Nursing Conference we would find an eclectic group standing outside, with a range of interests, gifts, medical issues, views and dancing skills. In the same way, people with IDD are not a homogenous group; neither are people with the label of challenging behaviour.

Challenging behaviours range widely in how they look and in the environmental, psychological and biological processes underpinning them. The reason people engage in behaviours varies between and within individuals, therefore one approach to intervention should not be applied to all individuals who exhibit topographically similar challenging behaviour. In settings where a number of people whose behaviour challenges live or work, standard responses to everyone (for example, token economy) will be unlikely to meet everyone's best learning interests all the time. From this it is clear that the most important aspect of working with such behaviours is to understand why the individual person engages in the behaviour at a given time.

The definition of any given behaviour as 'challenging' tends to be influenced by its impact (Baker, 2002). Defining behaviour as challenging is influenced as much by the perceptions of people around the person as the behaviour itself (Zarkowska and Clements, 1994). We will come back to this point later. A good place for a busy LDN to start is to ask a straightforward question: Whose problem is it anyway? To define behaviour as an issue, consider:

- Is the behaviour itself or its severity inappropriate given a person's age and level of development?
- Is the behaviour dangerous either to the person or others?
- Does the behaviour constitute a significant obstacle by interfering with learning or by excluding the person from important opportunities?
- Does the behaviour cause significant stress to the lives of those who live and work with the person?
- Is the behaviour contrary to social norms? (Zarkowska and Clements, 1994).

The final point, of whether or not the behaviour is contrary to social norms, needs to be considered carefully. Conceptualising the phenomenon as partly a social construction supposes such behaviour may in reality be adaptive for the person, given their abilities and the understanding of the supporting environment: not all people might define withdrawing from activities as challenging, but some may well define it so. Who defines what is appropriate in some locations and not others? The decision to define behaviour as challenging needs careful consideration: a service provider may define a behaviour as challenging whereas the same thing may be interpreted by the LDN as an act of self-determination (complaining about a lack of the right kind of support). The idea of behaviour as (in part) a social construction in no way belittles the experiences of people facing daily the personal struggle of supporting an individual whose behaviour is challenging: such experiences are exhausting and frustrating, stressful and isolating. Watching someone you love or support hurt themselves or others is not easy to experience.

If we were to investigate the huge amount of research available and listen to experienced skilled practitioners, we would create a list such as the one reproduced in *Table 11.1*.

Effects of challenging behaviour

Seriously challenging behaviours may well impact on the physical, emotional and social well-being of the person and the people associated with that person. Serious self-injurious behaviour, for example, can result in

- infections
- malformation
- loss of sight or hearing
- neurological impairments
- death of the person

    while seriously aggressive behaviours may result in

- injury to others
- injury to the person him or herself as a result of defensive or restraining action of others.

But these immediate effects are only part of the story. The feelings of people working or living with people who challenge needs to be sensitively considered, as does how they account for the behaviour they experience. Behaviour is shaped by the responses received and inadvertent reinforcement can strengthen the behaviour our interventions are intended to reduce. Supporting individuals whose behaviour challenges is hard work, and the impact of the behaviour influences not only how people

---

Table 11.1. Some broad conclusions about challenging behaviour

- The reasons for similar looking behaviours appearing within individuals varies according to time, place and state (I jump up and groan when my leg cramps, I do the same when I see a smart young couple holding leaflets opening the garden gate; I raise my hand to be excused, you raise your hand to gain attention)
- Challenging behaviour as a category of human behaviour is a social construction (challenging behaviour does not lie within the person: people do not carry it around with them in a bag. Challenging behaviour is a feature of the interplay between the individual and the understanding and ability of the environment to respond to the needs of the person)
- Defining behaviour as challenging is usually a product of the behaviour's impact and the understanding of those around the person
- Challenging behaviours range widely in their appearance and the psychological and biological processes which underpin them: they have varied personal and social consequences
- Interventions reported as effective tend to be constructive (they teach a functionally equivalent replacement behaviour), socially valid (interventions deal with socially important issues in socially appropriate ways), and use low-aversive technology (avoiding punishers – as Donnellan and colleagues, 1988, note it is often more useful to reinforce the behaviour you want than to punish the behaviour you do not want), and meet the person's needs

---

conceptualise but how they respond to the behaviour (Noone et al, 2006). The use of mechanical restraints and protective devices can lead to muscular atrophy, demineralisation of the bones and shortening of tendons as well as other injuries. There is also the risk of degrading psychological treatments. People whose behaviour is considered challenging may also find themselves excluded and neglected and deprived of opportunities (Murphy, 1994).

People with long histories of behaviour considered challenging may find themselves regularly moving home, or in 'challenging behaviour' settings, because sometimes the view is taken that only specialist provision has the answer. Specialist provision is often robust and able to provide secure environments, but this is no guarantee of happiness or quality of life. Another effect is that of pathological thinking: if behaviour is persistent, it may be tempting to view it as inherently part of the person, and as such, we may overlook practical changes in how we organise the ecology that might reduce or alter the behaviour (McBrien and Felce, 1992). The over-prescription of medication has also been widely reported.

Influences on behaviour

Different professions may view the same behavioural event as meaning different things: a psychiatrist may interpret behaviour in one way (say, evidence of an internal emotional disorder), a psychologist another (depending upon which 'school' of psychology they have been trained within), a speech therapist a third (frustration due to communication deficits within the person and ecology), and an LDN may see physical issues as of paramount influence (feeling unwell, biological factors, etc.) when trying to account for incidents of challenging behaviour. All these perspectives may be useful in themselves but it is seldom the case that one conceptual model explains all. With LDNs often in co-ordinating or lead roles, listening to a myriad of theories or explanations accounting for certain behaviours is often a common experience. Behaviour is fluid and changing, and conceptually we often have to run to keep up with the 'behavioural stream' (Dillenburger et al, 1997) of evolving insights from applied research. The responsibility for working in the field of challenging behaviour does not reside with any single professional group but LDNs can bring skills to help in the valid and reliable assessment of complex situations when working in collaboration with other professionals.

With challenging behaviour, it does seem rare indeed to find a single simple cause in IDD regardless of what research may suggest (Durand and Crimmins, 1988). It tends to be a combination of factors (McGill et al, 1996), including biological variables (sensory, genetic, feeling unwell), social and environmental issues (learning opportunities, relationships, type of support), emotional factors (well-being, coping skills), and cognitive issues (problem solving, communication ability, skills), 'some of which are more important than others in individual cases' (Emerson et al, 1994: 6). Remember, challenging behaviour is not unique to people with IDD.

Biology

We cannot cite IQ as a causal predictor of challenging behaviour (Sigafoos et al, 2003), and neither can we cite gender, although certain forms of behaviour might be more prevalent in males. You do not have to be diagnosed as having IDD to be labelled with challenging behaviour, but the greater the impact of the IDD, the fewer the likely adaptive skills, and as the severity or impact of the intellectual and developmental disability increases we tend to see an increase in additional challenges, such as seizure disorders, physical issues, communication difficulties and so forth.

It has been established that the basic health needs of people with IDD have often not been wholly recognised and physical causes of 'distress' need to be thoroughly considered before reaching for your 80-page behavioural

Table 11.2. Health issues that may influence behaviour

- Seizure disorders
- Pain
- Infection
- Sleep disturbances
- General well-being
- Allergies
- Constipation

- Hunger
- Skin complaints
- Otitis media
- Sensory impairment
- Medication toxicity
- Rhinitis
- Ulcer, etc.

assessment protocol. Basic health screening and health facilitation is a vitally important area of work for LDNs working with individuals whose behaviour challenges. This is not to imply that just the presence of seizure activity will automatically predict challenging behaviour, but anything impacting upon physical well-being may influence people's ability to manage with demands and may affect emotional well-being. The mind, after all, is not something separate and distinct from the body. So while we need to consider physical issues as influencing behaviour, it may be wrong to suggest a causal role. As will be discussed later, physical well-being (and emotional well-being), might act as 'setting events' for behavioural incidents. *Table 11.2* provides an at-a-glance list of physical health issues that may influence people's behaviour.

Certain conditions are reported to have higher incidence of some behaviours than you would expect, and thus some conditions are considered to be risk factors for challenging behaviour. These gene–behaviour correlations are studied as behavioural phenotypes. Examples include Lesch-Nyhan, Cornelia de Lange, and Smith-Magenis syndromes. Although rare, there are over 750 genetic conditions described, and it is likely that, as our understanding increases, we will identify more and, with this, describe apparent correlations with functioning and behaviour. Some behaviours do seem related to certain conditions (Prader-Willi with hyperphagia and food ideation; Down syndrome and autism with better visual than auditory receptive abilities; Rett syndrome with 'hand wringing' stereotypic movements, etc.). However, we are moving from a model known as total specificity, which suggests behavioural phenotypes result in specific behaviour in specific conditions (condition X always results in behaviour K and you seldom see behaviour K in any other circumstances) (Flynt and Yule, 1994), toward a probabilistic, partial specificity model (Hodapp, 1997), where the presence of certain genetic omissions, translocations, repeats, etc, result in the probable increase of certain characteristics, including certain patterns of behaviour. Simply put, many, but not all people with a given condition will show a behaviour, and people with the specific condition show variations in the behaviour, and not everyone with the condition tend to show all the characteristic behaviours. Not everybody with these conditions shows challenging behaviour, in the same way that not everyone with the condition of 'humanity' shows the benefits of common sense, and not everybody who shows challenging behaviour has an identified condition (Dykens and Hodapp, 1999; Dykens et al, 2000).

It is important to remember the following: genetic diagnosis and behaviour phenotypes should not lead to a biological-deterministic view because the impact of genetics is not immutable (consider the use of dietary intervention for phenylketonuria), and knowing likely sensory characteristics arising from the neurological outcomes of autistic spectrum conditions inform interventions that can impact on functioning. 'The new genetics', so called because it deals with understanding genetics at the molecular as opposed to consequence level (Comings, 1980) should be welcomed insofar as it offers insights into potential influences upon behaviour and functioning: the fear remembered from the eugenic movement is salutary, but it must not blind us to the benefits of understanding the impact of genetics on behaviour. Genetic disorders are rarely determinative in their direct or indirect effects on behaviour. Here, it is likely the assessment and advocacy skills of LDNs can often come to the fore, balancing the large number of influences on behaviour and agendas of those involved in suggesting intervention and support into a coherent formulation and summary of just what is occurring in regard to an individual's behaviour.

Emotional health

Research over the last 20 years has recognised the existence of psychiatric disorders or emotional health difficulties in people with IDD (Meltzer et al, 1994; Department of Health, 1998; Gravestock, 1999). A number of possible explanations have been proposed for the high prevalence of psychiatric disorders in people with IDD including communication difficulties; an absence of competent coping mechanisms and social, interpersonal and recreational adaptive skills; low self-esteem; experience of failure or rejection; controlling environments; a lack of choice; and organic damage (Goldberg and Huxley, 1980; Holt et al, 1995; O'Hara and Sperlinger, 1997). Yet identification and treatment of emotional health problems in people with IDD remains poor (White et al, 1995; Russell, 1997; Moss et al, 2000) and despite the high risk factors in the population it is clear the population is at greater risk than many groups in developing emotional health issues (Reed, 1997). Like all people, individuals with IDD who experience emotional health problems face serious consequences (Caine and Hatton, 1999).

There are a number of difficulties in recognising emotional health issues in people with IDD, including communication deficits of both service user and professional (Rodgers, 1994), and the reliance on third party awareness (Moss, 1999; Fraser and Nolan, 1994). Some may view behaviours potentially symptomatic of emotional health difficulties erroneously as 'part of the disability'. Murphy (1994) suggests that when working with individuals with intellectual or developmental disabilities and serious communication deficits, psychiatric diagnoses are at best unreliable and at worst unhelpful labels. Challenging behaviour by itself does not indicate a specific pathological psychiatric disorder: presenting problems may rather reflect ecological dynamics (Sturmey, 1999). Poor environments do not particularly help our emotional well-being.

The prescription of psychotropic medication and major tranquillisers has been examined in some studies, including that by Molyneux et al (1999). This study suggested that 66% of people with severe learning disabilities had been prescribed antipsychotic medication despite the absence of any first-rank symptoms. Medication was therefore primarily used for general tranquillisation. It is possible that prescribing is influenced as much by the characteristics of the client's environment and the practitioner's views and training as by the client's own behaviour (Intagalia and Rinck, 1985). One study found 40.2% of people with an IDD in hospital were prescribed psychotropic medication for challenging behaviour, compared with 19.3% in group homes, and 10.1% in family homes (Clarke et al, 1990). For many years, psychiatrists have continued to prescribe antipsychotic medication to people with IDD despite concerns about lack of efficacy, side-effects, tardive dyskinesia and effects on learning ability (Branford, 1996). More recent research suggests some of the benefits of psychoactive medication on the behaviour of people with IDD perceived by staff and carers may be questioned (Tyrer et al, 2008).

It is suggested that before raising the spectre of emotional health problems a consideration of ecological factors should occur. An understanding of the person's unique needs, gifts and functioning can thus be arrived at, based on clear assessment. Such an approach requires the experimental single-case model (Morley, 1989) to be dominant – where each case is treated as an individual experiment in which hypotheses are tested against data. This is a step towards a more person-centred approach. Such an approach will require close collaboration between psychologist, psychiatrist, and LDN. (For informed cohesive guidance, see *Challenging Behaviour: A Unified Approach*, produced by the Royal College of Psychiatrists, British Psychological Society and the Royal College of Speech and Language Therapists in 2007). In conclusion, people with IDD need good mental health services at least as much as the general population, yet access remains poor. Service intervention should focus on mental health rather than mental distress (Hare and Leadbetter, 1998; British Psychological Society, 2000).

Learning

The science of behaviour suggests that what we do is a product of the interaction between evolving genetics, the individual and ecology. As Mahayana Buddhists noted centuries ago, our lives, our minds and our actions of today are the result of our behaviour, thoughts and experiences of yesterday. Here, challenging behaviour might usefully be considered a problem of learning (e.g. Halle, 1994). This suggests we may need to think about possible interventions aimed at the ecology: if someone cannot read we teach them to read, if someone cannot speak we teach alternatives, if someone engages in self-injurious behaviour we teach them and those around them not to need to rely upon such behaviour to gain or avoid things, but to use other safer and more socially acceptable behaviours. Application requires sophistication though.

The behaviour we determine to be challenging has in all likelihood been 'taught' to the person: an appropriate attempt to gain attention may have been ignored while behaviour not considered appropriate may have evoked a response. Behaviour meets a need for the individual however odd or inappropriate it seems to us (Cooper et al, 1987). Challenging behaviour is behaviour that is adaptive in that it serves a function for the person (and sometimes the people around that person) (Durand, 1990).

We behave in certain ways to achieve an end. A busy waiter may not respond to your complaint about the quality of the soup arriving at your table in a hectic restaurant if you are not considered worthy of such attention, but try throwing a table or writing a negative review, and that waiter will come running. As Halle (1994: xii) notes: 'We have unwittingly taught those referred to as having disabilities… to behave in socially maladaptive ways to secure their entirely human wants and needs.' Why is this? As Risley (1996: 426) says: 'What behavioural practitioners know is that people immediately respond, almost without fail, to actions that are dangerous, disgusting, or disruptive. Because consumers who develop challenging behaviours are usually dependent and often considered otherwise unimportant, little else they do is unfailingly responded to by others…' Therefore '…our goal must change from the elimination of problem behaviours to understanding their function so that we can craft an intervention designed to teach a new form of behaviour that is at least as successful in achieving the identified function as the old, more coercive form' (Halle, 1994:.xii). This is at the heart of what is termed positive behaviour support, which is discussed below.

Not only do individuals influence the world, the world changes individuals. In the majority of cases behaviour is influenced by a convoluted mixture of internal and external factors and is a learned response to the situations people find themselves in (Horner et al, 1996). Most people are aware of the three-term contingency, antecedent (A), behaviour (B), consequence (C), model. This basic but elegant model might be thought of as a time machine, in that it enables us to consider not just what the behaviour looks like, but also what follows the behaviour and very importantly, what occurs before. This is not as easy as it sounds. To understand why behaviour occurs, one needs to take multiple examples to look for patterns or functional relationships between antecedents (signals that certain behaviour will be reinforced), behaviour and consequences. Looking at one example shows no pattern over time and means it is difficult to predict probable future occurrences or to establish functional relationships between events. A defect of the applied use of ABC charts and analysis of these is that they tend to focus on limited 'slots of time'. It is a little like looking at a road through a letterbox, observing passing cars. It may be logical but fundamentally flawed to conclude, after three or four observations, that the exhaust is caused by the preceding headlights. As a real example, many people will have experienced the same antecedent (asking someone to help clear the dishes, say) with different behaviours following (i.e. throwing the dishes at them, or clearing the dishes). How can the three-term contingency account for this?

What research (and experience) tells us is that while consequences to behaviour are vitally important, things called setting events often influence the selection of certain behaviours (*Figure 11.1*). Setting events set the scene by altering the 'motivation' or susceptibility of the person to antecedents. For example, if someone is feeling unwell, they may be less likely to respond positively to being asked to do the washing up than they would if they felt physically fine. So looking beyond the three-term contingency toward setting events can be very helpful for anyone trying to establish when any given behaviour is likely (McGill, 1999).

As a very rough guide, the functions of operant behaviour (why people do what they do) could be considered to fall broadly within four main categories:

- To gain tangibles (such as foodstuffs).
- To gain or maintain social interaction/attention.
- To gain automatic sensory stimulation (it feels good).
- To avoid or escape aversive situations or interactions.

For many people with IDD and communication difficulties, behaviours can have a communicative intent applied to them over time by those around them, even if the challenging behaviours have an organic basis (Carr and McDowell, 1980; Carr and Durand, 1985). Challenging behaviour may fundamentally be telling us we are not meeting people's needs, but paying closer attention to the function of behaviour may offer us an opportunity to

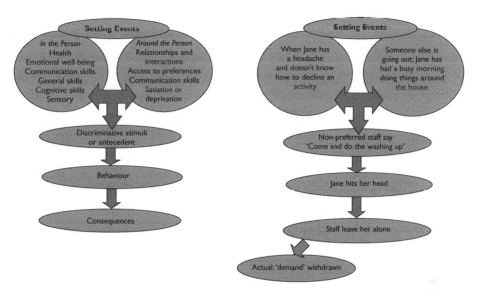

Figure 11.1. Where setting events fit.

work pro-actively with the person, by considering behaviour as potentially communicative. Challenging behaviour seeks to obtain universally human outcomes: escape, attention, stimulation, and satisfaction. This challenges us to alter our view of something that has historically been viewed as merely a problematic behaviour, something to be stopped, something to be managed.

Exotic communication

Communication skills and challenging behaviour are often correlated with each other (Kevan, 2003) although not always, and most authors would agree there is a the need for constructive interventions (developing skills) to address communication issues when working with challenging behaviour: influence the communication skills and you tend to influence the occurrence of challenging behaviour (Carr et al, 1993, 1994; Dunlap and Fox, 1996). This could be through enabling functionally related behaviours (offering alternatives that can result in needs being met) or equivalent behaviours (offering an alternative behaviour that has the same function as the challenging behaviour). In effect, strengthening communication skills can 'replace' some behaviours. The reduction in behaviour might also be a product of the inherent changes required in developing a reciprocal communication relationship: responding and listening to people with IDD can change our perception of the person, a positive rapport can develop between the person with IDD and those around him or her.

Communication can be defined as an intended sending of information to another person sharing the code. This can often pose problems when working with individuals who communicate ambiguously. Using this strict definition, it is difficult to make challenging behaviour qualify as a form of communication, but the communication hypothesis is very useful nonetheless. A somewhat extreme but useful summary of the concept of behaviour as communication is shown by Ephraim (1998: 211–12) when he writes, '...let me suggest there is no such thing as challenging behaviour. What we have is exotic communication... A punch in the face is an act of communication which is very difficult not to hear.' This may well be the case, but ascribing meaning to all behaviour may be just as unhelpful. A sneeze means a sneeze, not that I dislike your perfume. Not all behaviour is intentional, but meaning can be developed or shaped over time.

The communication hypothesis states that problem behaviour often functions as a primitive form of communication for people who do not possess more sophisticated modes of communication. In this view, 'adaptive communication' and problem behaviour both result in a variety of desirable outcomes for the person (reinforcement). The communication hypothesis does not mean that people who do not talk will use problem behaviour to influence others and it does not state individuals systematically and intentionally use their behaviour to influence others. Communication requires at least two; behaviour, to have meaning applied, also requires at least two. Behaviour can be shaped and it can acquire meaning to individuals or those around them. The communication hypothesis is useful because it suggests a constructive and educative way of functionally addressing problem behaviours.

We can make the challenging behaviour less effective by reinforcing replacement behaviour (communication) powerfully. The replacement behaviour should meet the same function as the challenging behaviour and be more efficient (less effort). In effect, we aim to teach the person a better way of getting what he or she wants. Functional communication training is an example of this (Durand, 1990).

Person-centred planning and person-centred action

Person-centred planning (PCP) has arrived (at least in name), in the UK after a prolonged development in North America (O'Brien and Lovett, 1992; O'Brien et al, 1997; O'Brien and O'Brien, 2000; O'Brien, 2002), and while much research and comment around it has occurred from that continent (Smull, 1996; Holburn et al, 2000; Holburn and Vietze, 1999, 2002) initial UK research and comment is beginning to emerge (Robertson et al, 2005). Beyond the rhetoric, real successes are occurring (Sanderson, 2002), although perhaps not yet as often as it might be hoped (Mansell and Beadle-Brown, 2005). The focus needs to be on the number of person-centred plans completed as opposed to the outcomes for people receiving services as a measure of implementation success.

PCP and person-centred action can improve the quality of life of some individuals, but they may not positively reduce challenging behaviour; indeed, people with the label of behaviour that challenges are often less likely to receive support to develop a cohesive person-centred plan, and if they do, the plan may not result in major increases in social networks or activities or contact with family or friends. PCP implementation and outcome does seem dependent on leadership and both personal and professional commitment. It might be that people with reputations for severely challenging behaviour are less likely to benefit from the factors shown to increase the chances of receiving person-centred planning, such as living near to family and having an environment that is receptive to the individualistic principles of PCP (Robertson et al, 2005). LDNs will often be invited to attend or even lead the meetings to develop person-centred plans given their often long-term relationship with the individual. PCP is not likely to hurt in the process of developing an understanding of why people's behaviour challenges, but it is person-centred action that is more helpful in delivering what a person requires. Spending time with people as equals is humanising and informative when finding out what people enjoy and what they seek to avoid: being person-centred only strengthens our understanding of 'the other'.

Positive behaviour support

Very useful guides to positive behaviour support (PBS) it can be found elsewhere (e.g. Koegel et al, 1996; Allen et al, 2005), but briefly, PBS involves basing life-enhancing constructive interventions upon functional assessment or analysis of the difficulty. PBS is the ethical, person-centred and scientific application of applied behaviour analysis: science and values used to address real problems in real situations. Good PBS practitioners ask straight questions, such as, do service systems or schools or families supporting people labelled as 'having challenging behaviour' suit the requirements of the person? Most provision for challenging behaviour still expects the person to fit the service (Lovett, 1996).

Person-centred behavioural support is primarily directed at creating responsive systems and environments rather than attempting to 'fix' the person. It is aimed at supporting individuals with challenging behaviour to make their own way in the world, at reducing challenging behaviour constructively (teaching new skills), as well as applying behavioural science to overcome individual difficulties of learning (Carr et al, 1999). Today it is beginning to be recognised that good behavioural assessment and support can be augmented by person-centred planning.

Here, functional assessment means establishing the functioning through talking with people who know the individual, direct observations of the situation, indirect observations, and record examination. Functional analysis requires all the above plus the experimental manipulation of variables to confirm the assessment (often called analogue conditions). Functional assessment can be thought of as a method of describing, categorising and verifying. The functional assessment process is discussed elsewhere in detail, such as, O'Neill et al (1997) and Emerson (1998, 2001).

The results of the functional assessment are used to develop an intervention plan that usually consists of teaching replacement behaviours, making changes to the ecology and altering antecedents and consequences. Most situations in which challenging behaviour occurs have evolved over time and it is not uncommon to find that the response made is maintaining the behaviour. Therefore changes are usually needed in the environment, including the way that people think about and work with the person. Emerson (2001) suggests practitioners of behavioural approaches need to consider the following issues:

- Intervention goals should be developed with all stakeholders.
- The form of the intervention should take account of existing culture, value and skills.
- Intervention should enmesh with existing routines and activity patterns.

An example of a multi-element approach to intervention can be found in the work of LaVigna et al (1986), which will suffice to illustrate the themes found in many such models, but it should be noted that a number of alternative methods for intervention organisation have been published and discussed. LaVigna et al recommend four broad categories of intervention domains when interventionists seek to respond positively to challenging behaviour. First, ecological changes 'smooth the fit' between the individuals' needs and their environment, which means addressing conflicts between service users' needs or preferences and requirements and the environment. It could include things such as having a predictable routine, how the person is spoken to, reducing noise levels, etc. Second, positive programmes provide opportunities for the individual to learn new skills, including new ways of communicating needs, specific teaching opportunities to increase general skills and skills directly related to the behaviour, for example anger management. Third, focused supports are designed to reduce the frequency, strength and duration of the challenging behaviour, and this may involve techniques such as differential reinforcement schedules. Reactive strategies are the final element, and provide guidelines to help all concerned to cope with the behaviour when it occurs (Donnellan et al, 1988; Baker et al, 1998).

There is a huge amount of evidence showing modern behavioural approaches can be effective in enabling significant short and medium-term reductions in challenging behaviour, yet there are real challenges in consistently applying the technology in the real world for many people, not least because of the lack of informed practitioners. Ironically, there is little evidence for antipsychotic medication being effective in the treatment of challenging behaviours, although many individuals whose behaviour challenges have such prescriptions. It is ironic then that the latter is the most common form of intervention for challenging behaviour, while the evidence-based behavioural support is often not available.

The challenging demands faced by the nurse specialist

The actual job title varies between locations but the primary function of nurse specialists in challenging behaviour is to assess and intervene in the lives of people with IDD who are considered to have challenging needs. Often such assessment and intervention work requires practitioners to look beyond the pathological view (where the 'disorder' lies within the person) towards an ecological-behavioural perspective (behaviour occurs in functional relationships to ecology, both environmental and biological). In effect, the nurse specialist searches beyond the medical model without dismissing its usefulness.

A by-product of being known as working within the field of IDD and challenging behaviour may be that nurse specialists' expert opinion and involvement is sought in problematic situations by those responsible for commissioning. Nurse specialists may find themselves suitably positioned to influence the architecture of general service provision, as well as the teams within which they operate and they may often become involved in operational management. The issue of clinical governance and professional accountability are of vital importance but are even more relevant when working with seriously challenging behaviour, since the advice given by LDNs to families, schools or services will likely be seized on enthusiastically. While being viewed as an 'expert on behaviour' does carry kudos, it also carries risks and responsibilities: effective, detailed clinical supervision (often separate from operational management) is often beneficial and should be provided by experienced and qualified professionals.

When referrals are first received, it is not uncommon for nurse specialists to complete an initial screening assessment. This provides invaluable information often not provided within the referral. It also helps ensure eligibility criteria are adhered to and that resources are equitably provided. Such initial assessments may show alternative pathways to services or advice for the person referred: not everyone referred is demonstrating behaviour of such high intensity, duration or frequency that they require specialist nurse involvement.

It might be helpful to provide less intense consultation arrangements or mentoring arrangements whereby nurse specialists are able to guide other less experienced practitioners, providing clinical governance issues are addressed. People making referrals to nurse specialists may have many less obvious motivations in addition to the presenting behaviour (funding, accessing training, approval for existing interventions, seeking recommendations about placement suitability, etc.), so careful screening is vital (see the section on challenging behaviour above). The story of Mary may help illustrate some of the points discussed.

Case study: Mary

Mary lives alone in an isolated house in a small village, where there are at least two support staff working at any one time. It is a five bed house and a lot of the house is sealed or locked to her. Mary knows it is there but cannot get access, in case, the service said in a risk assessment, she damages the property. Prior to being moved to the house, Mary shared a house for six years in a town eight miles away with five men: like Mary, all had a diagnosis of autistic spectrum condition and intellectual disabilities. Mary has lived in the house for around 11 months. Her move was an emergency response by the service providing Mary's housing and support to Mary's increasing aggressive behaviours aimed at the men living in the service. Mary had been saying she didn't like it at the old house, and that it was too noisy. After putting her arm through a window and hitting two residents during a five hour incident, the service felt they had to act.

Following a quiet four months in her new home (two staff known to Mary followed her to the new house, but the other eight staff were new), Mary's behaviour began to give concerns. She started hurting herself by punching her legs, and could be heard screaming, 'Go away!', 'Stop laughing!', 'Bad girl!', when alone in her room. Mary complained of noise, even when, according to the staff, there was no TV or radio, and no traffic noise. The local community learning disability team were asked to come and give advice due to the behaviour, but only after the staff had tried to support Mary through seven months of increasingly disturbed behaviour. Because the referral was quite imprecise about exactly what was being sought, an initial assessment was conducted by a registered learning disability nurse, and she was shocked at the level of aggression and self-injury reported. She was also concerned about how staff responded to the challenging behaviour and how the situation was being managed. In effect, the placement was now under threat.

What appeared to be a routine screening visit became much more complex.

Desni, the RNLD, had been qualified for a little over a year and although she had had limited experience of challenging behaviour in her new role, she had previously worked as a support worker. In this role, Desni had acquired a huge amount of practical experience of working with people in crisis and distress. Working in a team, Desni was able to gain support from more experienced nurse colleagues and other practitioners, most notably a speech therapist and psychologist. In completing her initial assessment, Desni had worked hard to collate the 'war stories' of staff and bring together the often contradictory views about Mary from staff, operational managers, and Mary's worried family. It felt to Desni that everyone had their own views and agendas, and that Mary had become 'lost' in the confusion. Just completing the initial assessment took two long visits because everyone wanted to explain to Desni what it was like working with Mary. The service provider demanded immediate strategies and risk assessments for the seven or eight incidents each day. Although Mary herself appeared calm whenever Desni visited, and Desni had no difficulty communicating with Mary, one thing was clear: staff seemed frightened of Mary, and Mary seemed wary of staff. Mary enjoyed Desni's presence, smiling at her and showing Desni her room, but Mary did not want to speak about how she felt. Whenever Desni asked Mary about how she felt, Mary shouted. After gaining consent, Desni used video to record events and Mary liked to watch herself (Desni gave the video to Mary at the end).

The learning disability team agreed to open Mary as an active case with immediate effect after listening to the results of Desni's initial assessment. Desni agreed to co-ordinate the input, with advice from the team's psychologist. Desni's other cases were reduced in number (through colleagues taking over specific tasks), and a memorandum of understanding was agreed between the service provider and the team. This, in itself, took some negotiation. Finally, it was agreed Desni would complete a functional assessment within five weeks, and this document would outline precisely the behaviours of concern, when they were likely to appear and the function or reason Mary behaved in the way she did. The service agreed to co-operate fully. As a specialist provider of challenging behaviour and autism services, they felt they did not have a lot to learn about Mary, and they did not want any training – they just wanted Mary to stop the behaviour and 'be happy'. Staff said to Desni, 'It's like we've lost Mary.' During a functional assessment interview, the operational manager said the service had serious doubts about their ability to manage Mary 'within existing resources', despite the placement costing care management several thousand pounds each week.

Desni first agreed to refer Mary to the psychiatrist to review the cocktail of medication Mary took each day, and then referred Mary to the speech therapist, for his expert view on the communication exchanges between staff and Mary. Meanwhile, Desni began to visit the service and Mary twice a week, with each visit lasting up to three hours. During one visit, Desni observed staff locking themselves in the kitchen away from Mary for two hours 'because she's not happy and might hit out' and the risk assessment written by the service specified this action (although not the criteria of when to lock the door). Desni spoke at length with staff, exploring with them how Mary might interpret this, and it was clear staff felt that if they kept engaging with Mary and ignored the risk assessment, should they be assaulted by Mary, there would be no support from management because they had not followed the risk assessment. After a couple of weeks, Desni had accumulated about seven hours of direct observations, measuring how much interaction Mary received, and what type of behaviour was being shown. Desni's data showed Mary received staff attention and interaction for less than 7% of the time.

Examination of the ABC records suggested that most incidents of aggression followed periods of inactivity and a lack of engagement. Self-injury usually occurred when Mary was alone in her room for long periods or just before a telephone call to her parents (she had telephoned them every third day at 9p.m. precisely), but Desni was not convinced of the reliability of the ABC data, as there were big gaps in the records. Desni also had concerns about the communication partnerships that were operating: most communication from staff was complex and verbal, and staff tended to make deals with Mary about what might happen over the next two weeks, e.g. 'If you're good we'll go to the shopping centre...' Such imprecise statements seemed contrary to good autism practice, but more importantly, Desni noticed a lack of consistency in the staff group: deals would be made and then not followed through. When she raised these with the home manager, he said that all staff were consistent and had been trained by autism professionals. The home manager seemed to take the discussion as an implied criticism of his management. He had introduced a two team approach, splitting the staff team, some seven months previously (this coincided with an increase in reported behavioural disturbances).

Over the next two weeks, Desni recorded more incidents of 'miscommunications', even less activity and interaction, and an increase in self-injurious behaviour and Mary 'talking to herself'. The service sought a hospital admission under the Mental Health Act. The psychiatrist liaised with Desni and the psychologist: the team suspected the lack of activity and structure and the overly complex communication, had led to the increasing behaviour, which resulted in less and less engagement. A downward spiral of inactivity and emotional distress seemed to be occurring but the service was convinced the difficulty was mental illness, despite the contrary psychiatrist's views. Things were happening fast and Desni felt there were different agendas operating: she called a case conference to review what was known about Mary's behaviour. Desni also discussed the situation with the local adult protection coordinator, who invited himself to the case conference.

The case conference took place six weeks after Desni began her work, and she had by now completed the brief functional assessment: the hypothesis Desni had arrived at was supported by the psychologist and the speech therapist. The three had spent two hours creating a formulation, also known as a contingency diagram, a pictorial representation of all the things that Desni's work had suggested might be influencing Mary's behaviour. Desni had spoken to most of the staff, Mary's parents, and had asked Mary to talk (Mary said 'Don't talk, don't talk'- so Desni had to interpret Mary's behaviour). Desni's work showed a clear link between environmental issues (low levels of support and engagement, a focus on restrictive containment, fearful staff), physical well-being (when Mary was in pain or discomfort her tolerance toward staff was lower than at other times, which her family put down to 'too many pills'), the way communication occurred, and challenging behaviour.

On arrival, the service announced they had given notice to Mary, and commissioners had 28 days to find alternative accommodation. The service accused the team of failing Mary by not coming up with quick and effective solutions. The service also stated they 'had to give notice' to ensure Mary received the psychiatric help she needed. Desni and her colleagues explained functional assessment work was time consuming, but the conclusions they had reached reflected the service conclusion – but for completely different reasons. The team felt the service's inability to look at their own approach had left few options but to find a planned alternative, through the judicious use of person-centred planning and needs assessment. Desni and her colleagues had planned a support intervention to keep the service going while commissioners found an alternative placement, but this plan would be impossible to implement given the service resistance.

Care management asked Desni to help them identify a temporary placement, which she did, but out of area. Desni and the family visited the more structured environment, and took photos to show Mary, who asked to visit. Desni supported the family to write a plan outlining how they would support Mary during the visit. Following the visit, Mary asked to move to the new placement. Care management commissioned an independent facilitator to develop with Mary, her family, and those Mary chose, a person-centred plan, which would in turn help them develop a local placement. Mary did not want to attend the meetings, but she did write out for her family a long list of things she wanted. She also made use of video. Because Mary was now out of area, Desni was unable to keep Mary open on her caseload for more than two months. Eight months later, care management created a supported living model for Mary, and Mary visited her new flat. Desni met her and they went for a coffee. Desni will recommence her involvement with Mary, contributing to the induction Mary and her family and care management have designed. Desni has learned a lot and will start specialised training to learn more about both person-centred planning and behaviour analysis: colleagues said she was a natural.

Mary's mother reported that on a brief family trip to the beach, Mary wrote on the sand, 'I do have a good heart'. The family is hopeful but nervous, and Desni will ensure the new provider keeps Mary's family aware of service issues. 'Even so,' Mary's mother noted, 'I do wonder who taught my daughter she didn't have a good heart in the first place.'

A common part of the nurse specialist's role is to help people understand why some people with IDD may sometimes engage in behaviours deemed challenging, as well as what to do about it, using evidence-based methods. A general training or mentoring function is not uncommon within this brief, and could be equated to a broad information sharing function. Nurse specialists aiming to intervene with individuals will often need to intervene in mediator (staff, family, co-worker) behaviour, and arrange appropriate contingencies to support maintenance and generalisation of new skills. Direct observations are vital, often after a more informal 'look see' at what seems to be occurring. In specific cases, general awareness training or workshops will likely be insufficient to change mediator thinking. Nurse specialists are likely to provide targeted training and mentoring in specific cases, to families, schools, services and so forth, and provide real examples to others by showing how things can be achieved.

There are likely to be a myriad of factors affecting service performance: such issues directly influence the lifestyle and skills development and behaviour of people living within the provision, and the LDN will often need to take these into account or at the very least be sensitive to their existence (McGill and Mansell, 1995; Mansell, 1996; Mansell and Elliot, 2001). These include, but are not limited to, the values, skills and understanding of the staff or family members, the organisational culture and procedures, and forces operating on the service from other agencies and Government policy (Emerson et al, 1994). So informed application of the principles of PBS will require the nurse specialist to consider the systemic contexts within which the behaviour occurs (Sailor, 1996). Nurse specialists will be aiming to understand cultures as well as addressing behavioural challenges (Hastings, 2005).

Nurse specialists tend not to work in isolation: working alone is risky, clinically speaking. It is likely that specialists will be part of a multidisciplinary team, and as such their work will fit with other viewpoints. Much of the challenging behaviour training available is likely to be drawn from psychological technologies, but a fundamental consideration when working with behaviour that challenges is that of communication (see the section on exotic communication above). Close links between nurse specialists and other professionals are essential. The nurse specialist will be uniquely placed to be able to consider both fundamental health influences upon behaviour as well as psychological influences. It is still the case that medication plays a large part in the 'management' of challenging behaviour, right or wrong (Clarke, 1999), and the nurse specialist may well be involved in mediating between the views of services, users, families and psychiatric professionals. Taking pills or undertaking ad hoc behavioural programmes is no substitute for having service, family or school focus their efforts on supporting the person to gain a lifestyle we ourselves would value (O'Brien, 1987; Clements, 1992, 1997), and the nurse specialist may often have to resist the demands for quick solutions to difficult problems.

The development of behavioural support plans is neither simple nor bound to result in success, and nurse specialists will be required to assess carefully the capacity of the environment to implement their advice faithfully and in a valid manner. As such, much time will be spent collecting, collating and interpreting quantitative and qualitative data in order to gain baseline and post-intervention evidence of efficacy. Competent PBS requires careful assessment of the behaviour and the nurse specialist will collect reliable and valid data often using computers and videos. The completion of a functional assessment or analysis is just one option: from clinical experience addressing basic lifestyle issues is often effective, through, for example, essential lifestyle planning or interaction skills, and the changing of non-aversive contingencies operating in the environment. This can often lead to an increase in quality of life (and skills), and a reduction to some degree in reported levels of behaviour, without the need to resort to functional assessment.

Here, the approach is for people with IDD to get on with their lives and see how things progress (Risley, 1996), to develop respectful working, ensuring access to reinforcing events and interactions are available, rather than to reach immediately for the functional assessment. The greater the amount of experience the nurse specialist gains, the finer her 'clinical intuition' develops as to what approach is indicated in any given situation. This in no way should be interpreted as advocating for avoiding functional assessment, but sometimes it does not take a scientific sledgehammer to crack a social deprivation nut, given that much research suggests that, for many people with IDD, quality of life remains poor, and power differentials remain a real feature of many people's lives, particularly for individuals whose behaviour challenges the system (Clements and Martin, 2002: 30).

Beneath the spin we operate in a society that sees people with disabilities as a threat in need of control, sometimes benevolent, sometimes malevolent, but always control... Of all the issues that arise, behavioural issues stimulate a power-base response. Now the subtext rises to the surface, the gloves are off. Those who should be humble and grateful for our kindness have stepped out of line. They have failed to show proper respect for their betters. They need to be taught a lesson. Frequently, they are... and all in the name of treatment... If the behaviour guy says I have to earn soda rather than just have it in the fridge that's what happens. If the legalised drug dealer says that I should take this pill then that is what will happen. If I spit it out it will be buried in my ice cream. That is, if I'm allowed ice cream and haven't been put on a diet by a bunch of overweight suits calling themselves the team.

If a functional assessment or analysis route is taken, this should be viewed not as an end in itself but as a pre-cursor to the focus of the nurse specialist's work, that of implementing life-enhancing interventions (Emerson, 1998). Here, our nurse specialist will need to demonstrate high levels of skills indeed. Getting people to change how they work with someone is not as easy as it first seems: people have their own values and, despite the nurse specialist writing some wonderful evidenced and logical intervention plans that make sense to everyone else, if the staff or family do not 'buy into it', it will remain a pristine, wonderful, evidenced and logical plan lying on a dusty office shelf. Sometimes, being focused upon delivering a humane service to a particular person may lead us to forget that carers have their own viewpoints which can make or break our ideas. Nurse specialists, because they work intensively with a handful of people, may even so not be the primary provider of hands-on support; they will rely upon mediators – people doing the day-to-day work. Hence, in addition to analytical skills, nurse specialists will need to hone their presentations and their interpersonal, facilitation and implementation management skills.

Dare to hope to change

Given specialist training, a growing bank of experiences from which to draw, and ongoing professional development, the nurse specialist should, through reflection, consider the potential dangers of 'the institution of the mind', which Ericsson (2005) considers the final challenge of institutionalisation. Inclusion, independence, rights and choice, the fundamental outcomes all practitioners strive towards if adhering to the value-goals of *Valuing People*, all presuppose 'equality between the person with disability and those providing services' (Ericsson, 2005: 60). Therefore, regardless of training and continuing professional development, it is important for us all to remember that people with intellectual disabilities may inhabit the same physical world, but the social world they experience is often very limited: 'Most people have something to hurt about, but many people with intellectual disability are among the most devalued people in society and have a lot to hurt about'

(Cullen, 1999: 438). Compare the number of friends you have to the friends of someone you know with IDD. It is a sobering exercise.

This is a world we ourselves have little direct experience of living within. People with the label of IDD are often powerless, poor and ignored; things are done 'to them', albeit dressed up within prosaic 'best interest' arguments. Positive behaviour support, like person-centred planning, is not learned from a book, nor from shouting the slogans, but from doing and being with a fellow human, from listening to others and reflecting, and from thinking not only about technical procedures and clinical validity, but also from witnessing socially important outcomes such as growing friendships and increasing happiness. Do our assessments lead to interventions that result in improvements in quality of life? Do we dare to hope for such occurrences? Such outcomes are our business.

Professionals hold powerful roles and have opportunities to influence people's lives for the better or worse. Through the myriad of assessments and explanatory models around, never forget our purpose is to serve and understand a fellow human in acute distress. So seek to remain humane and open. This is a challenge to us all, regardless of profession: to be human and responsive to our companions in distress, regardless of their knowledge, ability and social value, and despite our training and roles.

Thanks are due to the following for their contributions: Des Clarke, Maria Hurman, Emma Osgood, and the many other nurses with whom I discussed real situations. I would also like to thank Peter McGill for his, as ever, constructive advice.

References

Allen D, Felce D (1999) Service responses to challenging behaviour. In: Bouras N (ed.) *Psychiatric and Behavioural Disorders in Developmental Disabilities and Mental Retardation.* Cambridge University Press, Cambridge

Allen D, James W, Evans J, Hawkins S, Jenkins R (2005) Positive behavioural support: Definition, current status and future directions. *Tizard Learning Disability Review* **10**(1): 4–11

Allen D, Lowe K (1995) Providing intense community support to people with learning disabilities and challenging behaviour: A preliminary cost–benefit analysis. *Journal of Intellectual Disability Research* **39**: 67–82

Baker P (2002) Confrontation or communication? Supporting people whose behaviour challenges us. In: Carnaby S (ed.) *Learning Disability Today, Key Issues for Providers, Managers, Practitioners and Users.*

Pavilion, Brighton: 189–202

Baker P, LaVigna G, Willis T (1998) Understanding and responding to challenging behaviour: A multi-element approach. In: Fraser W, Sines D, Kerr M (eds.) *Hallas's Caring for People with Learning Disabilities* 9th edn, Butterworths, Oxford

Blunden R, Allen D (1987) *Facing the challenge: an ordinary life for people with learning difficulties and challenging behaviour*. King's Fund, London

Branford D (1996) Factors associated with the successful or unsuccessful withdrawal of antipsychotic drug therapy prescribed for people with learning disabilities. *Journal of Intellectual Disability Research* **40:** 4

British Psychological Society (2000) *Recent advances in understanding mental illness and psychotic experience*. BPS, Leicester

British Psychological Society (2004) *Psychological interventions for severely challenging behaviours shown by people with learning disabilities: Clinical Practice Guidelines*. BPS, Leicester

Caine A, Hatton C (1999) Working with people with mental health problems. In: Emerson E, Hatton C, Bromley J, Caine A (eds.) *Clinical Psychology and People with Intellectual Disabilities*. Chichester, Wiley

Carr EG, Durand VM (1985) Reducing problem behaviour through functional communication training. *Journal of Applied Behaviour analysis* **18:** 111–26

Carr EG, Horner RH, Turnbull AP, Marquis JG, Magito-McLaughlin D, McAtee ML, Smith CE, Ryan KA, Ruef MB, Doolabh A (1999) *Positive Behavior Support as an Approach for Dealing with Problem Behavior in People with Developmental Disabilities: A Research Synthesis*. American Association on Mental Retardation Monograph Series

Carr EG, Levin L, McConnachie G, Carlson JI, Kemp DC, Smith CE (1994) *Communication-based Intervention for Problem Behavior: A User's Guide for Producing Positive Change*. Paul H Brookes, Baltimore

Carr EG, McConnachie G, Levin L, Kemp DC (1993) Communication based treatment and severe behavior problems. In: Van Houten R, Axelrod S (eds.) *Behavioral Analysis and Treatment*. Plenum Press, New York: 231–67

Carr EG, McDowell JJ (1980) Social control of self injurious behaviour of organic etiology. *Behaviour Therapy* **11:** 402–9

Chief Nursing Officers of the United Kingdom (CNOUK) (1991) *Caring for People – Mental Handicap Nursing (the Cullen Report)*. CNO(91)5.

Department of Health, London

Clarke D (1997) Towards rational psychotropic prescribing for people with learning disability. *British Journal of Learning Disabilities* **25:** 2

Clarke D (1999) Treatment and therapeutic interventions: The use of medication. *Tizard Learning Disability Review* **4:** 2

Clarke D, Kelley S, Thinn K, Corbett J (1990) Psychotropic drugs and mental retardation. Pt.1: Disabilities and the prescription of drugs for behaviour and for epilepsy in three residential settings. *Journal of Mental Deficiency Research* **34:** 169–80

Clements J (1992) I can't explain... 'challenging behaviour': Towards a shared conceptual framework. *Clinical Psychology Forum* **39:** 29–37

Clements J (1997) Sustaining a cognitive psychology. In: Stenfert Kroese D, Dagnan D, Loumidis K (eds.) *Cognitive Behaviour Therapy for People with Learning Disabilities.* Routledge, London

Clements, J, Martin N (2002) *Assessing Behaviours Regarded as Problematic for People with Developmental Disabilities.* Jessica Kingsley Publishers, London

Comings D (1980) *Presidential Address*: American Society of Human Genetics 31st Annual Meeting, New York

Cooper J, Heron T, Heward W (1987) *Applied Behaviour Analysis.* Merrill Publishing Co, Columbus

Cullen C (1999) Contextualism in intellectual disability research: The case of choice behaviour. *Journal of Intellectual Disability Research* **43**(6): 437–44

Davidson PW, Cain NN, Sloane-Reeves JE, et al (1995) Crisis intervention for community based individuals with developmental disabilities and behavioural and psychiatric disorders. *Mental Retardation* **33:** 21–30

Department of Health (1993) *Services for People with Learning Disabilities and Challenging Behaviour or Mental Health Needs.* HMSO, London

Department of Health (1998) *Signposts for Success in Commissioning and Providing Health Services for People with Learning Disabilities.* HMSO, London

Department of Health (2001) *Valuing People: A New Strategy for Learning Disability for the 21st Century* (Cm 5086). HMSO, London

Dillenburger K, O'Reilly M, Keenan M (eds.) (1997) *Advances in Behaviour Analysis.* University College Dublin Press, Dublin

Donnellan AM, LaVigna GW, Negri-Schoultz N, Fassbender L (1988) *Progress without Punishment.* Teachers College Press, New York

Dunlap, G., Fox, L., (1996) Early intervention and serious problem behaviours: A comprehensive approach. In: Koegel L, Koegel R, Dunlap G (eds.) *Positive Behaviour Support: Including People With Difficult Behaviour in the Community*, Paul H Brookes, Baltimore, 31–50

Durand VM (1990) *Severe Behaviour Problems: A Functional Communication Training Approach.* Guilford Press, New York

Durand VM, Crimmins DB (1988) Identifying the variables maintaining self-injurious behavior. *Journal of Autism and Developmental Disorders* **18:** 99–117

Dykens E.M, Hodapp RM (1999) Behavioural phenotypes: Towards new understandings of people with development disabilities. In: Bouras N (ed.) *Psychiatric and Behavioural Disorders in Developmental Disabilities and Mental Retardation.* Cambridge, Cambridge University Press: 96–108

Dykens EM, Hodapp RM, Finucane BM (2000) *Genetics and Mental Retardation Syndromes: A New Look At Behaviour and Interventions.* Paul H. Brookes Publishing, Baltimore

Emerson E (1995) *Challenging Behaviour: Analysis and Intervention in People with Learning Difficulties.* Cambridge University Press, Cambridge

Emerson E (1998) Working with people with challenging behaviour. In: Emerson E, Hatton C, Bromley J, Caine A (eds.) *Clinical Psychology and People with Intellectual Disabilities.* John Wiley and Sons, Chichester: 127–53

Emerson E (2001) *Challenging Behaviour: Analysis and Intervention in People with Intellectual Disabilities* 2nd edn. Cambridge University Press: Cambridge

Emerson E, Cambridge P, Forrest J, Mansell J (1993) Community support teams for people with learning disabilities and challenging behaviours. In: Kiernan C (ed.) *Research to Practice? Implications of Research on the Challenging Behaviour of People with Learning Disabilities.* British Institute of Learning Disabilities, Kidderminster

Emerson E, Felce D, McGill P, Mansell J (1994) The nature of the challenge. In: Emerson E, McGill P, Mansell J (eds.) *Severe Learning Disabilities and Challenging Behaviour: Designing High Quality Services.* Chapman and Hall, London: 1–16

Emerson E, Forrest J, Cambridge P, Mansell J (1996) Community support teams for people with learning disabilities and challenging behaviours: Results of a national survey. *Journal Of Mental Health* **5**(4): 395–406

Emerson E, Kiernan C, Alborz A, Reeves D, Mason H, Swarbrick R, Mason L, Hatton C (2001) The prevalence of challenging behaviours: A total population study. *Research in Developmental Disabilities* **22**: 77–93

Emerson E, McGill P, Mansell J (1994) *Severe Learning Disabilities and Challenging Behaviour: Designing High Quality Services.* Chapman and Hall, London

Ephraim G (1998) Exotic communication, conversations and scripts – or tales of the pained, the unheard and the unloved. In: Hewitt D (ed.) *Challenging Behaviour: Principles and Practice.* David Fulton Publishers, London

Ericsson K (2005) The institution of the mind – the final challenge. *Tizard Learning Disability Review* **10**(1): 57–61

Flynt J, Yule W (1994) Behaviour phenotypes. In: Rutter M, Taylor E, Hersov L (eds.) *Child and Adolescent Psychiatry: Modern Approaches* 3rd edn. Blackwell Science, London: 666–87

Fraser W, Nolan M (1994) Psychiatric disorders in learning disability. In: Bouras N (ed.) *Mental Health in Learning disability.* Cambridge University Press, Cambridge

Goldberg D, Huxley P (1980) *Mental Illness in the Community.* Tavistock Publications, London

Gravestock S (1999) Adults with learning disabilities and mental health needs: Conceptual and service issues. *Tizard Learning Disability Review* **4**(2): 6–13

Halle JW (1994) Forward. In Carr EG, Levin L, McConnachie G, Carlson JI, Kemp DC, Smith CE (eds.) *Communication-based Intervention for Problem Behavior: A User's Guide for Producing Positive Change.* Paul H Brookes, Baltimore

Hare D, Leadbetter C (1998) Specific factors in assessing and intervening in cases of self-injury by people with autistic conditions. *Journal of Learning Disabilities for Nursing, Health and Social Care* **2**: 2

Hastings RP (2005) Commentary: Staff training in positive behaviour support: Research into practice. *Tizard Learning Disability Review* **10**(1): 31–3

Hodapp RM (1997) Direct and indirect behavioural effects of different genetic disorders in mental retardation. *American Journal of Mental Retardation* **102**: 67–79

Holburn CS, Jacobson J, Vietze P, Schwartz A, Sersen E (2000) Quantifying the process and outcomes of person centred planning. *American Journal on Mental Retardation* **105**: 402–6

Holburn CS, Vietze P (1999) Acknowledging the barriers to person centred planning. *Mental Retardation* **37**(2): 117–24

Holburn S, Vietze PM (2002) *Person-Centred Planning: Research, Practice and Future Directions*. Paul H Brooks

Holt G, Kon Y, Bouras N (1995) *Mental Health and Learning Disabilities: A training pack for staff working with people who have dual diagnosis of mental health needs and learning disabilities*. Pavilion, Brighton

Horner RH, Vaughn BJ, Day HM, Ard WR Jr (1996) The relationship between setting events and problem behaviour. In: Koegel L, Koegel R, Dunlap RL, Dunlap G (eds.) *Positive Behavioural Support: Including People with Difficult Behaviour in the Community*. Paul H Brookes, Baltimore: 381–402

Intagalia J, Rinck C, (1985) Psychoactive drug use in public and community residential facilities for mentally retarded persons. *Psyschopharmacology Bulletin* **21:**

Jukes M, Bollard M (2003) *Contemporary Learning Disability Practice*. Quay Books, Salisbury

Kay B, Rose S, Turnbull J (1995) *Continuing the Commitment. The Report of the Learning Disability Nursing Project*. Department of Health, London

Kevan F (2003) Challenging behaviour and communication difficulties. *British Journal of Learning Disabilities* **31:** 75–80

Koegel LK, Koegel RL, Dunlap G (eds.) (1996) *Positive Behavioural Support: Including people with difficult behaviour in the community*. Paul H. Brookes Publishing Co, Baltimore

Kushlick A, Trower P, Dagnan D (1997) Applying cognitive-behavioural approaches to the carers of people with learning disabilities who display challenging behaviour. In: Stenfert Kroese B, Dagnan D, Loumidis K (eds.) *Cognitive-Behaviour Therapy for People with Learning Disabilities*. Routledge, London

LaVigna GW, Willis TJ, Donnellan AW (1986) The role of positive programming in behavioural treatment. In: Cipani E (ed.) *Behavioural Approaches in the Treatment of Operant Behaviour*. AAMD, New York

Lehr DH, Brown F (eds.) (1996) *People with Disabilities who Challenge the System*. Paul. H. Brookes, Baltimore

Lovett H (1996) *Learning to Listen. Positive approaches and people with difficult behaviour*. Paul Brookes Publishing Co, Baltimore

McBrien J (1994) The Behavioural Services Team for People with

Learning Disabilitics. In: Emcrson E, McGill P, Manscll J (cds.) *Severe Learning Disabilities and Challenging Behaviours: Designing High Quality Services*. Chapman and Hall, London

McBrien J, Felce D (1992) *Working With People Who Have Severe Learning Difficulty and Challenging Behaviour: A practical handbook on the behavioural approach*. BILD Publications, Clevedon

McGill P (1999) Establishing operations: Implications for the assessment, treatment, and prevention of problem behavior. *Journal Of Applied Behavior Analysis* **3**(32): 393–418

McGill P (2000) Ten years of providing intensive support services for people with learning disabilities and challenging behaviour. *Tizard Learning Disability Review* **5**(3): 23–5

McGill P, Clare I, Murphy G (1996) Understanding and responding to challenging behaviour: From theory to practice. *Tizard Learning Disability Review* **1**: 9–11

McGill P, Mansell J (1995) Community placements for people with severe and profound learning disabilities and serious challenging behaviour: Individual illustrations of issues and problems. *Journal of Mental Health* **4**: 183–98

Maguire K, Piersel W (1992) Specialised treatment for behavioural problems of institutionalised persons with mental retardation. *Mental Retardation* **30**: 227–32

Mansell J (1996) Issues in community services in Britain. In: Mansell J, Ericsson K (eds.) *Deinstitutionalization and Community Living: Intellectual Disability Services in Britain, Scandinavia and the USA*. Chapman and Hall, London

Mansell J (2005) *Beyond the Unit and The Team: Meeting the Needs of People with Challenging Behaviour in Community Based Service Systems*. Tizard Centre, Canterbury

Mansell J, Beadle-Brown J (2005) Person centred planning and person-centred action: A critical perspective. In: Cambridge P, Carnaby S (eds.) *Person Centred Planning and Care Management with People with Learning Disabilities*. Jessica Kingsley Publishers, London

Mansell J, Elliot T (2001) Staff members' prediction of consequences for their work in residential settings. *American Journal on Mental Retardation* **106**(5): 434–47

Meltzer H, Gill B, Petticew M (1994) The prevalence of psychiatric morbidity among adults aged 16–64, living in private households in Great Britain. *OPCS Surveys of Psychiatric Morbidity in Great Britain Bulletin 1*. OPCS, London

Mitchell D (2004) Keynote review: Learning disability nursing. *British Journal of Learning Disabilities* **32:** 115–8

Mobbs C, Hadley S, Wittering R, Bailey NM (2002) An exploration of the role of the community nurse, learning disability, in England. *British Journal of Learning Disabilities* **30:** 13–8

Molyneux P, Emerson E, Caine A (1999) Prescription of psychotropic medication to people with intellectual disabilities in primary health care settings. *Journal of Applied Research in Intellectual Disabilities* **12:** 1

Morley S (1989) Single case research. In: Parry G, Watts F (eds.) *Behavioural and Mental Health Research: A Handbook of Skills and Methods*. Laurence Erlbaun Associates, Hove

Moss S (1999) Assessment of mental health problems. *Tizard Learning Disability Review* **4**(2): 14–9

Moss S, Emerson E, Kiernan C, Turner S, Hatton C, Alborz A (2000) Psychiatric symptoms in adults with learning disability and challenging behaviour. *British Journal of Psychiatry* **77:** 452–6

Murphy G (1994) Understanding challenging behaviour. In: Emerson E, McGill P, Mansell J (eds.) *Severe Learning Disabilities and Challenging Behaviours: Designing High Quality Services*, Chapman and Hall, London: 37–68

Murphy G, Oliver C, Corbett J, Cayton L, Hales J, Head D, Hall S (1993) Epidemiology of self-injury: Characteristics of people with self injury and initial treatment outcome. In: Kiernan C (ed.) *Research into Practice? Implications of Research on the Challenging Behaviour of People with Learning Disabilities*. Hester Adrian Research Centre, University of Manchester, Manchester

Newman I, Emerson E (1991) Specialised treatment units for people with challenging behaviours. *Mental Handicap* **19:** 113–9

Noone JS, Jones SSP, Hastings RP (2006) Care staff attributions about challenging behaviours in adults with intellectual disabilities. *Research in Developmental Disabilities* **27:** 109–20

Nursing and Midwifery Council (2004) *The NMC Code of Professional Conduct: Standards for Conduct, Performance and Ethics*. NMC, London

O'Brien J (1987) A guide to life-style planning: Using the activities catalog to integrate services and natural support systems. In: Wilcox B, Thomas Bellamy G (eds.) *A Comprehensive Guide to the Activities Catalog: An alternative curriculum for youth and adults with severe disabilities*. Paul H. Brookes Publishing Co, Baltimore, 175–90

O'Brien J (2002) Numbers and faces. The ethics of person centred planning. In: Holburn S, Vietzc PM (cds.) *Person-Centred Planning: Research, Practice and Future Directions*. Paul H Brooks, Baltimore, 399–414

O'Brien J, Lovett H (1992) *Find A Way Toward Everyday Lives: The Contribution of Person Centred Planning*. Pennsylvania Office of Mental Retardation, Harrisburg

O'Brien J, O'Brien CL (2000) *The Origins of Person Centred Planning: A community of practice perspective*. Responsive Systems Associates

O'Brien J, O'Brien CL, Mount B (1997) Person centred planning has arrived... or has it? *Mental Retardation* **35**: 480–4

O'Hara J, Sperlinger A (1997) *Adults with Learning Disabilities: A Practical Approach for Health Professionals*. Wiley, Chichester

O'Neill RE, Horner RH, Albin RW, Sprague JR, Storey K, Newton JS (1997) *Functional Assessment and Program Development for Problem Behavior: A Practical Handbook*. Brooks/Cole, Pacific Grove, CA

Reed J (1997) Understanding and assessing depression in people with learning disabilities: A cognitive-behavioural understanding. In: Stenfert Kroese B, Dagnan D, Loumidis K (eds.) *Cognitive Behaviour Therapy for People with Intellectual Disabilities*. Routledge: London

Risley T (1996) Get A Life! Positive behavioral intervention for challenging behaviour through life arrangement and life coaching (Ch. 18). In: Koegel, Koegel, Dunlap (eds.) *Positive Behavioral Support: Including people with difficult behavior in the community*. Paul Brookes Publishing, Baltimore

Robertson J, Emerson E, Hatton C, Elliott J, McIntosh B, Swift P, Krijnen-Kemp E, Towers C, Romeo R, Knapp M, Sanderson H, Routledge M, Oakes P, Joyce T (2005) *The Impact of Person Centred Planning*. Institute for Health Research, Lancaster

Rodgers J (1994) Primary health care provision for people with learning disabilities. *Health and Social Care* **2**: 11–7

Rose J (1995) Stress and residential care staff: Towards an integration of research. *Mental Handicap Research* **8:** 220–36

Rusch RG, Hall JC, Griffin HC (1986) Abuse-provoking characteristics of institutionalized mentally retarded individuals. *American Journal of Mental Deficiency* **90:** 618–24

Russell O (1997) Hidden Meanings. *Community Care* **6**(12): 18–9

Sailor W (1996) New structures and systems change for comprehensive positive behavioural support. In: Koegel LK, Koegel RL, Dunlap G (eds.) *Positive Behavioural Support: Including people with difficult behaviour in the community*. Paul H. Brookes Publishing Co, Baltimore

Sanderson H (2002) A plan is not enough: Exploring the development of person centred teams. In: Holburn CS, Vietze PMeds. *Person Centered Planning: Research, practice and future directions*. Paul H. Brookes, Baltimore

Sigafoos J, Arthur M, O'Reilly M (2003) *Challenging Behaviour and Developmental Disability*. Whurr Publishers Ltd, London

Smull M (1996) *Person Centred Planning: Should we do it with everyone?* Support Development Associates, Maryland

Stewart D, Todd M (2001) Role and contribution of nurses for learning disabilities: A local study in a county of the Oxford–Anglia region, *British Journal of Learning Disabilities* **29:** 145–50

Sturmey P (1999) Classification: Concepts, progress and future. In: Bouras N (ed.) *Psychiatric and Behavioural Disorders in Developmental Disabilities and Mental Retardation*. Cambridge University Press, Cambridge

Toogood S, Bell A, Jaques H, Lewis S, Sinclair C, Wright L (1994) Meeting the challenge in Clwyd: The intensive support team. *British Journal of Learning Disabilities* 22: 18–24.

Turnbull J (2004) *Learning Disability Nursing*. Blackwell, Oxford

White M, Nichols C. Cook R, Spengler P, Walker B, Look K (1995) Diagnostic overshadowing and mental retardation: A meta-analysis. *American Journal on Mental Retardation* **100:** 293–8

Zarkowska E, Clements J (1994) *Problem Behaviour and People with Severe Learning Disabilities: The STAR approach*. Chapman and Hall, London

CHAPTER 12

Forensic learning disability nursing practice

Anne Kingdon

Introduction

In the UK forensic nursing can be traced back to the opening of Broadmoor hospital in 1863 (Burrow, 1991). Much has been done to understand and articulate the roles of forensic mental health nurses but relatively little, as yet, has been done to study learning disability nursing roles in secure services in any depth. Practice development, particularly in community-based services, is therefore still in its infancy. There are no nationally agreed definitions or standards upon which learning disability nurses can draw to articulate their roles and, while the evidence base for learning disability forensic practice is growing, evidence that relates specifically to nursing practice remains limited.

The purpose of this chapter is to explore the scope and position of learning disability forensic nursing and identify some of the key factors that have driven and influenced role and practice developments. The chapter will draw on literature relating to mental health nursing to provide a description of forensic learning disability nursing. The characteristics of the client group, the settings and contexts in which practice takes place, and some of the key components of practice will be explored. Learning disability nurses in forensic roles are faced with many complex issues and dilemmas, and it has not been possible to cover all these within the limitations of the chapter. This chapter therefore provides a taster of what forensic learning disability nursing practice is about and readers who wish to learn more are signposted to other sources of information and texts for further reading.

What is forensic nursing?

The widespread popularity of crime fiction and TV crime drama has brought the word 'forensic' into common use and most people would now identify this term as having an association with dead bodies and the investigation of death as a result of criminal activity. The *Concise Oxford Dictionary* defines forensic as an adjective that, when applied to other terms, denotes a connection with courts of law. In practice the word forensic is now used as an adjunct to many disciplines and professional groups to denote a connection between the work or practice area concerned and the processes of criminal investigation and the law.

A strong relationship exists between medicine and the law and doctors fulfil many different 'forensic' roles including the provision of expert and professional opinions in the court arena, direct and indirect roles in criminal investigations, roles directly related to police procedures and psychiatric roles relating to the care of mentally disordered offenders. This long-standing 'medico-legal' relationship is based on very formal arrangements for doctors that include stringent postgraduate education requirements and clear career pathways for those wishing to specialise in forensic care. Increasing recognition of the relationship between criminal justice and healthcare systems has resulted in the development of forensic-specific roles for other professional groups who are involved in the delivery of healthcare to both offenders and victims of crime.

Forensic nursing roles can now be found in most countries across the Western world. It is clear from the available literature (for example, see Evans and Wells, 2001; Kettles et al, 2001) that there is considerable role diversity and significant variations in practice both nationally and internationally. In the USA, where there is formal recognition of the role, there are a number of practice areas in which forensic nursing roles exist (Saunders, 2000). Some of these roles, including sexual assault nurse examiners, death investigators and nurse coroners, focus on the provision of nursing care to the victims of crime, including those who survive or are killed as the result of trauma. Other practice areas where forensic nursing roles have been established focus on the needs of offender populations; these include correctional nurses, whose role is to provide nursing care to meet the physical and mental health needs of prisoners, forensic psychiatric nurses, whose role is to bridge the gap between the criminal justice and mental health systems, and legal nurse consultants, whose role is to provide assistance to the legal system.

In the UK forensic mental health nursing roles are now well established and posts can be found across secure environments, including hospital services and prisons, and in the community, including criminal justice settings. It is clear from the literature that there are still considerable difficulties with these roles. An agreed definition of the role remains elusive and some researchers have asked fundamental questions about the visibility, status, scope of practice, education and regulation of forensic nurses (Kettles et al, 2001; Peternelj-Taylor, 2001; Baxter, 2002). A major study focusing on nursing in secure environments (UKCC, 1999) identified that the use of the term forensic in the UK health sector implies that care is provided to mentally disordered offenders but also identified that many of the patients in secure care have not been convicted of offences and have not been in contact with the criminal justice system. Only some of the nurses who fell within the scope of the UKCC study were formally identified as forensic nurses in their job titles, while others undertaking the same work roles with the same client group were not. Later studies (Evans and Wells, 2001; Kettles et al, 2001) replicated these findings and identified that there are still no clear career pathways and no standardisation in relation to preparation for practice. Evans and Wells (2001) identified that this raises questions about the recognition of forensic practice as a specialism and the unification of forensic nurses as a group, and argued that this must cause confusion within the nursing community. Kettles et al (2001) stated this concern more strongly, arguing that the 'lack of vision and career pathways into forensic care is stifling a growing profession'.

Is forensic nursing a specialism?

Specialisation in nursing is still an issue for debate. It is clear from the literature that the issue of regulation and preparation for practice is a serious concern in relation to forensic mental health nursing. In an international study by Evans and Wells (2001) half of the 58 respondents, all of whom considered themselves to be in forensic nursing roles, had no forensic-specific qualifications. There are currently no statistics available relating to this issue in learning disability nursing but it seems likely that a considerable number of nurses in forensic roles may have no formal relevant post-registration qualifications. While many learning disability nurses who work with offenders may consider themselves to be in specialist roles, this practice area is not formally recognised as a nursing speciality. There are no standard post-registration educational requirements and no clear career pathways for learning disability nurses who want to pursue a forensic career. These issues are a challenge to the nursing profession. In the absence of role clarity, definition and regulation, it will be difficult to achieve formal recognition as a specialism.

What is forensic learning disability nursing?

There is currently no information regarding how many forensic learning disability nursing posts exist and it is more difficult still to estimate how many learning disability nurses would identify themselves as forensic nurses. In common with mental health services it is clear that the forensic role of many nurses is not recognised in their job titles and the number of nurses in clearly recognised forensic posts remains relatively small.

Rather than any reliable and defining differences between the work activities of nurses in forensic roles and their non-forensic counterparts it appears that the factors that define forensic nursing roles are derived from the practice setting and the characteristics of the client group. This in turn introduces a range of issues and dilemmas that give rise to particular knowledge and skills requirements in practice.

There appear to be three broad groups of nurses who might be identified as being in forensic roles or engaged in forensic practice. Posts may fall into one, two or all three groups:

- Setting: Learning disability nurses who work in secure forensic settings, including high secure care and low and medium secure services in the NHS and independent sector. These nurses currently constitute the biggest group but often remain largely invisible and are often disconnected from 'mainstream' learning disability nursing colleagues. Learning disability nurses who work within prison environments including young offender institutions. It is probable that the roles of these nurses are rarely exclusively aimed at responding to the needs of people with learning disabilities.
- Client group: Learning disability nurses whose practice is focused mainly on working with offenders with learning disabilities, and those at risk of conviction (offending).
- Job title and job description: Learning disability nurses who are formally identified as forensic nurses in their job title (i.e. community forensic nurse, forensic liaison nurse, etc).

The development of forensic learning disability services: Key drivers

An understanding of the main drivers will assist nurses to put their practice into context, and to appreciate how and where the priorities and perspectives of the various agencies differ and the potential for conflict exists.

The policy drivers and other factors that have influenced and directed the development of forensic learning disability services have been generated on two broad fronts. Firstly the policy of community care has meant that people with learning disabilities are no longer admitted to hospital as a matter of course and the majority of people who lived in large institutions now live in community settings (Department of Health 1971, 1992a, 2001). Both Day (1993) and Lindsay (2001) recognised that this has resulted in small but significant numbers of people with learning disabilities, who may not have previously done so, coming to the attention of community-based health, welfare and criminal justice agencies because of concerns about their behaviour. Secondly the needs of the small number of people with learning disabilities who are considered to require care and treatment in conditions of security have been included in the wider agenda related to the development of services for mentally disordered offenders. (Department of Health and Social Security, 1975; Home Office, 1990, 2003; Department of Health, 1992b; Home Office and Department of Health, 1995). In combination these shifts in policy have resulted in re-provision of some hospitals to focus on the delivery of assessment and treatment in secure conditions, development of new secure services in the NHS and independent sector, the roles of some learning disability nurses working in in-patient settings acquiring a more forensic focus and the creation of community-based forensic teams and learning disability forensic nursing posts. For a more detailed exploration of the policy context see Beacock (in Riding et al, 2005).

The client group

As identified above the characteristics of the client group is one of the factors that defines the forensic role. Nurses will recognise that this issue is central to many debates about forensic work with people with learning disabilities, and one that often causes conflict between services and agencies. Learning disability nurses in this field must have an ability to critically consider this issue in order to make an informed contribution to the assessment process and the debates, and to identify the appropriate evidence base for their practice.

As we have already identified, forensic is normally used as an adjective which is then attached to other words and terms to indicate a connection to the law and legal processes. It could therefore be argued that this term should only be applied to people with learning disabilities when they are subject to the legal processes associated with the criminal law and the courts, including detention subject to the provisions in Part III of the Mental Health Act 1983 (Patients concerned with criminal proceedings and under sentence). The responses of the criminal justice system to people with learning disabilities however often seem arbitrary. The issues of responsibility for actions and criminal responsibility and culpability are always a consideration for this group and many people are, quite rightly, actively diverted away from the normal processes of law. In practice, therefore, our application of the term is much broader and clients who are referred to as having forensic needs often include people who have been diverted, not been dealt with through the courts, and are detained in secure 'forensic' services under Part II of the Mental Health Act (Compulsory admission to hospital and guardianship). While many characteristics may be more common across this client group than in other groups there are only two characteristics that are shared across the whole client group with any degree of reliability.

Learning disability

Despite the fact that the presence and significance of learning disabilities is often the subject of debate this is still one of the characteristics that defines the client group. Kearns (2001) argues that the term learning disability is a colloquial and political, rather than diagnostic, term and it is important to recognise that, in the context of the forensic agenda, learning disability is a mental disorder. In diagnostic terms the clinical label of mental retardation is still used as defined in the two internationally recognised systems of mental disorder (*International Classification of Diseases* and the *Diagnostic and Statistical Manual of Mental Disorders*). People who attract the forensic label, whether or not they are accommodated in secure services, are likely to be in the more able group (borderline or mild learning disabilities) hence the debates regarding significance. To a lesser extent the group includes some people with moderate learning disabilities. It is however not possible categorically to state that people with severe learning disabilities are never subject to the process of criminal law and will not be found in secure forensic services.

Behaviour

The other characteristic that is shared across the group is that of a behaviour problem/s. It is the behaviour of the person, which may be described as offending, anti-social, maladaptive or challenging (to name but a few), and the risks associated with it that provide the grounds for detention under the categories of mental impairment or severe mental impairment (as defined in Part I of the Mental Health Act). For some people the behaviour may have resulted in conviction for an offence/s but, as we have already identified, this will by no means be the case across the whole group. It is inappropriate, inaccurate and possibly slanderous to refer to people who have not been convicted of an offence as an offender/s and it is therefore not possible to state that all people who use secure forensic services are offenders. Most nurses in community-based forensic roles also work with people who have been convicted and those who are considered at risk of conviction (or offending).

Other factors that seem to increase the likelihood of a person with a learning disability acquiring a forensic label relate to the nature of the behaviour that is the main cause for concern. Regardless of the level of a person's learning disability, extreme violence resulting in very serious harm or death is likely to be dealt with through the criminal justice process and for a very small minority may be dealt with under the unfitness to plead or insanity procedures (see Stone, 2003). Particular behaviours that cause high levels of concern in the public domain, including arson and behaviours that cause sexual harm to children, also appear more likely to result in identification as a 'forensic' client. If the behaviour is also prolific and resistant to management the tendency to apply a forensic label appears to increase still further.

It is clear that we are not dealing with concepts that can be easily differentiated, compartmentalised or defined. All services work to some form of eligibility criteria but it is important to recognise that the process of labelling can be arbitrary and there are significant grey areas in relation to the labels and definitions that we attach to the services we provide, the people who use them, and behaviour. Many would also argue that, despite the complications that this would cause in services, the application of a forensic label should be strictly limited to those who have been subject to the process of criminal law and dealt with via the courts.

Guiding principles for practice development

Effective learning disability nursing practice comes in many guises, all of which require the application of a sound value base and a broad range of knowledge, skills and capacities. Learning disability nurses who fulfil specific or specialist roles must build on the knowledge and skills gained from their learning disability nurse training and remain true to the core values of their discipline and profession. This is particularly important for nurses in forensic roles who can all too easily become isolated from non-forensic colleagues, subsumed in the agendas and perspectives of other disciplines and agencies, and may be working with others who have a very limited understanding of the learning disability agenda or the wider needs of people with learning disabilities.

In terms of continuing professional development, nurses in forensic roles may well be drawn towards forensic-specific courses and qualifications. Many of these will not consider the needs of people with learning disabilities, and what is learnt may need significant adaptation in order to be applied in practice. In addition to forensic-specific learning, it is absolutely essential that continuing professional development encompasses contemporary issues and the developing evidence base relating to the needs of people with learning disabilities. This balance may be enhanced through networking with nursing and other colleagues outside the forensic arena, and the use of creative approaches to practice development, for example role shadowing and short-term work placements in mainstream and non-secure learning disability services.

Role clarity is absolutely essential in forensic practice. Nurses who undertake forensic work must always work strictly within the boundaries of their role and competence and must be suitably trained if they are taking on extended roles (for example, involvement in the delivery of psychological interventions). The forensic process is adversarial and nurses may often feel pulled in many different directions and experience serious conflicts between their caring and custodial/public protection roles. The understandable temptation to identify with one of the other professions to the exclusion of one's own must be avoided (Hammer, 2000).

Some aspects of forensic work, for example the provision of opinions and advice and the preparation of reports for use by the probation service, police or courts, should only be undertaken by nurses who have a good understanding of the terms of such an undertaking. Nurses in all forensic roles, and particularly those at the interface with the criminal justice system, must understand that they may be called upon to justify any opinions they express in the legal arena, and they will need to develop the necessary knowledge and skills to enable them to function in this environment. All nurses in forensic roles must consider the risks associated with forensic practice and ensure that they have the full support of their employers for all aspects of their practice.

Practice issues

Many of the activities that make up nursing practice can be described under the headings of assessment and intervention. The description below, which emerges from the literature regarding mental health forensic nursing, also identifies the management component of the forensic nursing role. If we accept that offenders with learning disabilities are part of the group referred to as mentally disordered offenders, with some adaptation this could provide a useful general description of learning disability forensic nursing:

> *Forensic (psychiatric) nursing is about the assessment, treatment and management of mentally disordered offenders across a spectrum of secure environments, including the community.*
> *(UKCC, 1999; Chaloner and Coffey, 2000; Peternelj-Taylor, 2001).*

The remainder of this chapter considers some of the specific areas upon which forensic learning disability practice is focused, and some of the issues that are of particular concern to nurses in forensic roles.

Dilemmas

The perplexing problems and moral dilemmas associated with forensic practice are well recognised and relate to the many potential areas where apparently conflicting agendas exist. In an international study by Kettles et al (2001) mental health nurses identified dilemmas associated with forensic practice including, for example, treatment versus punishment, patient versus offender, motivation to change versus compulsion, and need for protection versus need for control.

Perhaps the most frequently encountered dilemma faced by nurses has been described by many researchers and is particularly well articulated by Peternelj-Taylor (1999) who said, 'nurses who practise in this [the forensic] domain face a dual obligation – one of social necessity and one of social good'. The dual obligations of security/public protection and therapy means that nurses need very good interpersonal skills in order to achieve the delicate balancing act necessary to successfully fulfil both aspects of their role. Despite these apparently conflicting demands, a nurse in secure services and other forensic roles, can often be one of a very few people with whom some clients have been able to achieve a sustained or therapeutic relationship. In order to cope with the inherent dilemmas in forensic practice, nurses must find a way to separate the client from certain aspects of their behaviour and maintain values that are based on the belief that all clients can achieve change.

Joint working and collaboration

Peternelj-Taylor (2001) says, 'the practice of forensic nursing is collaborative and interdisciplinary by its very nature', and while the level and frequency of contact that nurses have with colleagues from other disciplines, services and agencies will vary, the model of multidisciplinary team working forms the basis of most modern service delivery. Effective team working can be difficult to achieve under any circumstances and can be particularly problematic in a forensic context. The issues and problems faced by multidisciplinary teams are often complex and, at times can seem irreconcilable. The diverse nature of these teams will almost certainly give rise to tensions related to mission, philosophy and procedure (Hammer, 2000). A study by Dale and Storey (2004) found that many nurses in secure mental health services felt isolated and reported the belief that they lacked the authority to influence the work of the team. Despite this, few of the professionals involved in multidisciplinary teams will have received specific training in effective team working and there is rarely the time or the resources available to undertake the kinds of activities that would assist a group to come together as a team. Given the complexities and gravity of the decisions that fall to these teams, interdisciplinary tension must be recognised and managed and all involved must make the necessary investment in time, resources and commitment to achieve effective team working. Many of the skills needed for joint working (for example, listening, negotiation, conflict resolution) will also assist staff in their direct work with clients.

There is no doubt that the success of nursing roles that involve working across service and organisational boundaries, including those at the interface with criminal justice, depend heavily on the credibility of the nurses and their ability to build effective working relationships with others. In this context role clarity and the particular contribution nurses can make to achieve a coherent joint response to the needs of the client are absolutely essential. It could be argued that the other agencies should be able to achieve this without additional support but the prevailing reality is that people with learning disabilities who get into trouble with the law constitute a small minority group and are not a high priority for the criminal justice system. Professionals whose roles are entirely focused on the needs of this group must therefore develop the confidence and credibility to take on a lead role in achieving collaboration.

Risk assessment and risk management

There is a vast amount of literature relating to the assessment and management of risk, some of which relates specifically to risk and offending, and to a lesser extent offending behaviour in people with learning disabilities. A great many decisions hinge on the outcome of risk assessments and most forensic services would consider risk management and risk reduction to be their core aims. Learning disability nurses in forensic roles across all settings will be required to contribute to the assessment of risk, and in some roles will play a lead role in facilitating the process. They must therefore have a good understanding of the theory relating to risk assessment, the various approaches to risk assessment and management, and the systems and mechanisms that have been developed and/or adopted in their own services. Nurses working in community-based roles may also be called upon to contribute to risk assessment processes led by the police, the probation service and social services using systems and processes specific to these agencies.

Recognition of the power that nurses can wield on decisions about risk management, which can result in the loss of liberty or ongoing restrictions for clients, is essential to enable nurses to make a balanced contribution and ensure that any information they contribute to the process is based on factual evidence and informed opinion. For further general reading on risk assessment and management see Sellars (2005). For more detailed information about risk assessment and management as they apply to people with learning disabilities in a forensic context see Turner (in Riding et al, 2005).

Security

For people in secure services, including staff and patients, the imposition of restrictive measures aimed at managing risk is a high priority and the focus of a great deal of attention. It is absolutely essential that nurses working in secure settings are familiar with the various forms of security (for a useful definition of physical, relational and procedural security see Collins et al, 2003), and that they understand the reactive nature of externally imposed security and the contribution that security makes to overall risk management. Nurses who are responsible for the imposition of security must be familiar with policies and procedures for the use of all forms of security, and the mechanisms for decision making.

The use of close, special or one-to-one observation and/or supervision is perhaps one of the more common risk management procedures in secure hospital settings, and one in which nurses are routinely involved. A review of the literature about special observations (Bowers and Park, 2001) identified that little has been done to evaluate the effects this procedure, and its use is based mainly on pragmatism and tradition. Many studies have identified the negative impact of the procedure, but some researchers have recognised the potential for therapeutic value. This review provides food for thought for nurses who are called upon to implement such restrictive and intrusive interventions.

The use of physical intervention as a reactive strategy to manage behaviour is a feature of learning disability nursing practice in many settings. It is likely, however, that nurses who work in secure settings will encounter and be involved in this more frequently than their non-forensic counterparts. Secure services normally have clear protocols and provide standardised training in the use of physical intervention and associated techniques for the management of aggression and violence (for example, de-escalation, conflict resolution, de-brief). Within the 'cope with anything' culture that often prevails in secure services, the psychological effects of these restrictive interventions on the staff who are involved in their implementation may well be underestimated. It is important that staff support needs associated with this intervention, and that the imposition of all restrictive and compulsory external controls are recognised and addressed. A study by Sequeira and Halstead (2004) explored the psychological effects of physical restraint on nursing staff and discussed the possible implications of these in practice.

Mental health law

The pathway diagram (*Appendix 12.1*) demonstrates the stages where the provisions in Part III of the Mental Health Act 1983 (*Appendix 12.2*) may be applied. Nurses in forensic roles may also be working with people who are detained under the provisions of Part II or subject to other community-based legal provisions. They will therefore need a good working knowledge of these provisions, mental health law in general and the many complexities involved in its application to people with learning disabilities. Wiseman (in

Riding et al, 2005) provides a useful overview of mental health law from a clinical perspective.

Amendments to the Mental Health Act, which came into law in November 2008, include flexibilities that allow nurses and other professional groups to take on roles relating to the application of the Act that were previously reserved for social workers and psychiatrists. Nurses in forensic roles should pay particular attention to the development of these roles within their own organisations.

Communication

Communication is a core role for all nurses and a particularly important role for learning disability nurses. Learning disability nurses, whose roles often involve a great deal of direct contact with their clients, are in a very good position to support people with learning disabilities to understand their own situations and the decisions that others have made, and to enable their clients to participate in the decision making process. To fulfil this role effectively, nurses working in the forensic arena need sufficient knowledge of the various systems and processes, including criminal justice processes, mental health law and processes for decisions about treatment and management (including restrictions associated with physical, relational and procedural security) to enable them to translate this information and communicate it in a form that the client is able to understand. Einstein is reputed to have said that he did not consider that he had an adequate understanding of anything unless he could explain it to his mother; perhaps nurses could usefully apply a similar test to measure their own understanding against their ability to explain what is happening, why and how to their clients/patients.

Criminal justice liaison

Burrow (1993) proposed that the intersection between mental health care and legal systems creates an exclusive domain for a nursing speciality. Roles that involve the provision of advice directly into the criminal justice system have historically been limited to psychiatrists and psychologists but this situation is changing and nursing roles have now been developed in some areas to work at the interface between the various services and agencies who may be involved when a person with learning disabilities gets into trouble with the law. Decisions about whether, how and when the criminal justice process will be applied to people with learning disabilities are often extremely complex and weighty for those involved as each decision may have a life changing effect on the person with a learning disability, and in some cases can set precedents that will have wider effects.

Colleagues in the criminal justice system need advice and guidance to assist them in their decisions, and support to help them work directly with the people with learning disabilities with whom they come into contact. The pathway diagram (*Appendix 12.1*) illustrates the points at which there is an interface between specialist learning disability health services and the criminal justice system and the points at which diversion is a possibility. The grey boxes indicate where and how the services of specialist health professionals could support the decision making process and the client. Riding and Bullivant (in Riding et al, 2005) give an in-depth description of the criminal justice liaison model and how this can provide a way of working with offenders with learning disabilities.

Therapeutic approaches

The variety and range of forensic nursing roles encompass a broad spectrum of practice across both secure and community settings. Many nurses in forensic roles, and particularly those who work in secure services, are involved in the delivery of psychological interventions to individuals and groups using a variety of therapeutic models. Other roles include the provision of day-to-day nursing care and behavioural support to detained patients in secure services, roles focused on supporting clients to access mainstream services to address their offending behaviour and other problems, and other roles that have a greater focus on general behavioural analysis and intervention.

In broad terms therapeutic work can be taken to include all the activities that make a contribution to enabling the client to make different, and pro-social choices about their behaviour and lifestyle. In practice all nursing interventions should be clearly described and included in care or treatment plans so that the impact of the day-to-day therapeutic work that nurses undertake can be recognised and the impact of this input can be evaluated.

An entire book would be needed in order to consider the diversity of the problems presented by the client group and the range of interventions in which nurses are involved. For useful reviews see Lindsay and Macleod (2001), Lindsay (2002) and Beail (2002). The *Handbook of Forensic Learning Disabilities* (Riding et al, 2005) includes individual chapters that consider assessment and intervention in relation to the three main groups of offending behaviours (violence, sexual offending and arson) and approaches to working with deliberate self-harm.

Conclusion

The Government's policy in 1990 (Home Office, 1990) that 'Wherever possible mentally disordered persons should receive care and treatment from health and social services' has remained unchanged. While there has been a shift away from a belief that diversion is necessary for all people with mental disorders it is clear that many people with learning disabilities cannot be considered criminally responsible for their actions, that they are vulnerable in the criminal justice system, and need care and treatment rather than custody and punishment.

There is increasing recognition on the need to return people to their local areas from secure out-of-area placements (National Development Team, 2006) and it seems probable that the next few years will see the creation of more low secure learning disability services and further growth in the number of community-based posts to support this transition. High secure care for people with learning disabilities provided at Rampton Hospital is undergoing a major service re-provision and improvement programme and it also seems inevitable that there will be increasing discussions, as advocated by Kearns (2001), relating to the perceived need for long-term secure care facilities for some people with learning disabilities. The evidence base for practice is growing and learning disability nurses make an important contribution to forensic services. Despite the many challenges that are faced by nurses working in the forensic field these are important roles that can offer a stimulating and satisfying career choice for learning disability nurses.

References

Baxter V (2002) Nurses' perceptions of their role and skills in a medium secure unit. *Mental Health Nursing* **11**(20): 1312–9

Beail N (2002) Constructive approaches to the assessment, treatment and management of offenders with intellectual disabilities. *Journal of Applied Research in Intellectual Disabilities* **15:** 179–82

Bowers L, Park A (2001) Special observation in the care of psychiatric in-patients. A literature review. *Issues in Mental Health Nursing* **22:** 769–86

Burrow S (1991) The special hospital nurse and the dilemma of therapeutic custody. *Journal of Advances in Health and Nursing Care* **1**(3): 21–38

Burrow S (1993) An outline of the forensic nursing role. *British Journal of Nursing* **2**(18): 21–38

Chaloner C, Coffey M (eds.) (2000) *Forensic Mental Health Nursing: Current Approaches.* Blackwell Science, Oxford

Cullinv M, Dunion S, Ashmull C (2003) Meeting patients' needs in secure forensic psychiatric units. *Nursing Standard* **17**(49): 33–4

Dale C, Storey L (2004) High, medium and low security care: Does the type of care make any difference to the role of the forensic mental health nurse? *NT Research* **9**(3): 168–84

Day K (1993) Crime and mental retardation: A review. In: Howells K, Hollins CR (eds.) *Clinical Approaches to the Mentally Disordered Offender*. Wiley, Chichester

Department of Health (1971) *Better Services for the Mentally Handicapped*. HMSO, London

Department of Health (1992a) *Services for People with Learning Disabilities and Challenging Behaviour or Mental Health Needs*. HMSO, London

Department of Health (1992b) *Review of Health and Social Services for Mentally Disordered Offenders and Others Requiring Similar Services. Volume 7. People with learning disabilities (mental handicap) or with autism*. HMSO, London

Department of Health (2001) *Valuing People: A New Strategy for Learning Disability for the Twenty First Century*. The Stationary Office, London

Department of Health and Social Security, Home Office (1975) *Report of the Committee on Mentally Abnormal Offenders* (Butler Report). HMSO, London

Evans AM, Wells D (2001) Scope of practice issues in forensic nursing. *Journal of Psychosocial Nursing* **39**(1): 38–45

Hammer R (2000) Caring in forensic nursing: Expanding the holistic model. *Journal of Psychosocial Nursing and Mental Health Services* **38**(11): 18–24

Home Office (1990) *Provision for Mentally Disordered Offenders*. Circular 66/90. Home Office, London

Home Office (2003) *Mappa Guidance: Multi-agency Public Protection Arrangements*. Home Office, London

Home Office and Department of Health (1995) *Mentally Disordered Offenders: Inter-agency Working*. Circular 12/95. HMSO, London

Jones R (2008) *Mental Health Act Manual*. 11th edn. Sweet and Maxwell, London

Kearns A (2001) Forensic services and people with learning disability: In the shadow of the Reed Report. *Journal of Forensic Psychiatry* **12**(1): 8–12

Kettles AM, Peternelj-Taylor C, Woods P, Hufft A, Van Erven T, Martin H, Donisch-Siedel U, Kuppen A, Holmes C, Almvik R, Hatling T, Robinson DK (2001) Forensic nursing: A global perspective. *British Journal of Forensic Practice* **3**(2): 29–41

Lindsay WR (2002) Integration of recent reviews on offenders with intellectual disabilities. *Journal of Applied Research in Intellectual Disabilities* **15**: 111–9

Lindsay WR, Macleod F (2001) A review of forensic learning disability research. *British Journal of Forensic Practice* **3**(1): 4–10

Peternelj-Taylor C (1999) Forensic psychiatric nursing: The paradox of custody and caring. *Journal of Psychosocial Nursing and Mental Health Services* **37**(9): 9–11

Peternelj-Taylor C (2001) Forensic psychiatric nurse: A work in progress. *Journal of Psychosocial Nursing and Mental Health Services* **39**(9): 8–11

Riding T, Swann C, Swann B (eds.) (2005) *The Handbook of Forensic Learning Disabilities*. Radcliffe, Oxford

Saunders L (2000) Forensic nursing: Formalising a new role or recognising existing practice. *Australian Nursing Journal* **8**(3): 49–50

Sellars C (2005) *Risk Assessment in People with Learning Disabilities*. Blackwell, Oxford

Sequiera H, Halstead S (2004) The psychological effects on nursing staff of administering physical restraint in a secure psychiatric hospital; "When I go home it's then that I think about it". *British Journal of Forensic Practice* **6**(1): 3–15

Stone N (2003) *A Companion Guide to Mentally Disordered Offenders*, 2nd edn. Shaw, Kent

United Kingdom Central Council and University of Central Lancashire (1999) *Nursing in Secure Environments*. UKCC, London

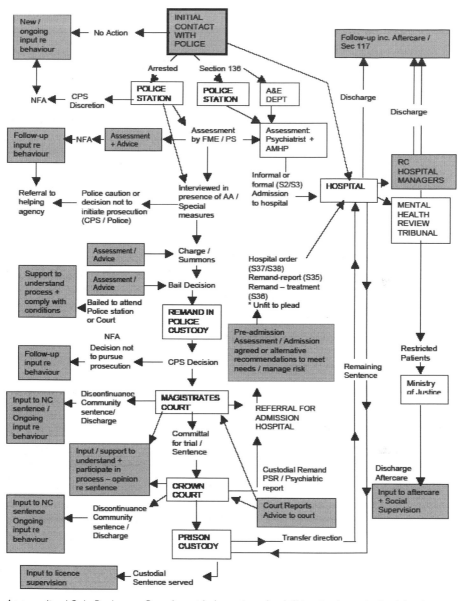

Appendix 12.1. Pathway: People with learning disabilities in the criminal justice system (shaded items indicate specialist learning disability team contributions).

AA: *appropriate adult*
AMHP: *approved mental health professional*
ASW: *approved social worker*
CPS: *Crown prosecution service*
FME: *forensic medical examiner*
Section 136: *Removal to a place of safety*

NC: *Non-custodial*
NFA: *no further action*
PS: *police surgeon*
PSR: *pre-sentence report*
RC: *responsible clinician*

Appendix 16.2: Mental Health Act 1983

Section 136:	Care and control of persons found in a public place. The power of a constable to remove a mentally disordered person found in a public place and in need of immediate care and control to a place of safety (usually an accident and emergency department or a police station).
Section 35:	The power of a court (Magistrates and Crown Courts) to order an accused person to be detained in hospital for assessment.
Section 36:	The power of the Crown Court to order an accused person to be detained in hospital for treatment.
Section 37:	Hospital Order or Guardianship: The power of a court (Magistrates and Crown Courts) to order a convicted person to be detained in hospital for treatment of mental disorder, or to be taken into the guardianship of the local authority.
Section 38:	Interim Hospital Order: Power of a court (Magistrates and Crown Courts) to order a convicted person to be detained in hospital for treatment to establish whether it is appropriate to make a hospital order (Section 37 above).
Transfer Direction:	Power of the Home Office to order convicted persons to be transferred from prison to hospital for treatment of mental disorder.
Section 117:	Imposes a duty on the local authorities and health authorities to provide aftercare services for patients who have been detained under the Mental Health Act.

CHAPTER 13

Autism spectrum conditions

Jill Aylott

Introduction

The term, autism spectrum condition (ASC), describes a range of conditions on the autism spectrum including that of Asperger syndrome. This chapter considers issues that are relevant to both people with a label of autism and those with Asperger syndrome. However there are more specific support issues relating to employment and people with Asperger syndrome which have been discussed elsewhere (Aylott et al, 2008). The diagnosis of autism and Asperger syndrome is usually made by a trained professional with reference to the Diagnostic and Statistical Manual (DSM-IV-TR) (American Psychiatric Association, 2000). The DSM criteria are based on the work of Wing and Gould (1979), who developed the term, 'triad of impairments'. However, over the last two decades there has been an increasing attempt to describe and explain autism from a 'user' perspective (Cesaroni and Garber, 1991; Grandin, 1984, 1992; Williams, 1992; 1994; 1996a; Gerland, 1997, Lawson, 2001). This chapter will draw upon the user perspective of autism and propose an alternative definition to the triad of impairments. The user perspective definition of autism and Asperger syndrome will highlight three main elements of the user experience, namely: sensory processing, information processing and anxiety. Donna Williams (1996b:25) defines these issues as problems in three main areas: *Table 13.1*

The skills and knowledge required of the learning disability nurse to become more person centred in the support provided to people with ASC is explored in this chapter and the reader is introduced to the communication and sensory profile. The profile was developed by the author when working with individuals with complex needs and helped to identify specific support

---

Table 13.1. Williams' (1996b) problem areas in ASC

Problems of control	Anxiety and 'obsession'
Problems of tolerance	Sensory and emotional
	Emotional hyper-sensitvity
Problems of connection	Difficulties with information processing

strategies in different environments (Aylott, 2003). In addition, key elements of the Government White Paper, *Valuing People* (Department of Health, 2001a) will be examined with a discussion of how this paper relates to the lives of people with an ASC.

Alternative definitions of autism spectrum condition

Sensory processing difficulties

Understanding autism from a sensory perspective is not new and was originally proposed as a theory to explain autism in the 1960s (Creak, 1961; Delacato, 1974; Rimland, 1978). Reports in the literature document hyper or hypo sensitivity occurrences to either auditory or visual stimuli, taste, touch and smell. The person may experience stress, pain or discomfort from some environments as they are receiving information through their senses in a hypersensitive way. For example, Williams (1994: 41) illustrates the experiences of acute auditory hypersensitivity:

> *I discovered I could use cotton wool in my ears in order to tolerate the pitch and intonation of her voice, but it still set my nerves on end.*

Both Williams (1998) and Grandin (1995) explain autism as a sensory continuum. Without reference to the sensory continuum the behaviours presented by individuals with an ASC will often be responded to with the use of more traditional behavioural interventions. Such behaviours may also be labelled as challenging or difficult. Once a sensory understanding of autism is used as part of the theoretical underpinnings of a practitioner's support, the use of the word 'challenging behaviour' becomes unhelpful and redundant. The theoretical framework of the sensory continuum helps to interpret and understand that behaviour may have a sensory origin in relation to stimuli in the environment. It also takes as given that most people with an ASC will relate to their environment in a different way through their senses.

Williams (1998) describes the sensory continuum as being made up of three parts: sensory, literal and significant. Williams argues that all people with an ASC will start within the 'sensory' part of the continuum and will move to a greater or lesser extent towards the significant. Some will stay within the sensory and may fail to make the transition because of the 'barriers' in support, or barriers may be present within frightening environments. Others will make the transition and may ask a lot of questions as they make this transition, but may revert completely to the sensory if a situation, event or an environment leads them to experience a high level of 'anxiety'. It is the 'sensory continuum' that exists in the lives of people with an ASC, regardless of their intellectual ability. If the environment becomes too overwhelming they may retreat to the safe world of the sensory as a protective strategy to cope with the bombardment of their senses by stimuli or demands in the environment. It is the interplay between a person's senses and the environment that can cause the person to become disabled in one environment and not in another. It is the barriers in place that create a 'disability'.

People with Asperger syndrome can experience sensory overload in a way that disables them in a particular environment. Some individuals find that they cannot hold down a job for more than a few weeks because they are experiencing stress in the environment (Aylott et al, 2008). It is within the sensory continuum that a support strategy can be designed and developed to help the person develop strategies to cope with different environments and to develop self-awareness of the environment that is right for them.

Some environments may have too many stimuli within them and will flood too many senses all at once, while other environments may not be stimulating enough. Take for example Jason (not his real name, Aylott, 2003):

There were about nine children who had been sitting on benches around the hall, observing the netball game and not participating. Jason was given a netball shirt and asked to join in. The games were in the large hall and there was a lot of whistle blowing and running around, a lot of movement and excitement and Jason started to jump up and down, clapping and flapping his hands. He just became immersed in his environment and almost oblivious to those around him. The environment was causing a 'flooding' and there was too much stimulation and too much arousal. Just because he had the shirt on, he was never going to be included within the game as he was experiencing too much sensory arousal and stimuli from the environment.

Jason had learnt strategies to help him cope with difficult environments and there are ways that can help him to concentrate and achieve. He needs a quiet environment to concentrate on a focused activity. He learns well with the use of the computer on his own as having other people around him makes him too anxious to concentrate:

Jason needs thinking time for each of his sums but he seems confident to take his time to work through them. He has earphones on while the other children do not have theirs on. He seems relaxed and comfortable. I have not seen him rock or flap his hands or use any stereotypical behaviour. He types in his answer and then folds his arms waiting while the computer computes a result and a score. It looks like the earphones keep out any unnessary noise that would impede his concentration.

The behaviour presented in the first extract is not at all evident in the second. Jason's so-called or observed 'autistic type' behaviour was a direct response to the stimuli present in the environment. Hence this example provides some illustration as to why it is important to understand autism as a condition which is directly affected (or not, as the second extract demonstrates) by stimuli present in any environment.

Information processing difficulties

Some individuals have reported that autism can be defined as an information processing difficulty, a feeling of being overloaded with information (Cesaroni and Garber, 1991). When this happens it may result in behaviours which appear to the onlooker as strange or 'challenging'. Some of the strategies used by individuals to lessen this effect are to convert or translate information into visual images. Visual information is sometimes easier for individuals to process and will cause less anxiety if the person is able to understand what is expected of him or her. Grandin (1995: 33) gives an example:

> *I thought of peace as a dove, an Indian peace pipe or a TV newsreel footage of the signing of a peace agreement. Honesty was represented by an image of placing one's hand on the Bible in court.*

Visual thinking can take a longer time to process information and can be misinterpreted as 'non-compliance' or 'demand-avoidance' behaviour. Lawson (2001) argues that she and others have experienced 'monotropism' in relation to information processing, which is the inability to process information from more than one channel at a time. This is important to consider when supporting people with a label of autism, especially when a support person is trying to explain changes in routine, expectations, instruction or changes to medication or a summary from a health practitioner. Lawson is unable to listen and participate at the same time (without due time to process information). She needs time to move from processing information from one sensory channel to another.

Understanding ASCs from an information processing perspective has implications for day-to-day support and for longer-term planning. If the person is attending a day centre or adult education class, time will need to be built in to help the person make the transition from one environment to another and for the person to process information that is in the different environments. This should be made explicit in support plans. There should also be observations made as to how the person best processes information in different environments. People may be faster to process in their own home but they may take up to six seconds or longer to process an instruction in a new environment. The support person should also adapt his or her own communication. Potter and Whittaker (2001) found that when adults reduced the complexity of their speech and language, this increased the levels of children's engagement in interactions.

Anxiety

Autism has been explained as a neurological developmental disability which often becomes apparent in crowded or overwhelming environments. When individuals are in a crowded environment this may overwhelm their neurological system and make them feel threatened or overloaded. This can trigger a hormonal response that creates high anxiety. The high anxiety chemicals start pumping, resulting in the person exhibiting behavioural outbursts when a tolerance level has been exceeded. The neurological system then starts to shut down to protect itself from the aversive stimulation and in turn the system releases endorphins that are anxiety-reducing chemicals. When individuals reach this state there is very little they can do in relation to listening to instructions or giving an explanation as to what is happening. The only way to support the person at this point is to try to create an environment that will help the person come out of this heightened state of anxiety. For some people this will only happen if they are left alone, and they may engage in repetitive motor movements such as self-stimulatory behaviours, hand flapping, pacing up and down or rocking back and forth.

Blackburn (2000) talks about this behaviour as a 'coping strategy':

In order to create a distraction or cut off between me and 'out there', I will flick my fingers in front of my face. My attention is drawn to my fingers rather than what is going on beyond. I can focus on what is near and close to me and what is predictable and 'me controlled' rather than what is further afield, unpredictable and therefore threatening.

They may even resort to making guttural sounds where there had previously been speech. Richard (1997) argues that self-stimulatory behaviours play a double-positive role in people with an ASC. The sustained rhythmic, repetitive movement triggers the release of calming endorphins as well as providing vestibular stimulation to innervate the reticular formation to arouse the cortex to make sense of the world. Williams (1994: 151) explains how this feels:

The lights were damned bright. Adrenaline was running through my veins and noise was already climbing up through the roof, despite the cotton wool in my ears. It would have been so easy to 'disappear'. It would have been too easy. Being numb and unaffected, being someone other than yourself is simply too addictive when being affected is so difficult and so sensorially overwhelming.

The White Paper: *Valuing People*

The White Paper, *Valuing People: A New Strategy for Learning Disability for the 21st Century* (Department of Health, 2001b) is a significant policy document to guide service provision for people with a learning disability and to steer professional practice. It has four key principles that guide it: civil rights, independence, choice and inclusion, and these principles are evident in the paper's aim that 'people with a learning disability are to have as much choice and control as possible over their lives and the services and the support they receive'. The Government has invested finance in the development of advocacy services, and person-centred planning will be a vehicle for this. Learning disability nurses are likely to be 'health facilitators', a role outlined in the White Paper to ensure that people with a learning disability get the health care they need through their own health action plan.

It is not always easy to identify how this paper relates to the lives of all people with an autism spectrum condition. Initially people with a diagnosis of Asperger syndrome were excluded from the White Paper because such individuals were likely not to have intellectual learning disabilities. A test case of a boy with autism (Megarry *v* Chief Adjudication Officer 29.10.99) who was seeking to claim the higher rate of Disability Living Allowance was upheld by the Court of Appeal when the judge ruled that, 'A high intelligence quotient was not sufficient to deprive an autistic child of entitlement to disability living allowance' within the meaning of the social security regulations. This case highlighted the problem of IQ tests for people with an ASC who can sometimes score unusually highly just because they are being tested outside the real-life context. Success in IQ tests is not a true indication of what might be called their 'useful intelligence' or social functioning. An IQ result might give a misleading impression of the person's 'useful intelligence' and in some cases social impairment may be sufficiently equal to that of an impairment of intelligence. Social impairment or social communication difficulties as a feature of Asperger syndrome can disable individuals sufficiently to inhibit their quality of life and in some cases can lead to mental health problems. Pressure from the National Autistic Society and other lobby groups led the Government to produce supplementary guidance that makes it clear that people with Asperger syndrome or high functioning autism should have access to appropriate learning disability services (Department of Health, 2001a):

Adults with Asperger's syndrome or higher functioning autism are not precluded from using learning disability services, where appropriate, and may require an assessment of their social functioning and communications skills in order to establish their level of need.

The White Paper should then, in principle, have relevance to all people with an ASC, but the principles of civil rights, choice, inclusion and independence, which underpin the objectives of the White Paper may be experienced differently to people on the autism spectrum.

Civil rights

This includes all aspects of life that identifies people as citizens. It is about the right to relationships and a family life, the right to marry to have children and to participate fully in a local community. It also includes the right to employment, leisure and partaking in political processes, such as voting. For many people with an ASC the experience of sensory and information processing difficulties and the likelihood of anxiety occurring in new and different environments will make all of the above extremely challenging to achieve. Blackburn (2000) writes:

While I don't want friends for social reasons, 'cocktail talk' etc., I need people. In fact I need people more than the average person, as I am not able to decode social signals and pick up on things myself and learn as I go along.

Blackburn suggests that one of the answers to help provide the support is to have a 'circle' or a group of volunteers based in the community who could take it in turns to be 'on-call' for the person with autism should they wish to go out or should they have a problem, either in or outside of the home.

The learning disability nurse will need to help build a network of resource for the person with autism since, far too often, the support network can 'burn out' with very few people having knowledge of the person, especially in the absence of parents and extended family.

Choice

The principle and practice of 'choice' is now clearly entrenched in policy and practice of learning disability services, but this is less defined when exploring choice in services for people with an ASC. The bigger picture of choice in relation to housing and support has been comprehensively researched (Powell, 2002; Harker and King, 2004) but the smaller day-today issues in relation to choice for people with an ASC appears to create the most contention and debate.

It is often suggested that people with autism need to have limited choices in their life, as to give the person a wider choice would cause the person to experience 'anxiety'. It is clear that such a statement departs from current person-centred planning principles, yet there is some element of truth in this statement. Due to a person's information processing style the person may take time to process the information when being offered a choice. More than one choice may be overwhelming and cause an increase in anxiety levels. In the same way, choices being offered through the senses (for example personal care products), may take time to process if the person is experiencing monotropism (the ability to process information through one sensory channel at a time). Choice making plans must be clearly linked to the evidence (or knowledge) of the way the person: (a) processes information; (b) relates through his or her senses to the environment; and (c) experiences anxiety in different environments. Even if high levels of anxiety do exist, having choice can still be an important part of a person's everyday life. Identifying information about the person's anxiety levels (See *Table 13.2*) can help.

Having choices in life is one of the fundamental tenets of developing an awareness of self and developing communication skills. One of the limitations of some of the person-centred planning frameworks is to list 'likes and dislikes'. There is a tendency to limit opportunities to what is known on the 'likes and dislikes' list and choice may gradually decline from a person's life, particularly if he or she has non-verbal communication skills or limited communication abilities. One of the ways to safeguard this from happening is to introduce a 'choices inventory' for a period of two to three weeks. The aim of the choices inventory is to find out a person's response to a range of choices offered through the different senses (at least one choice offered in the morning and one in the afternoon). This is a particularly good exercise to undertake when new staff have been recruited or to find out more about the person for the person-centred planning process.

For example, this exercise was undertaken with Mary's support team and all the staff agreed to offer at least one choice each shift, to document how the choice was offered and to write down Mary's response. The following information emerged over a two week period:

- Gave Mary a manicure and started a hand massage with cocoa butter cream. I was massaging Mary's right hand and when I put more hand m on the same hand, Mary suddenly grabbed my hand directing it rds the hand cream and showed me her left hand. She wanted me the cream on her left hand.
  pulled out one of her cardigans (the blue one) from the still wet

laundry wanting to wear it. I explained to her that she could not wear it because it was still wet and told her that we could go upstairs into her room and choose a cardigan from her wardrobe. When upstairs she was happy to choose the same colour cardigan as the one downstairs.

- Mary chooses to drink from a mug rather than a glass. I tried to give her some milkshake in a glass, she refused it, but drank it when I transferred the drink into a mug.
- Mary took a cardigan off the peg but this time it was not hers. I explained to her that the cardigan was somebody else's and that we would go upstairs and choose one from her wardrobe. When upstairs by the wardrobe, Mary was laughing loudly and got one of her cardigans. I believe she was happy that I understood her need.

The above information helped the staff team to conclude that Mary definitely knows when she is making a choice, but needs time to build more confidence. She is more likely to choose by looking, tasting and touching rather than using her sense of smell. When Mary was offered bath oils and yoghurts to choose at bath and meal times she pushed both away, even though she enjoys yoghurts. Mary uses 'looking' a lot in her communication and has led the team to think about the use of photographs to aid the communication process.

Developing the choices inventory has helped raise a level of awareness of choice among the staff team and it has moved the team along in their support of Mary to develop her communication skills.

Inclusion

The primary difficulties for people with a label of autism are in relation to understanding a confusing social world, that is maintained and perpetuated by many social, communication and attitudinal barriers.

It has often been the experience of children with an ASC that an inability of their school to respond to their needs has resulted in their exclusion. In a report published by the National Autistic Society *Inclusion and Autism: Is it Working?* (2000) it was found that secondary schools needed to give more attention to social and life skills and that support staff should understand the specific needs of this group of children. These children make up the biggest single group of children excluded from school, with one in five children with a label of autism or Asperger syndrome having been excluded from school. This is nearly 20 times the national average. The reason for the exclusion is frequently the result of the lack of appropriately trained support staff.

There are now more children with a label of autistic spectrum disorders on their statement of special educational needs in special schools than any other impairment label. A report by the National Autistic Society *Autism in Schools: Crisis or Challenge?* (2002) reveals that one in three children in special schools have needs related to autism, yet 75% of schools in the survey reported that their teachers are inadequately trained.

It could then be argued that children with an ASC are being excluded from mainstream schools, not because of their 'impairment' but because of the barriers in place that continue to deny their access to education. Such barriers will continue to deny individuals choice, independence, civil rights and inclusion. A legal framework is in place to challenge discriminatory practice. The Special Educational Needs Code of Practice (Department of Education and Skills, 2001) implements the Special Educational Needs and Disability Act (2001). The Code of Practice replaced the 1994 code in England and was implemented in 2002. All schools, education facilities, health and social services must have regard to the Code of Practice:

> *Schools will be required not to treat disabled pupils less favourably for a reason relating to their disability and to take reasonable steps to ensure that they are not placed at a substantial disadvantage to those who are not disabled.*

In practice, the Special Educational Needs and Disability Act 2001 amends the Disability Discrimination Act 1995, to prohibit all schools from discriminating against disabled children in their admissions arrangements, in the education of its pupils or in relation to exclusions from school. There is a new emphasis in the Special Educational Needs Code of Practice on the rights of children with special educational needs to be involved in decisions and to be able to exercise choice. There is a whole chapter on pupil participation and recognition that the process of communication may well be varied and different for some children, the document argues:

> *Consultation with young children will necessitate a range of communication strategies, including the use of play, art, audio and video as well as verbal communication.*
> *(Special Educational Needs Code of Practice, 2001:28)*

This position places emphasis on the acknowledgement of the different communication styles, which becomes the starting point for developing pupil participation. It will be the establishment of a means and method of communication that will enable participation rather than communication difficulties being an excuse for the exclusion of some individuals from such a process. The Special Educational Needs Code of Practice has started to acknowledge the sensory difficulties of children with special educational needs. Although the document does not identify any particular children, there is a sentiment in the following extract that indicates that we may need to understand children in different ways:

> *It is important to avoid making assumptions about levels of understanding, particularly amongst very young children and older children with learning, communication or sensory difficulties. These children may need additional help to be able to make their views and wishes known and efforts should be made to arrange for this help to be provided where it is needed.*
>
> *(Special Educational Needs Code of Practice, 2001:31)*

Independence

It is only through the process of communication that a true picture can be built of the issues and concerns of children and young people with the label of autism. It is also only through a system of communication that the person can develop skills for independent living.

The Special Educational Needs Code of Practice (2001: 31) indirectly refers to barriers in their recognition that staff need skills to communicate with children with special needs. They argue this specifically in relation to learning support assistants:

> *Learning support staff have a critical role in supporting many children and their training should include an element on pupil participation and the development of communication skills.*

Research by Curcio and Paccia (1987) illustrates that support staff can break down barriers of communication between themselves and people with a label of autism. There was a direct correlation between the increase in facilitating features of adult utterances and the increase in adequate replies from the children. Facilitating features included yes/no questions, questions that were conceptually simple and questions that were semantically contingent on the child's topic. One of the negative findings from this research was that 64% of adults did not simplify their subsequent utterance following an inadequate reply from the child. The researchers found that there were many missed opportunities for adults to simplify their questions when children incurred a lapse in their turn to answer.

A focus on how barriers exist in the communicative/support relationship with people with a label of autism can enable professional development that can enhance the teaching and learning of individuals who work with those so labelled. The breaking down of barriers in social relationships is a much more useful, proactive and helpful strategy, as opposed to using behavioural management strategies to focus on 'impairments', 'deficits' and 'disorders', particularly when things start to go wrong. The training of staff in understanding autism is vital to ensure that people with an ASC have opportunities to develop their independent living skills.

Developing support and intervention strategies

Using the new definition to understand the experience of autism and Asperger syndrome, this next section outlines a communication and sensory profile to identify the support required in the areas of sensory processing difficulties, information processing difficulties and anxiety in environments.

Developing a communication and sensory profile

The aim of using the communication and sensory profile shown in *Table 13.2* is primarily to identify a way of breaking down barriers in the working relationship between the person and the practitioner. The profile can be used as a tool to learn how the person makes sense of the world, identifying what is important to the person (special interests) and how this may help the person's motivation to participate in interaction and activities. The most important aim of using the communication profile is to establish some consistency with the care/support team in how staff communicate with the person (for example, the use of personal space, tone and pitch of voice, use of body language or not, etc.).

The learning disability nurse will need to start from the premise of working out the extent of the person's communication abilities and his or her preferred style and method of communication. Even when a person has extensive language skills (which is often the case for people with Asperger syndrome) and is able to articulate well, they may not fully understand elements of this spoken language. Others, meanwhile, may communicate without language and find that there are barriers to prevent the support staff from understanding what they are communicating. The person may use vocal sounds and the communication profile can identify if different sounds have different meanings; do they, for example, convey emotion such as happiness, sadness, anger or frustration. The communication profile can be used in addition to a tape recording of sounds or a video/DVD to record communicative behaviours.

The communication and sensory profile in *Table 13.2* was developed with Sam (not her real name). I worked extensively with Sam and her parents after meeting them at a training event. Further details about the approach used with Sam is documented elsewhere (Aylott and Sell, 1997)

Table 13.2. The communication and sensory profile

Verbal communication Does the person use verbal communication? If yes, how is this used to communicate with others?	Sam uses some verbal communication, only when she chooses to do so. She uses key words mainly nouns. When communicating verbally her words are clear and concise. She has a limited vocabulary but is capable of communicating her needs and choices but needs to trust the people around her.
The meaning of words Does the person have his/her own words for things that are different to the ones we would normally use? Their word is ..... it means......	Sam uses her own words, i.e. nanurk (this means nanna, who is deceased, and means she wants her photograph book to look through), dadan (means daddy) ergan (means horse riding, and was the name she had for the first horse she went on), and funky (means fudgecake)
Non-verbal communication What non-verbal communication does the person use and how effective are they in putting the message across?	Sam uses lots of non-verbal communication, it is one of the main ways that she communicates what she wants to do and when she doesn't want to do something.
The meaning of non-verbal communication What is the meaning of the person's non-verbal communication? When they do .... it means	When there is too much sound in the room she will put her hands over her ears and move away to the quietest corner of the room Shakes head when she doesn't want to do something Gestures to the window or door when wanting to go out
Communication through the senses How does the person communicate through: Touch, sight, hearing, movement, taste, smell	Touch – likes to touch on her terms. If others touch her she will usually recoil Sight – likes to look at her photograph

Table 13.2 continues

Table 13.2/cont

	album and pictures in the catalogue Hearing – can hear well and is able to respond to instruction but her hearing is impaired when there are other sounds in the room or from outside traffic Movement – Sam walks with an awkward gait and this can sometimes unsettle her balance. She has some scoliosis of the spine and her walking is sometimes slower if she is in pain Taste – Sam likes to taste hot and spicy foods and enjoys trying new tastes Smell – not observed as a particular sense that she relates to
Communicating emotion How does the person communicate emotions such as happiness, anxiety, sadness, being scared and frightened, feeling excited	Happiness – When Sam is happy she will squeal and give out a loud laugh, usually this is accompanied by rocking back and forth Anxiety – When anxious her facial expression looks stern and she has increased eye contact. She becomes more vocal and makes a guttural sound at the back of her throat Sadness – she gets her photograph book and starts to sob loudly, she appears lethargic Frightened – Sam becomes withdrawn, makes whimpering noises, seeks closeness with the people she trusts and backs away from the source of fear Feeling excited – Sam becomes very loud, clear speech, sobs with laughter, similar and this is very similar to when she is happy

Table 13.2 continues

Table 13.2/cont

Anxiety levels	
Does the person's communication change when his/her anxiety levels increase? If yes then how does this change?	When anxious, Sam will increasingly rock back and forth and she is unable to listen to any request or instruction She may start to scratch her arms and cry and then she may bite her hands. Moans in distress

Developing a support strategy for a person with an autism spectrum condition

Managing the environment to prevent anxiety	
What needs to be in place in the environment to prevent the person from feeling anxious (e.g. furnishings, pictures on the wall and other landmarks of familiarity). Also a need to consider how the person relates to environments through his/her senses	Sam needs a structure and needs to know what she will be doing 'now' and 'later'. She needs to be communicated with and engaged with so that she understands what is required of her. She likes to have her photograph book to hand and she likes to have a quiet environment around her. If there is too much noise in her environment she gets distressed and starts to get anxious
What support is required to prevent anxiety	
For example the physical distance between the person and the staff member needed to communicate, introducing new staff and planning a change in routine	All new staff to keep their distance and not to make demands of Sam until she understands who they are and what they will be doing with her. Sam will become anxious and distressed if there is not a period of introduction with her before an activity starts
Special interest	
What do staff need to do to share a dialogue with the person around his/her special interest?	Sam likes paper and cutting and making hats from the paper. She will bring the paper to you and expects you to create a hat from the paper. This activity helps her to relax and helps to build a positive working relationship

Table 13.2 continues

Table 13.2/cont

What is likely to motivate the person to get involved in an activity?

Is it possible to build the person's special interest into the activity in some way?	Use the makaton sign for 'later' to communicate the making of hats and show Sam a picture of the activity and sign 'now'. As soon as the activity has finished show her that the making of hats becomes the activity for 'now'

How should staff communicate to the person?

For example, the use of language, tone, the use or non-use of particular words	Staff should use simple language, key words instead of sentences. Staff need to avoid conversations with each other in front of Sam as she finds this confusing and it creates a level of anxiety with her

---

What can staff do to help the person better understand what is about to happen to him/her? (Information processing)

The use of pictures, diagrams, the building on the person's current level of understanding of similar issues	Sam loves to look at photographs so the camera should be used as often as possible to take pictures of places and activities that she likes. The photographs can be used to help to explain what is going to happen 'now' and 'later'

How do you recommend that information be presented in a visual way? How would you use photographs, pictures, drawings, symbols or objects?
See above

Describe how you show the person what it is you want him/her to do? Describe the process

When giving Sam a choice of activities or tasks offer her three photographs and explain what each one is using speech in a clear way. Make sure you carry out the task with the person. Try not to use too much communication as this will overload her information processing abilities and create confusion. Using one or two words helps to aid her understanding.

The communication and sensory profile provides a starting point to engage with the person and his or her family. It will not provide all the answers and sometimes the information will be contradictory. It is hoped that it may go some way to help build consistent support for people with autism and Asperger syndrome and make some small inroad into breaking down some of the barriers in an unpredictable and confusing social world.

Knowledge and skills for a specialist nurse practitioner in autism

Reflecting on my own career as a learning disability nurse, I can recall many examples of meeting service users who were not diagnosed with an autism spectrum condition, but their behaviour could now be explained by such a diagnosis. I can remember a young man, Doug, on a locked ward of a hospital (only in his early 20s). He communicated in repetitive sentences and needed to keep people a certain distance from him. If people stepped into his space without announcing their intention to come closer to him he would jump up and bite or pull the person to the ground by their hair (a sensory processing difficulty). The staff were often at a loss of how to work with him and he spent a lot of his time rocking back and forth engaging in sensory self-stimulating behaviours.

At the same hospital on the mental health/learning disability (locked) ward a young woman, Amy, was described by staff as 'volatile'. It was often said that she would 'explode' and smash furniture, and self-injure for 'no apparent reason'. What was key for this young woman was that she had an information processing difficulty and often misunderstood information that was given to her by the staff. She was an able and independent woman and this often led staff to communicate with her in long sentences without checking her understanding.

There are numerous examples of people like Doug and Amy but for many people their diagnosis of a learning disability overrode any recognition of an autism spectrum condition. This did very little to help and support them to find strategies to cope with often very complex and demanding environments. A diagnosis of an ASC is about helping people make sense of their environments and to create practical strategies that will help them adapt and cope with a confusing world. It is also about signposting people to other support services and helpful information.

One of the major steps for a learning disability nurse is making the transition from the 'medical' to the 'social' model of understanding disability. There is a lot of information and instruction on how to work with people with autism written from a medical perspective and this can often misdirect and mislead learning disability nurses. The most useful framework to use when working with people with autism are the skills teaching frameworks (understanding how to teach new skills, Bereweeke system), and understanding theories on how people learn. In addition it is important to recognise that people with autism and Asperger syndrome will have a different cognitive process (explained by Happe, 1994, and illustrated by Grandin in her book *Thinking in Pictures*, 1995). Learning disability nurses have excellent skills in working in partnership with people with a learning disability to promote advocacy, and these skills are excellent when transferred to working with people with autism. It is the listening skills that matter the most, listening for things that may not have been spoken. Finally, there is an attitude required which is about not having an ego. It is about being laid back, being humble and letting the person be your teacher. Not all learning disability nurses or nurses in other specialties have a history of presenting with this particular attitude, as the profession overall has reigned using power and control. Working with people with autism is for the unassuming, it is for staff who have nothing to prove but everything to learn. Sometimes you think you might have cracked it (when understanding a person's behaviour) only to learn the next day that things have changed.

Coping with stress and building in support structures for staff is essential as the demands of working with these individuals are high. It is about thinking through the processes of everyday support through the eyes of a person with autism and this can be very draining. It is about seeing with new eyes and opening up all possibilities when building bridges of trust in communication.

References

American Psychiatric Association (2000) *Diagnostic and Statistical Manual of Mental Disorders (DSM-IV)*. American Psychiatric Association, Washington

Aylott J (2003) *Developing a Social Understanding of Autism Through the 'Social Model'*. Unpublished PhD thesis, Sheffield Hallam University

Aylott J, Philips K, McLimens A (2008) 'They would have sacked me anyway': The real barriers to employment for people with Asperger syndrome. *Good Autism Practice* 9(1): 32–9

Aylott J, Sell I (1997) Gentle teaching as an empowering approach to challenging behaviour. *British Journal of Nursing* 6(8): 442–6

Blackburn R (2000) 'Within and Without autism' *Good Autism Practice Journal* 1(1): 2–8

Cesaroni L, Garber M (1991) Exploring the experience of autism through first hand accounts. *Journal of Autism and Developmental Disorders* **21**(3): 303–13

Creak M (1961) The schizophrenic syndrome in childhood. *British Medical Journal* **2:** 889–90

Curcio F, Paccia J (1987) Conversations with autistic children: Contingent relationships between features of adult input and children's response adequacy. *Journal of Autism and Developmental Disorders* **17**(1): 81–93

Delacato C (1974) *The Ultimate Stranger.* Doubleday, New York

Department of Education and Skills (2001) *Special Educational Needs Code of Practice.* DfES/581/2001. HMSO Stationary Office, London

Department of Health (2001a) *Valuing People. A New Strategy for Learning Disability for the 21st Century.* Department of Health, London

Department of Health (2001b) *Supplementary Guidance to the White paper Valuing People.* Department of Health, London

Gerland G (1997) *A Real Person – Life on the Outside.* Translated by J.Tate. Souvenir Press, London

Grandin T (1984) My experiences as an autistic child and review of selected literature. *Journal of Orthomolecular Psychiatry* **13:** 144–74

Grandin T (1992) An inside view of autism. In: Schopler E, Mesibov GB (eds.) *High Functioning Individuals with Autism.* Plenum Press, New York

Grandin T (1995) *Thinking in Pictures.* Vintage Books, USA

Happe F (1994) *Autism: An Introduction to Psychological Theory.* University College London Press, London

Harker M, King N (2004) *Tomorrow's Big Problem: Housing Options for People with Autism: A Guide for Service Commissioners, Providers and Families.* National Autistic Society, London

Lawson W (2001) *Understanding and Working with the Spectrum of Autism: An Insider's View.* Jessica Kingsley Publishers, London

National Autistic Society (2000) *Inclusion and Autism: Is it Working?* National Autistic Society, London

National Autistic Society (2002) *Autism in Schools: Crisis or Challenge?* National Autistic Society, London

Potter C, Whittaker C (2001) *Enabling Communication in Children With Autism.* Jessica Kingsley Publishers, London

Powell, A (2002) *Taking Responsibility: Good Practice Guidelines for Services – Adults with Asperger Syndrome.* National Autistic Society,

London

Richard GJ (1997) *The Source for Autism*. Lingui Systems, Ilinois

Rimland B (1978) Savant capabilities of autistic children and their cognitive implication. In: Serban G (ed.) *Cognitive Defects in the Development of Mental Illness*. Bruner/Muzel, New York

Williams D (1992) *Nobody Nowhere*. Doubleday, New York

Williams D (1994) *Somebody Somewhere*. Republished by Jessica Kingsley Publishers, London (1999)

Williams D (1996a) *Like Colour to the Blind*. Republished by Jessica Kingsley Publishers (1999)

Williams D (1996b) *Autism – An Inside Out Approach*. Jessica Kingsley Publishers, London

Williams D (1998) *Autism and Sensing*. Jessica Kingsley Publishers, London

Wing L, Gould J (1979) Severe impairments of social interaction and associated abnormalities in children: Epidemiology and classification. *Journal of Autism and Developmental Disorders* **9:** 129–37

CHAPTER 14

Development of services for children

Owen Barr

Introduction

The last 20 years have seen a major change in the abilities and needs of children with learning disabilities. On one hand, improved healthcare and opportunities for education have enabled many more children with learning disabilities to live healthier and more fulfilling childhoods (Department of Health, 2001). On the other hand, the numbers of children with complex physical healthcare needs has increased as neonatal and paediatric services have been able to support an increasing number of children who would previously not have lived into adulthood. Many of these children will have life-limiting conditions and will require intensive support throughout their childhood, at times being dependent on technology to receive adequate nutrition and medication and, possibly, help with breathing. In many ways this group of children are a 'new' group of children in community settings who previously would have spent longer periods in hospital care and probably died at a younger age.

There is also an increasing recognition of the mental health needs of children and young people with learning disabilities. This has led to mental health promotion and responses from health, social services and education professionals to the emerging mental health difficulties children may experience (Foundation for People with Learning Disabilities, 2002).

The changing demography of children with learning disabilities, together with changing policy objectives and priorities, has resulted in the need to review how services are planned and delivered to children and the role of professionals in services, including registered learning disability nurses.

The need for an integrated approach to children's services

The need to provide services for all children that allow opportunities for them to develop to their individual potentials and which recognises their value as people has been repeated with varying degrees of vigour and funding at regular intervals as a key Government objective over at least the past three decades (Department of Health and Social Security, 1976). The need to deliver services that made the needs of the child paramount, child-centred and focused on responding to the individual needs of children was a key strand of the Children's Act (1989) and corresponding legislation introduced in other countries in the UK during the 1990s. The need to provide child-centred services has been most recently restated within the *National Service Framework for Children, Young People and Maternity Services* (Department of Health, 2004). This framework once again emphases the need for effective interdisciplinary and interagency communication and integrated working that focuses on the needs of the child and family, rather than the needs of the service or professionals within the services.

The development of this framework was heavily influenced by the findings of the Victoria Climbie Inquiry, perhaps one of the most graphic illustrations of the failure of systems to protect a child in the UK, and a report which should be read by all health and social care professionals. The vision of future services, as outlined in the National Service Framework, is that they should be developed under the banner of 'Every child matters' which has been heralded as a 'new approach to the well-being of children and young people from birth to age 19, with the stated aim of 'every child, whatever their background or their circumstances, should have the support they need to: be healthy, stay safe, enjoy and achieve, make a positive contribution and achieve economic well-being'. The recommendations from this report have implications for services provided to all children, including children with learning disabilities.

Children with learning disabilities: An overview of policy direction

Since the mid 1970s there have been calls to recognise the childhood of people with learning disabilities and respond in an integrated and child focused manner. The Court Report (Department of Health and Social Security, 1976) stated that children with learning disabilities had more in common with other children, because of their childhood, than adults, because of their common disability. This position was emphasised in 1977 when the National Development Group stated that service planning should be underpinned by the view that children with learning disabilities were 'children first' and learning disabled second (NDG, 1977: 2).

Similar perspectives are evident within the recent reviews of policy for people with leaning disability across the UK, with policy objectives including, 'To ensure that disabled children gain maximum life chance benefits from educational opportunities, healthcare and social care...' (Department of

Health, 2001: 30), and to achieve 'a world in which children with a learning disability will have equal choices and equal value' (Department of Health, Social Security and Public Safety, 2005: 35).

The overarching policy for all children in England is presented within the *National Service Framework for Children, Young People and Maternity Services* (Department of Health, 2004). Children with learning disabilities are included and given specific attention within the standard on 'Disabled children and young people and those with complex health needs'. This standard relates to 'children and young people who are disabled and/or those with complex health needs, including children and young people with learning disabilities, autistic spectrum conditions, sensory impairments, physical impairments and emotional/behavioural disorders' (Department of Health, 2004: 4).

The vision presented for services provided to children with disabilities as part of the National Service Framework includes (Department of Health, 2004: 5):

- Children supported to participate in family and community activities and facilities.
- Health, education and social care services organised around the needs of children and young people and their families, with co-ordinated multi-agency assessments leading to prompt, convenient, responsive and high-quality multi-agency interventions that maximise the child's ability to reach his or her full potential.
- Children and young people and their families actively involved in all decisions affecting them and in shaping local services.

Furthermore, the Framework states that the standard for the evaluation of services is the degree to which children with learning disabilities receive co-ordinated, high-quality child and family-centred services which are based on assessed needs, which promote social inclusion and, where possible, which enable them and their families to live ordinary lives. Although the Framework is specific to England it has influenced policy documents written in relation to children with disabilities across the United Kingdom.

The changing nature of service structures

The vision and policy aims contained within the specific reviews of learning disability policy and those within the Framework will involve four key shifts in emphasis within service provision; firstly, children with learning disabilities should have access to the same range of opportunities, support and services as other children. The presence of learning disabilities should not be seen as a reason for restricting access to opportunities (Scottish Executive, 2000; Department of Health, 2001; Department of Health, Social Security and Public Safety, 2005)

Secondly, and in a large part influenced by the need to provide increased access to services, children with learning disabilities now often have contact with a wider range of health, social care and educational service professionals than previously. During the 1980s and into the 1990s most professionals that children with learning disabilities had contact with were located within learning disability service systems. However, with the emphasis on rights to access services and the inclusion of children with learning disabilities in legislation such as the Children Act (1995) in England and equivalent legislation in the other devolved countries within the UK, as well as the development of a Common Assessment Framework there has been a resultant increased access to the wider range of services outside of learning disability services that are available to other children. It is likely that the number of professionals who may become involved in the lives of children with learning disabilities and their families will continue to develop as newer services for children become more established and seek to undertake more work with children with learning disabilities.

Thirdly, there is a growing emphasis on the need to seek to communicate actively and directly with children as individuals with less reliance on establishing children's needs by communicating through with their parents. Children are increasingly viewed as having something to say and there is a need to take steps to give them a stronger voice. There is increased acknowledgement of the ability of children to provide accounts of their lives including the expression of interests, preferences and choices. It has been argued that children have 'a unique perspective which differs from that of adults and are active in shaping their own lives' (Stalker and Connors 2005: 192). There is now an expectation that children with disabilities, including those with learning disabilities, and their families will have the opportunity to contribute to the development of policy that may impact on their lives, such as the development of children and young person plans which are now required in England and Wales as a result of the Children Act (2004).

Finally, the structures of services are required to change with all areas in England and Wales developing NHS Children's Trusts, with other areas of the UK also taking steps to improve the co-ordination of services to children through more unified structures. This has already resulted in a reconfiguration in some NHS trusts of previous service structures which focused on where and by whom services were delivered (e.g. primary care, learning disability, mental health or acute services) rather than who used the services. The revised structures are being designed to focus on the needs of children and their families and will in turn lead to different referral pathways and care journeys for children with learning disabilities who access services. The above changes are being implemented with the aim of improving the co-ordination of child and family-centred services for children with learning disabilities. The degree to which this is achieved will only become clear over the next 10 years.

However, one thing that is already apparent is the need for learning disability nursing services to engage with the process of developing new services for children, in order that children and their families will continue to have access to learning disability nursing services when these are required. In so doing learning disability nurses need to respond to 'a growing sense of frustration that the skills, knowledge and experience of learning disability nurses are not always used to best effect with children and their families' (Northway, 2004), and a reduction in the involvement of community nurses in learning disabilities with children (Barr, 2006).

A process of adaptation

There is no denying that having a child with learning disabilities in the family can have a major impact on individual family members and the family as a whole. Becoming parents of a child with learning disabilities can create tension as family members seek to reconcile their desire to be a 'normal' family, yet accommodate the differences in their situations and the roles they will expect to fulfil. Much has been written about how parents of children with disabilities adapt, although less has been written specific to children with learning disabilities and complex health needs, their siblings and other members of the extended family. The models that have been developed to explain the process of adaptation outline a series of stages that parents are considered to pass through as they progress from the initial shock and confusion to a state of successful adaptation or adjustment to their new situation (Miller et al, 1994; Grant et al, 2003). As families move through the process of adaptation they have to grapple with 'changed expectations for the child, altered perceptions for the future and an acknowledgement of being a different family' (Manthorpe, 1995: 118).

Maintaining one's physical and mental health as well as the health of a family unit requires an ongoing process of adaptation to changing circumstances in individuals and across family members. As the child grows, new challenges and opportunities arise for parents and other family members as there is a realisation of what this means in practical terms for the people involved and the family as a unit (Grant et al, 2003).

Progression is not always linear, and family members may find themselves oscillating between different stages at times of transitions or difficulty. In addition, adaptation is lifelong in response to the changing abilities and needs of the child and the composition of the family in which that person lives and as family developmental goals evolve (Maxwell and Barr, 2003; Wilgosh and Scorgie, 2006).

Children, parents and other family members may experience particular stresses at times of transition, when they find they need to permit other people to provide care for their child without their supervision (Miller et al, 1994), for instance when the child is preparing to enter pre-school education services, and moving from familiar nursing services to new services, or when transferring from child to adult services.

The conceptualisation of families as working through a process of adaptation is also consistent with the emerging view of families as resilient, which highlights their ability to cope successfully given the necessary opportunities. From this perspective the aim of intervention is empowerment of family members and professionals involved, which has been defined as the 'increased ability to meet the needs and goals while maintaining autonomy and integrity' (Patterson, 1995). Such a model requires professionals to work in partnership with families and to facilitate their development. This is in sharp contrast to the view of parents and families within a 'pathological' model, which places emphasis on the difficulties they experience in coping with their situation and highlights the need for professionals to advise and support families often in a directive manner. Within such a perception, families were viewed as 'in need' of services rather than striving towards independence (Scorgie et al, 1999; Wilgosh and Scorgie, 2006).

The needs of children and families

The extent to which the abilities and needs of children with learning disabilities, their parents and other family members are accurately identified and effectively met by formal and informal sources of support can have a considerable impact on their experience of adapting to their situation.

Two approaches to defining needs appear in the literature, firstly the identification of needs through a structured assessment, the components of which appear to have been largely derived with a professional framework. The second approach involves asking children and young people, as well as their parents and carers, what they believe their needs are. Limited work has been reported which has sought to establish the needs of children with learning disabilities through talking with them directly, and much of the information reported on the needs of children with disabilities has been gathered from a wider range of children with 'complex health needs' including physical, learning, emotional and sensory disabilities.

However, there is some convergence on the key areas that consistently emerge across a number of studies of children with disabilities, including

Table 14.1. Needs important to young people with complex health problems

- The need for information
- The need to be listened to
- Access to peer support
- Access to education

- Accommodation and support
- Communication needs
- Access to leisure and employment

children with learning disabilities. Following interviews with children who have learning disabilities, Stalker and Connors (2005) reported that they were able to articulate the importance to them of relationships with family members, including their extended family, and friends. They also reported their desire to be involved in a similar range of activities to their non-disabled peers. Their accounts of educational opportunities highlighted the importance they attached to learning and the pride they gained from their achievements. The children with learning disabilities also had thoughts about what they wanted to achieve in the future, and looked forward to having a job.

Morris (1999) focused on the issues young people with a wider range of 'complex health and support needs' felt were important. The needs identified are shown in *Table 14.1*.

Children and their families recognised the need to receive health services, but qualified this, as with other services such as education, housing and leisure services, by stating these should be of a high quality. The needs identified by children highlight the importance of developing effective communication and opportunities for education as necessities if children and young people are to become more involved in decisions about their care and their lives.

The clear message arising from previous research on the needs of children with complex health problems is that they want to be involved in decisions about their care and require the information, education and support necessary to do so. A recurring point in the literature is the necessity to recognise the human rights of children and young people with complex health needs and use these as a benchmark in recognising the needs of the child. Despite having complex physical health needs and in some instances being dependent on technology, children and young people can demonstrate resilience in the way they seek to manage and respond to their situation, how they continue to look forward and to have future goals.

The list of needs and aspirations identified reflects the holistic way in which children view their future, and how they do not appear to perceive themselves as overly restricted by their complex health needs, rather they are characterised by the forward looking resilience. It is important to acknowledge the perspective of childhood that children bring to their situation (Stalker and Connors, 2005). Kerr (2001) emphasised how important it is for health professionals to recognise the wider needs of children, including the issues associated with ethnicity and cultural aspects, and not to become overly focused on technological needs.

The needs of family members

Parents

On reviewing the published research on the needs of parents of children with complex health needs five key areas are prominent:

- The need for increased certainty and control.
- The need for information.
- The need to acquire knowledge and develop skills in caring for their child.
- The need for co-ordinated services.
- The need for respite care.

The need for increased certainty and control

Perhaps the overarching need of children, their parents and family members is the need for increased certainty, leading to a degree of increased control of the future, and the other needs identified as contributing to achieving this. The presence of complex health needs in a child will be a major challenge for parents and not what they had anticipated when looking forward to the birth and development of their child. When such needs are identified, parents will find they enter a largely unfamiliar world involving a wide range of professionals, acute care settings, community health and social services, special educational arrangements and the need to make major changes to their home and family environment. Parents will find this a difficult experience and feel they are faced with much uncertainty (Morris, 1999).

As noted earlier, children with complex physical health needs, their parents and other family members often find themselves in situations characterised by uncertainty. This is often compounded by a feeling that they have limited influence over many of the decisions, which directly affect their child and family, with these decisions being outside their control. They are subjected to a number of forces outside the family, a scenario which adds further to their stress (Ratliffe et al, 2002). Parents often strive to maintain a feeling of control and 'normality' as a family through seeking information to plan for their child's future (Hall, 1996).

The need for information

The availability of appropriate and timely information is crucial if parents are to develop the necessary knowledge to navigate and manage in the new situation they find themselves in. It is only through having access to information that parents will learn more about their child's condition, the professionals who can assist, and other resources available to their child and them. Without access to appropriate information parents will not be able to become as fully involved in decision making, nor be able to work in a collaborative partnership with professionals or plan as effectively for their child's care.

Parents are often focused on receiving a diagnosis for their child's condition. If available, the more specific the diagnosis, the more accurate a prognosis and the clearer the likely development and health of the child will be. This, in turn, may reduce uncertainty about the future for family members and give a focus to their interactions with the child. However, depending on the diagnosis it may also confirm parents' fears of a serious degenerative condition and remove hope of their child's recovery.

The precision of a diagnosis can vary from the confirmation of the presence of a specific condition, for instance a congenital condition, to a much broader diagnosis of complex physical health needs with no specific condition identified. A broad non-specific definition can leave considerable uncertainty about the future and provide less focus for interventions. It is anticipated that as both our understanding of genetics and ability to undertake genetic diagnosis increases more confirmed diagnoses will be available. While this may provide more specific information for parents and family members, it can also lead to added difficulties with parental and family relationships (Ward, 2001; Barr and Millar, 2003). Even then genetic tests cannot predict the degree of complexity of the physical health needs with complete accuracy, and for this reason a conclusive statement relating to eventual achievement or the possible degree of disability cannot be made. A major determinant of the eventual level of functioning of all children is their environment after birth.

The manner in which the diagnosis of complex health needs is communicated with children and their families is often a pivotal point in the story of parents. The memory of how a diagnosis was arrived at and shared with parents as well as the support they received at that time remains in their minds for many years. The prospects of active family involvement can be damaged in the short term, and possibly for several years, if these interactions are not carefully prepared for and conducted appropriately (Department of Health, Social Security and Public Safety, 2003).

Parents also need information on services and other resources available to their child and them in their specific circumstances, such as information on specialist and other community resources that their child may use to meet his or her physical, emotional, social and intellectual needs, such as, preschool groups, schools, leisure services, as well as local health and social services (Hall, 1996). Many parents will also wish to have information on financial aspects of having a child with complex physical health needs, as they may have had to reduce the hours they work (FPLD, 2004), give up work completely, or have had a change to their benefit entitlement, yet encounter increased costs in caring for their child (Roberts and Lawton, 2001; Sloper and Beresford, 2006).

Parents are clear about the type and format of information they desire and six key criteria have been identified against which available information could be evaluated:

- The provision of information that is up to date, easy to read and in straightforward language.
- Written information to take away, supplemented by a verbal explanation and the opportunity to ask questions.
- Information should be available in different levels and depth, in order that it can be provided to people at relevant points in their circumstances.
- Information is considered more accessible if it is available in everyday places.
- Key information should be provided by an individual who is knowledgeable, approachable and also understanding and respectful of different families' situations and coping strategies.
- Information should be comprehensive and provide an overview of how different departments work together (Mitchell and Sloper, 2002).

Although there is no doubt that parents receive a lot of information, particularly in the early stages of their child's diagnosis, it appears this is not the information they felt they needed at that stage of their adaptation process. They have reported a lack of access to information in a manner that they can understand and use it, at a time when they needed it, and often highlight that information is received too late to be helpful to them (Mitchell and Sloper, 2002).

Overall, less is known about the experience of fathers of children with complex needs in comparison to mothers. Recent research has highlighted that fathers often report they have less access to information from health professionals than their partners and this has an impact on their ability to understand what is happening for their child, particularly at appointments with health professionals (Foundation for People with Learning Disabilities,

2006). It has been acknowledged by some fathers that they may contribute in part to their feeling of isolation by holding self-perceived ideas about the need to remain 'in control' of their emotions and provide support to the rest of the family. This can result in the deeply felt needs of fathers going undisclosed, unnoticed and hence leading them to feel less supported (Dale, 1995; Rendall, 1997).

The need for services and individual professionals to take active steps to engage with fathers, particularly in the provision of information, is now considered to be an important part of health and social services for children. Professionals should actively seek to engage with fathers and provide opportunities to meet with them face to face and avoid stereotyping them as hard to reach or difficult to engage (Daniel and Taylor, 2001). In supporting families it is important that professionals recognise the limitations of working almost exclusively with mothers. Therefore, it is necessary, when providing information, to ensure both parents have access to the information rather than communicating with one parent through the other.

Knowledge/skills about the care of the child, the equipment they use

In addition to the need for information about their child's condition, parents also identified the need for knowledge and skills training specific to caring for their child. The specific needs of parents will be related to their child's situation; however, overall, parents identified the need to receive education and develop skills to use technological equipment, such as feeding pumps, infusions, dialysis, or ventilators. Depending on the extent of a child's needs, they may be using more than one piece of equipment about which they need to receive training (Heaton et al, 2005).

Most parents managed to master the equipment, so much so that some felt they were then 'left to get on with it', when they felt some level of continuing support would have been helpful (Heaton et al, 2005). The need for training is also necessary in relation to care procedures that do not involve technology, for instance the admission of emergency or routine medication. Although it may not be possible to continue providing intense ongoing support for all parents, such comments do highlight the need for a phased reduction in support to parents (Gibson, 1995).

Parents accepted the need for much of the equipment their child required, but also recognised the extra restrictions this can place on their children's educational and social activities, and family routines may have to be planned around equipment. They also felt at times, when children were dependent on technology, that the need to attend to the equipment placed some restrictions on the choice of employment opportunities parents may be able to take up (Heaton et al, 2005; Foundation for People with Learning Disabilities, 2006). Having acquired skills and knowledge, together with awareness of the child, parents stressed the need for their skills to be recognised and their concerns about changes in their child's health to be investigated. Many parents came to view themselves as 'experts' in the care of their child and the management of their equipment, at times having to explain it to other health professionals (Roberts and Lawton, 2001).

Co-ordination of service and support to the child and family

On a practical level, the need for coordinated services is required if the difficulties caused by perceived bureaucracy, delays in the provision of services and wasteful use of resources through duplication and gaps in services are to be avoided. The lack of co-ordination has also been reported by parents in respect of overlapping appointments, or failure to group appointments together requiring them to make multiple journeys, and the need to repeatedly share the same information with professionals. On occasions this can extend to educating health and other professionals about equipment used by their child or other aspects of the child's condition, because some professionals or support staff do not have the necessary knowledge, skills or confidence to work with the child (Roberts and Lawton, 2001).

Three crucial points of the co-ordination of services are the transition points between hospital and community services when discharging a child from hospital, the co-ordination of the support for the child when commencing education, and the transition between child and adult services. In these situations parents often highlight the lack of co-ordination.

In the first scenario the child may remain in hospital longer than is necessary and severe delays may be experienced in getting the child home (Noyes, 2002).

The commencement of education is a major point of transition for parents and the child as this is a new phase of the child moving outside of the family home to receive services on a regular (daily) basis and usually without the parents supervising the care provided (Miller et al, 1994; Lacey and Ouvry, 1998).

Finally, as more young people with complex physical health needs live into adulthood they may move to be cared for by 'adult' services. This is often a difficult transition for the child and parents who have built up trust and confidence in the staff and services they are familiar with (Morris, 1999) When this process of transition is not adequately planned in advance it may arise within a crisis situation, only becoming an issue when a young person becomes ill and needs admission to hospital. It is at this crucial and difficult time for parents that children's and adults' services may debate where the person should be admitted to, thus delaying access to services and increasing the distress of the child, parents and other family members.

The effective coordination of services for children at home will only be possible when parents and professionals across health, social services and education work together in a spirit of partnership and in a manner that seeks to empower parents of children (Gibson, 1995). This is in contrast to the regular reports of parents (and at times children) who feel they are not listened to and describe their relationships with professionals as a 'battle' and talk of 'the need to fight for everything' (ACT, 2003).

The provision of information and opportunities to develop the knowledge and skills noted above are pre-requisites to effective and empowering collaboration. All parents of children with complex physical health needs have the potential to work in partnership with health professionals and vice versa (Hornby, 1995). However, it often takes time to establish sufficiently trusting relationships and to have the confidence to renegotiate roles in caring (Kirk, 2001; Swallow, 2001). Professionals should remain cognisant of the needs of mothers and fathers as carers, while also engaging in discussions about how they wish to contribute to the child's care.

Coordination is required at all stages of the care planning process, from assessment through to evaluation. Within such a relationship all people can learn from each other and the expertise of parents in caring for their child is recognised and acknowledged, as is the presence of tension and possible conflict between parents and professionals (Dale, 1996). The focus of parents, other family members and professionals within health, social services and education is often on seeking to provide the best support possible for the child with complex health needs. Alongside this the needs of other family members and the family unit have to be responded to. This often leads to parents feeling they are pulled in different directions and need to prioritise their actions. Professionals have to work with finite resources and also have to make decisions about what support can be provided. As with teamwork the presence of conflict is not of itself a negative aspect, although it needs to be managed within agreed ground rules; however it is often a by-product of trying to get a number of people from different backgrounds, and possibly with different agendas, to reach agreement and be prepared to engage in the discussion rather than be passive (West, 2004).

Respite or short breaks

The need for respite care or short breaks from caring is frequently highlighted by parents of children with a range of complex health needs, including complex physical needs. The rationale for the provision of respite care services is that children will be able to be cared for at home over a longer period of time if parents receive a regular break from caring.

Respite care may involve different combinations of support for parents; at one end of the continuum it may involve a carer coming into the child's home to look after them for a few hours, either with the parents still in the home (perhaps with their other children) or when the parents are not present. Alternatively, it may involve the child leaving the family home for a few hours to be cared for in another carer's home or a statutory service. Finally it may involve the child moving to a specialist service such as nursing facility or children's hospice for an overnight stay or for several nights. Respite care is likely to be most useful when provided in a planned and predictable manner, yet there is also the need to be flexible enough to change the arrangements in order to respond to the changing needs of the child and family.

Families report that the break from caring for their child is beneficial to them as parents, the child him or herself, siblings and the overall family unit. It provides opportunities for parents to undertake activities with their partner as a couple or to spend time with other children or with other family members. At a practical level it can provide parents with the chance to 'recharge' their batteries and to have a full night's sleep, something that is often disrupted due to the need to care for the child during the night (Heaton et al, 2006). The opportunity for respite care also provides parents and other family members with a break from the need for constant supervision and the opportunity to undertake activities that would not be possible or very difficult if their child with complex physical health needs was present.

Respite care is frequently raised as an unmet need for parents and children, and one which they feel needs more emphasis. However, it has also been reported that parents and some professionals may have differing opinions as to what is desirable respite care. Whereas some professionals may feel it is preferable for the respite care to be provided in the child's home, parents at times perceive this as providing little respite and may view growing numbers of people entering their home as an intrusion on their privacy. When considering options for respite care, such issues need to be openly discussed (MacDonald and Callery, 2004).

Siblings

The need for information about their brother or sister's condition is a key need of siblings. Siblings too are directly impacted upon by the lack of co-ordinated services in a number of ways, primarily because this lack of service will require parents to spend more time meeting with or 'fighting' for services. The reality for many families and siblings is that the focus of family routines needs to be planned around the use of technology, which will in turn require more advanced planning, restrict places that can be visited as a family and may lead to parents having to split themselves between their different children, doing less activities as a family unit. Parents frequently highlight their concerns that their other children receive less attention and they regret that (Heaton et al, 2005)

Uncertainty can also be a major factor in the lives of siblings as the complexity of their sibling's needs may result in unexpected changes to family routines and increased stress and strain with the family. This has been reported to have an adverse impact, in particular if it results in siblings having to take time off school to assist at home, or when the increased difficulties occur around an examination period (Noyes, 2006). Siblings can find the increased tension and arguments among parents that may be witnessed as distressing and may lead to concerns about the future of their parents' relationship.

Siblings may also have concerns about aspects of their own future, which may be heightened if their brother or sister developed their complex needs after an earlier period of healthy development, for instance in the case of cancer or a degenerative condition. Older siblings may have concerns about risks to their current or future children if a condition is known to be genetic or be uncertain about their role in providing the future care of the sibling, yet these concerns are often not directly raised with parents (Evans et al, 2001).

The presence of a child with complex physical health needs in the family does not always result in totally negative consequences for siblings, who, like their parents, may develop knowledge and skills that they would not have otherwise had an opportunity to develop. Siblings may also develop a level of compassion, tolerance of difference and awareness of the needs of people with disability that may not have otherwise occurred. The experience of individual siblings will be influenced by their own circumstances and also by the support provided to them (Barr, 2003).

Professionals involved in supporting families should be aware of the abilities and needs of the siblings of a child with complex physical health needs and, as with fathers, make plans to engage directly with them in order that children have the opportunity to talk directly to professionals rather than having to communicate through their parents. It is important that siblings are provided with up-to-date information about their brother or sister and have opportunities to discuss their concerns and contribute to decisions taken in the family (ACT, 2003; Burke, 2004).

Other family members

Through ongoing contact and providing support to relatives with complex physical health needs, family members often increase their knowledge, skills and understanding about the person. For example, they may become more tolerant of people with disabilities or develop an increased awareness of the difficulties they can sometimes face. Members of the extended family are often an important source of informal support to parents and siblings. They can be of practical assistance in providing child care or 'babysitting' that facilitates parents to maintain their employment to varying degrees, or spend time together, as well as undertake activities with their other children.

However, this degree of support cannot be assumed, even if relatives live nearby it is possible that difficulties may arise for some members of the extended family due to feelings of awkwardness about visiting the child, because they are not sure what to say or do. They may also be embarrassed or have mixed emotions of guilt and frustration about some aspects of the behaviour of the child. Members of the extended family may also not be aware of the nature of the complex physical health needs, or may diminish the impact of its presence, which can lead to difficulties for parents, for example in visiting the homes of relatives or going to social activities at which they may be present. These uncertain emotions can result in disagreements and conflict within families that can further compound feelings of isolation (Maxwell and Barr, 2003).

Responding to the needs of the child and the family

The impact of having a child with complex physical health needs in the family is a combination of positive and negative consequences. Kearney and Griffin (2001) describe it as a combination of joy (at achievements however limited) and sorrow (from missed opportunities and distress experienced). Many parents and siblings demonstrate tremendous resilience and develop a range of effective coping strategies that help them to respond to the challenges they encounter. Although nurses must remain mindful of the observation by McCormack (1992: 15) that even for the parents who appear to be coping very well and demonstrating considerable resilience, even for these families 'it never gets easy'. Similarly, Gibson (1995) highlights the need for professionals to remain alert to the risk that mothers who appear empowered may find they receive less support and become overburdened with responsibility.

The impact on the family spans physical, psychological and social domains, and therefore to be effective, interventions by professionals must do the same. The needs of families, as reported in the literature, are shown in *Table 14.1*. Bearing these in mind it is not surprising that in reviewing services for children with disabilities the most successful attributes were:

- Listening to disabled children and young people.
- Providing information and advice.

- Having positive attitudes and a co-ordinated approach.
- Providing flexible support services that are tailored to individual children's and families' needs.
- Having more money – children and parents.
- Measuring the actions of all statutory and voluntary agencies against the human rights of disabled children.

Despite the identification of clear policy direction for services that seek to support children and their families, and the apparent agreement on the broad needs of families as well as the attributes of successful services, there has been little success in making these changes happen consistently. Some families still report struggling to receive services and often characterise their relationships with professionals as a 'fight' for services. This clearly highlights the need to respond more effectively to meeting the needs of children with disabilities and their families.

Service development and the implications for the future role of the registered learning disability nurse

It has been asserted strongly that learning disability nurses do have the skills, knowledge and experience to assist children and young people with learning disabilities and their families and carers. They should have access to such support and should have learning disability nurses available right from the start (Northway, 2004). In accepting the thrust of this argument, the challenge is that if learning disability nurses are indeed to be a valuable component of future services for children, they must take active steps to demonstrate, in practical terms, what they can provide for children with learning disabilities and their families. It is necessary to recognise that existing services have not served this group effectively and therefore change is necessary. This will require action by learning disability nurses in two main areas.

The abilities and needs of the child as an individual within the family context

The focus for nurses should be on the child with learning disabilities and in so doing it is necessary to view children as individuals who have their own abilities, needs, and desires for the future. At the same time nurses need to acknowledge that children are members of a family within which parents and other siblings also have abilities, needs and desires for their futures.

Access to information for parents is crucial in understanding their situation and being able to plan ahead. However, before providing 'advice' and information nurses need to take time to obtain a clear understanding of how the child and all family members perceive their situation, and the coping strategies employed by individuals and the family as a functional unit (Barr, 2007). In so doing, a more accurate picture of family interactions and priorities can be gained, and consequently support can be targeted to facilitate family adaptation (Hilbert et al, 2000; Todd and Jones, 2003). In providing support, nurses need to actively recognise the expertise that parents and other family members may have in caring for their own child and to work with them as equal partners. This can be further enhanced by assisting parents and other family members to identify their current and future training needs. Nurses can then respond to the identified needs by providing necessary training if possible, or locating the relevant training opportunities for parents.

At times this can be difficult, particularly if parents are undertaking a procedure or providing care which is not consistent with the recognised guidelines, for instance, moving and handling or feeding. Nurses need to explore with parents their reason for providing the care the way they do and then discuss the strengths and limitations of doing it that way. Parents may have carefully thought out reasons for what they are doing, or it may be due to a lack of training in relation to the procedure. It is necessary for nurses to discuss and negotiate a way forward, it is not appropriate to expect automatic compliance with the way the nurse feels it should be undertaken, after all there is the potential for nurses to learn new procedures from parents and other families.

Nurses should maintain frequent contact with children and families on their caseload and be in a position to provide 'hands on' care and emotional support when it is needed. In so doing they will have opportunities to gain the trust of the person with learning disabilities and the family members. This also provides opportunities to relieve parents of the requirement to be the only person providing care, as well as giving older children and young adults with learning disabilities opportunities for privacy that they may wish to have in relation to aspects of their personal care. Providing 'hands on' care to the child also creates opportunities for nurses to discuss aspects of health and development with the child and to directly explore their views on the care they receive, in contrast to relying totally on feedback from parents and other family members.

If nurses find they are visiting children and their families infrequently, for instance less than monthly, and are not actively involved in their care, then it is necessary to review openly with the child and parents the need for continued nursing involvement. Nurses should establish if the input is still necessary and if needs have altered, including the possibility of discharging the child. It is important not to add to the difficulties parents experience from a larger number of professionals than necessary visiting their home. Many parents clearly recognise that nurses and other professionals cannot solve many of the child's difficulties; nurses need to be mindful of not making a difficult situation worse through ineffective support and unnecessary continuation of visiting. In essence, the usefulness of the nurse's contribution should be judged against what their involvement continues to achieve for the child and the family, rather than by the belief that the child should have a named nurse or may need a nurse at some time in the future, in which case visits should continue 'just in case'.

Key to successfully developing and supporting resilience in family members is forward planning to identify and provide information and training, which builds on existing family strengths and provides opportunities to obtain the necessary information and skills that make it possible for children and their parents to remain actively involved in discussions and decisions about their son or daughter as equal partners.

The need to develop new knowledge and skills to respond to the changing needs of children

Developments in medical, surgical and nursing care together with advances in services delivered by allied health professionals have resulted in more children with complex health needs living longer and increasingly into adulthood. While learning disability nurses will have the skills and knowledge to respond to many of these needs, increasingly children often require complex interventions in terms of detailed care regimes for nutrition, feeding, mobility, psychological support and may be dependent on technology or emergency medication in order to meet their physical or mental health needs.

For some nurses in learning disability services the procedures involved in supporting children will be new to them in the form of the equipment, medication or therapy required, as they may have limited previous experience with children, depending on where they worked and when they undertook their nurse education. If nurses for people with learning disabilities wish to remain an integral part of future services for children, much will depend on their ability to undertake an increasing range of nursing procedures and work effectively with children with complex healthcare needs and life-limiting/ life-threatening conditions.

A major gap in service provision identified by many parents was the lack of practical skills held by nurses who were unfamiliar with working with their children. Therefore it is imperative that learning disability nurses review their existing knowledge and skills in the light of the changing requirements of children presently in their caseload or likely to be referred and take prompt action to obtain the necessary knowledge and skills. As noted above, nurses involved with children should have 'hands on' practical skills as well as supportive and listening skills. While parents are often happy to share knowledge with professionals who are supporting their children, parents should not be relied upon to provide training or update staff.

Given the complexity of some treatment approaches and the possible range of equipment being used, it is accepted that nurses may not be competent in all areas of nursing care, even when they have undertaken additional training. Therefore it is important that nurses also accept this and do not undertake activities that are not within their competence (Nursing and Midwifery Council, 2008). The lack of knowledge or skills should not serve as an excuse to withdraw nursing services from the child and discharge them from the learning disability caseload, rather it should be the catalyst to identify unmet training needs and seek relevant training. Once competence has been achieved nurses should also ensure they take action to maintain this competence and avail themselves of any necessary training updates.

Interdisciplinary and interagency collaboration

No single profession or group of professionals have all the necessary skills and knowledge effectively to support children with learning disabilities. Therefore the need for co-ordination of services across a number of professionals and agencies, including community nursing, respite care, education, social services, allied health professionals and possibly inpatient services, is an essential (rather than optional) element of effective services (Nursing and Midwifery Council, 2008). Yet a consistent issue identified by parents of children with disabilities is the additional problems they encounter as a result of lack of co-ordinated services and conflicting information provided by professionals within and between agencies (Mitchell and Sloper, 2002).

Effective collaboration does not require all the professionals involved to be working in one structured team. Often professionals can work effectively together while being based at different locations and separate teams, if the mechanisms for communication, and processes for managing the collaboration and any disagreements are adequately developed and monitored (Barr, 2008).

A first step in achieving effective collaboration is for nurses to know which other professionals are working with the child and family. This is the starting point and it is worth taking time to identify from family members which other professionals are involved and the support they provide. Once it is known who is involved, nurses should ensure these other professionals are made aware that nurses are also involved. This could be done by telling them in person, contacting them by telephone or sending a letter. Only when people know who is involved will it be possible for them to collaborate with each other.

In order to avoid duplication and minimise gaps in services it is necessary to be aware of the support being provided by each person/agency involved. Once this has been clarified it should be easier to identify the services that nurses can contribute to complement the existing services being provided. When several people are involved in providing services to children and their families it is advisable to have identified one professional as the co-ordinator or link person for the family and to set up regular meetings, (perhaps every 4–6 weeks) for those staff involved on a weekly basis. This provides opportunities for staff to get to learn about the roles they each have and how these can be co-ordinated to the best effect to support the child and family. There is a need to focus on the needs of the child and family and then consider how nurses can effectively meet these, rather than the focus being on prescribed roles and hierarchies. This will require nurses to have confidence in the services they can provide together with knowledge of and respect for the services provided by other individuals and agencies. Often nurses in learning disability services complain that other services do not have knowledge of or value their role, yet at times limited steps are taken to either communicate this role in an organised way or learn about the current roles of other professionals.

Finally, overall policy development for services for children with learning disabilities is increasingly influenced by wider policy for all children's services such as National Service Framework, rather than only specific learning disability-led or nursing-focused policies. Therefore it is necessary for learning disability nurses to be aware of wider policy development in children's services and contribute to discussions in developing these, either through committee membership or responding to consultation documents. As it is no longer necessary for all student nurses to undertake a placement with people with learning disabilities, many nurses may reach registration without having contact with learning disability nurses. In response, nurses for people with learning disability need to remain visible within services for children in order that children and their families can have access to services when required. This will require these nurses to develop more successful links with staff in children's services both in hospital and community settings (for example, children's wards, general practitioners, respite services, and special schools) in order that effective use of nurses can be made at an appropriate stage. Other professionals need to be aware of the services nurses for people with learning disabilities could potentially deliver, their contact details, and the referral process. This information should be kept up to date and nurses in learning disability services should actively create and take opportunities to liaise and network with other professionals in children's services. This will provide opportunities to demonstrate, through working collaboratively with children, their families and other professionals, the real contribution learning disability nurses can make to the lives of children and their families.

References

ACT (Association for Children with Life-Threatening or Terminal Conditions and their Families) (2003) *A Guide to the Development of Children's Palliative Care Services*. 2nd edn. ACT, London

Barr O (2006) The evolving role of community nurses for people with learning disabilities: Changes over an 11-year period. *Journal of Clinical Nursing* **15**(1): 72–82

Barr O (2007) Working effectively with families of people with learning disabilities. In: Gates B (ed.) *Learning Disabilities* 5th edn. Churchill Livingstone, Edinburgh: 567–97

Barr O (2008) Teamwork in community nursing. In Sines, D, Saunders, M, Forbes-Burford, J (eds.) *Community Healthcare Nursing*. 4th edn. Wiley-Blackwell, Chichester

Barr O, Millar R (2003) Parents of children with intellectual disabilities: Their expectations and experience of genetic counselling. *Journal of Applied Research in Intellectual Disabilities* **16**(3): 189–204

Burke P (2004) *Brothers and Sisters of Disabled Children*. Jessica Kingsley, London

Dale B (1995) Creating answers. In: Meyer DJ (ed.) *Uncommon Fathers: Reflections on Raising a Child with a Disability*. Woodbine House, Bethesda: 1–12

Dale N (1996) *Working with Families of Children with Special Needs. Partnership and Practice*. Routledge, London

Daniel B, Taylor J (2001) *Engaging with Fathers. Practice Issues for Health and Social Care*. Jessica Kingsley Publishers, London

Department of Health (2001) *Valuing People: A New Strategy for People with Learning Disability for the 21st Century*. Cm 5086. Department of Health, London

Department of Health (2004) *National Service Framework for Children, Young People and Maternity Services*. Department of Health, London

Department of Health and Social Services (1976) *Report of the Committee on Child Health Services (1976) Fit For The Future* (Court Report). HMSO, London

Department of Health, Social Services and Public Safety (2003) *Breaking Bad News... Regional Guidelines*. Department of Health, Social Services and Public Safety, Belfast

Department of Health, Social Services and Public Safety (2005) *Equal Lives: Review of policy and services for people with a learning disability in Northern Ireland.* Belfast: Department of Health, Social Services and Public Safety

Evans J, Jones J, Mansell I (2001) Supporting siblings: Evaluation of support groups for brothers and sisters of children with learning disabilities and challenging behaviour. *Journal of Learning Disabilities* **5**(1): 69–78

Foundation for People with Learning Disabilities (2002) *Count Us In.* FPLD, London

Gibson C (1995) The process of empowerment in mothers of chronically ill children. *Journal of Advanced Nursing* **21**(6): 1201–10

Grant G, Nolan M, Keady J (2003) Supporting families over the life course: Mapping temporality. *Journal of Intellectual Disability Research* **47**(4–5): 342–52

Hall S (1996) An exploration of parental perception of the nature and level of support needed to care for their child with special needs. *Journal of Advanced Nursing* **24**: 512–21

Heaton J, Noyes J, Sloper P, Shah R (2005) Families' experiences of caring for technology-dependant children: A temporal perspective. *Health and Social Care* **13**(5): 441–50

Heaton J, Noyes J, Sloper P, Shah R (2006) The experiences of sleep disruption in families of technology-dependant children living at home. *Children and Society* **20**: 196–208

Hilbert GA, Walker MB, Rinehart J (2000) In for the long haul: Response of parents caring for children with Sturge–Weber syndrome. *Journal of Family Nursing* **6**(2): 157–79

Hornby G (1995) *Working with Parents of Children with Special Needs.* Cassell, London

Hunt J, Elston S, Galloway J (2003) *Voices for Change: Current Perception of Services for Children with Palliative Care Needs and Their Families.* Bristol: ACT

Kearney P, Griffin M (2001) Between joy and sorrow: Being a parent of a child with developmental disability. *Journal of Advanced Nursing* **34**(5): 582–92

Kerr GR (2001) Assessing the needs of learning disabled young people with additional disabilities: Implications for planning adult services. *Journal of Learning Disabilities* **5**(2): 157–74

Kirk S (2001) Negotiating lay and professional roles in the care of children with complex health care needs. *Journal of Advanced Nursing* **34**(5): 593–602

Lacey P, Ouvry C (1998) *People with Profound and Multiple Learning Disabilities: A Collaborative Approach to Meeting Complex Needs.* David Fulton, London

MacDonald H, Callery P (2004) Different meanings of respite: A study of parents, nurses and social workers caring for children with complex needs. *Child: Care, Health and Development* **30**(3): 279–88

Manthorpe J (1995) Services to families. In: Malin N (ed.) *Services for People with Learning Disabilities.* Routledge, London

Maxwell V, Barr O (2003) With the benefit of hindsight: A mother's reflections on raising a child with Down syndrome. *Journal of Learning Disabilities* **7**(1): 51–64

McCormack M (1992) *Special Children, Special Needs. Families talk about living with mental handicap.* Thorsons, London

Miller NB, Burmester S, Callahan DG, Dieterle J, Niedermeyer S (1994) *Nobody's Perfect.* Paul H Brookes, Baltimore

Mitchell W, Sloper P (2002) Information that informs rather than alienates families with disabled children: Developing a model of good practice. *Health and Social Care in the Community* **10**(2): 74–81

Morris J (1999) *Hurtling into a Void: Transition to Adulthood for Young Disabled People with 'Complex Health and Support Needs'.* Brighton, Pavilion Publishing

National Development Group (1997) *Right From the Start.* NDG, London

Northway R (2004) Right from the start. *Learning Disability Practice* **7**(7): 3

Noyes J. (2002) Barriers that delay children and young people who are dependent on mechanical ventilators from being discharged from hospital. *Journal of Clinical Nursing* **11**(1): 2–11

Noyes J (2006) Resources use and service costs for ventilator-dependant children and young people in the UK. *Health and Social Care in the Community* **14**(5): 508–22

Nursing and Midwifery Council (2008) *The Code: Standards for Conduct, Performance and Ethics for Nurses and Midwives.* NMC, London

Patterson J (1995) Promoting resilience in families experiencing stress. *Pediatric Clinics of North America* **42**(1): 47–63

Ratliffe CE, Harrigan RC, Haley J, Tse A, Olson T (2001) Stress in families with medically fragile children. *Issues in Comprehensive Paediatric Nursing* **25**: 167–88

Rendall D (1997) Fatherhood and learning disabilities: A personal account of reaction and resolution. *Journal of Learning Disabilities for*

Nursing, Health and Social Care **1**(2): 77–83

Roberts K, Lawton D (2001) Acknowledging the extra care parents give their disabled children. *Child: Care, Health and Development* **27**(4): 307–19

Scottish Executive (2000) *Same as You: A Review of Services for People with Learning Disability*. Scottish Executive, Edinburgh

Sloper T, Beresford B (2006) Families with disabled children social and economic needs are high but remain largely unmet. *British Medical Journal* **333**(4): 9289–9

Stalker K, Connors C (2005) Children with learning disabilities talking about their everyday lives. In P Goward, G Grant, P Ramcharan, M Richardson (eds.) *Learning Disability: A Life Cycle Approach*. Open University Press, Buckingham

Swallow V (2001) Mothers' evolving relationships with doctors and nurses during the chronic childhood illness trajectory. *Journal of Advanced Nursing* **36**(6): 755–64

Todd S, Jones S (2003) 'Mum's the word': Maternal accounts of dealings with the professional world. *Journal of Applied Research in Intellectual Disabilities* **16**(3): 229–44

Ward L (2001) *Considered Choices? The New Genetics, Prenatal Testing and People with Learning Disabilities*. BILD, Kidderminster

West M (2004) *Effective Teamwork: Practical Lessons from Organisational Research*. London: Blackwell Scientific Publications

Section Three:

Further perspectives

CHAPTER 15

Challenges for the curriculum in learning disability nursing

Bob Hallawell

Introduction

Learning disability nursing has evolved in response to a series of challenges arising from people with learning disabilities; from carers; from service commissioners; from service providers; from professional bodies; and from new models and philosophies of care. The architects of nursing curricula have likewise been challenged by the need to deliver programmes of education that reflect a new range of demands within health and social care; an evolving professional role within learning disabilities nursing; and competence rooted in practice realities. As Norman (1998b: 439) stated, education needs to be set 'against the backdrop of new ways of delivering services to clients'.

This chapter seeks to illuminate some of the contemporary challenges within pre-registration nursing curricula with specific reference to programmes of preparation for learning disability nursing. Consideration will be given to the differential use of models of disability within curricula; the place of user involvement; and the presence or absence of a standardised curriculum within pre-registration nursing with reference to both policy and provision within the UK.

Models of disability

Learning disability nurses apply their knowledge and skills in a variety of emergent and transient health and social care arenas. History has seen the transition of learning disability service provision from custodial and isolated care environments to community-based and individualised settings. Nurses have similarly experienced transitions in role as new philosophies of care and societal thinking about disability have necessitated new forms of provision and new ways of working with people with learning disabilities. A contemporary employment and practice landscape necessitates that nursing curricula engender in learning disability nurses a knowledge and skill base that enables them to demonstrate competence in a varied economy of health and social care provision for people with learning disabilities. Changes in practice and education have, at their core, recognition of both the health and social care needs of people with learning disabilities. Hence the need for consideration of alternative models of disability that serve to illuminate the experiences of people with learning disabilities, and that underpin service philosophies and delivery. Matthews (2006) notes how a failure to improve the health of people with learning disabilities since the publication of *Valuing People* (Department of Health, 2001) may be the result of the ideologies that serve to underpin service provision. People with learning disabilities may exist in many realities (Symonds, 1998a) and one way of defining these realities, and of understanding the ideologies and beliefs that underpin them, is the use of models developed by service organisations and service users (Beresford et al, 2000).

Within Western healthcare bio-medical models of the person have traditionally been used by professionals to conceptualise the position of service users as patients. The focus of the bio-medical model is the 'patient' and his or her individual illness or impairment. In this model the role of the patient is to comply with treatment (Symonds, 1998b). Individuals are held to be disabled by physical or cognitive impairments (Drake, 1998; Nuttall, 1998). The search for causality and treatment interventions is aimed at individuals and their diseases/conditions and the professional is responsible for taking treatment decisions which may not necessarily involve the patient. The professional may hence act in the best interests of the individual, a principle that is to be found in healthcare legislation, policy and practice. The establishment of hospitals for people with learning disabilities during the 20th century saw the emergence of the medical model as the dominant foundation for care.

However, bio-medical models do not explain how social and economic factors impact on people's lives nor do they address social, physical and human barriers to disability (Brown, 2000) or the economic, political and social dependencies which people with learning disabilities share in their lives (Thompson, 1997). Medical praxis focuses on the diagnosis and treatment of physical symptoms and in doing so isolates these from the patient's complex social and environmental relationships (Nuttall, 1998). This shifts attention away from any structural inequalities in society, masks social concerns, and perpetuates existing power divisions (Kelly, 1998; Finlay, 2000). The notion that 'socio-structural barriers serve to disadvantage and exclude people with impairments '...sits comfortably within a Marxist and materialist interpretation of the world' (Thomas, 2004: 22). Thompson (1997) argues that within an individual or 'personal tragedy' discourse of disability people with learning disabilities are expected to adapt to society rather than society adapting itself to support people with learning disabilities. Powerful groups in society influence policy by controlling both policy agendas and the definitions employed to represent people with learning disabilities. As an example Richardson (2005: 38) notes how the scientific knowledge that underpins the medical model is '...protected by professional cartels and a virtual monopoly over the crucial element of diagnosis'.

As an alternative to bio-medical models a social model of disability looks beyond the individual impairment to examine what causes the disadvantaged status of disabled persons and their potential exclusion from society. Oliver (2004) asserts that the social model originated in the Union of the Physically Impaired Against Segregation (UPIAS) publication *Fundamental Principles of Disability* (UPIAS, 1976) although Thomas (2004) opines that it was Oliver himself who actually coined the phrase 'social model of disability'. The UPIAS publication argued that it was not the impairments of disabled people that were the main cause of their problems but rather the way that society responded to disabled people as an oppressed minority. The social model thus discriminates between the impairment of the individual and their 'disability' (the degree to which society allows the individual to be disadvantaged) and focuses on the presence of external barriers (Brown, 2000). Beresford et al (2000: 194) define it as 'the drawing of a distinction between individual impairment and social disablement'. Walmsley (2005: 725) further supports the UPIAS (1976) argument in writing that the 'social model of disability defines disability as the societal response to impairment'. People are disabled not by their impairment but because they encounter barriers to full participation in society (Walmsley, 2005). Thus 'capacities, potentials and adequacies are to be understood as socially constructed and ascribed ... rather than "objective" attributes of persons' (Jenkins, 1998: 1). In this manner it may be argued that intellectual 'competence ... is socially constructed in terms of the normative standards and evaluative judgements enforced by the wider society, official agencies and their front-line representatives' (Booth and Booth, 1998: 77). Competence may hence be seen as an attributed status that arises from the decisions of professionals rather than individual behaviour. Competence can be viewed as axiomatic within society but this presumption may be challenged and thus not extended to some or withdrawn from others. These individuals must strive to be competent or be seen to be competent or otherwise experience exclusion from the 'fellowship of competence' (Jenkins, 1998). People with learning disabilities may be constrained by an axiomatic presumption of incompetence.

The social model highlights how a non-disabled society creates disability through 'attitudinal prejudices, physical obstacles and social barriers' (Drake, 1998: 188). Medical interventions, which may be appropriate at times of illness or injury, should thus be superseded by social action and personal assistance (not care) when individuals are building their lives (Øvretveit, 1996). As Brown (2000) succinctly notes the social model shifts the focus away from personal inadequacies and towards the availability and adequacy of service provision. During the 1970s the social model challenged the supremacy of the medical model in the care of people with learning disabilities as well as the medical and nursing hierarchies that operated within institutions. Key policy papers, such as *Better Services for the Mentally Handicapped* (Department of Health and Social Security, 1971) and the Jay Report (Department of Health and Social Security, 1976) together with new philosophies of care, such as normalisation (O'Brien and Tyne, 1974), drew on the social model of care to suggest new forms of service provision and new ways of working for learning disability nurses and other professionals.

Key elements of the social model of disability, as applied to people with learning disabilities, may be summarised as a distinction between disability and impairment; an emphasis on environmental, attitudinal, physical and structural barriers; a pride in being disabled and the assertion of a positive disabled identity; and the key to social inclusion and citizenship is independent living, supported by assistance when necessary, that is controlled by disabled people (Walmsley, 2005: 728). Development of the social model of disability has enabled people with learning disabilities, amongst others, to '...reassess the roles and identity attached to them, the oppression they experience and ways in which their rights and needs are or, more often, are not met' (Beresford et al., 2000: 194). Similarly, it requires that professionals re-evaluate their role within services and reflect on the values that underpin their practice and education.

However, Thomas (2004) notes that while the social model of disability and social conceptualisations of disability have both broadened disability theory and offered a powerful means of political struggle there remains a need to sociologically conceptualise impairment and the relationship between this and disability. It is to be acknowledged that while impairment is not the root cause of disability it is the foundation upon which disability works. The specific nature of the impairment plays a crucial role in the formation and degree of disablism encountered. Hence, impairment should not be seen as insignificant or irrelevant. As such it is necessary that nursing curricula contain content that addresses both impairment and disability in order for students to understand the health and social needs of people with learning disabilities and the societal structures and processes that enable or disable them. In England a number of programmes have been developed which offer a curriculum leading to qualification in both nursing and social work but these are the exception rather than the rule. It is also not clear where the practitioners that emerge from such programmes may best utilise their knowledge and skills and they may thus end up employed in services that are almost exclusively either health or social care orientated but not both. This view was supported by Norman (1998b) whose research indicated that while shared learning was valued by individuals within learning disability services, joint training (courses leading to a joint qualification) was less so. Joint training was considered to 'fudge the issue' of what nurses are or should be doing. Curricula do though have to be reconciled with a policy agenda that has encouraged a distinction between health and social care in both financial and service systems and education commissioning agendas that centre almost exclusively on healthcare provision. Creating a distinction between health and social care financing and provision fails to recognise the interaction between health and social need and how this interaction ultimately influences the overall health of the person with a learning disability. It is thus necessary to think broadly about health and to give consideration to physical, intellectual, social, and emotional health in a manner that may lead to health being synonymous with 'well-being' (Matthews, 2006). Learning disability nursing curricula are required to reflect this view of health in order to prepare practitioners capable of delivering and developing a holistic pattern of care that may also encompass sexual and spiritual health. Matthews (2006) argues that such a view of health may lead to social care practitioners recognising their responsibilities for promoting health. Similarly it may also lead to nurses being less inclined to dismiss the meeting of social needs as the exclusive domain of others. Norman (1998a) reported that learning disability practitioners favoured specialist rather than generic preparation for nurses.

It remains important that learning disability nursing curricula continue to draw upon models underpinning both health and social care in order to ensure that practitioners receive a comprehensive education that is grounded in social sciences and biomedicine and which thus enhances the provision of holistic care to people with learning disabilities. In addition the use of diverse models may lead to diverse curricula that address the changing needs and requirements of learning disability services and those of the commissioners of nurse education. It is, though, also important that nursing curricula promote healthcare (health promotion, health improvement, health education, and promoting access to healthcare systems) as the foundation for learning disability nursing practice.

User involvement

The involvement of users within health services and nursing education has become both a policy imperative and a pragmatic reality. This section of the chapter explores how this has become the case and considers the implications for nursing curricula as well as some approaches to the involvement of people with learning disabilities in curriculum planning and delivery.

Clearly the involvement of service users has become important within health services (Wright, 1995; Department of Health, 1997; 1999, 2000, 2002) and the College of Health has had in excess of 2500 self-help and service user groups on its database (Sang, 1999). But while user involvement is now a policy imperative for the National Health Service (Barnes et al, 1999) a concern for user involvement is not a new phenomenon in health and social care. Indeed, there is some tradition within the voluntary sector of offering self-help or user-led alternatives to statutory health and social care services (Truman and Raine, 2002). In 1974 public involvement in health services was promoted via the establishment of community health councils (CHCs). However, Richardson (1983) noted how the establishment of these organisations had enabled political interests to square the need for greater participation without unduly tampering with the centralised planning systems present within healthcare at the time. During the 1980s three expert groups were set up to inform developments specifically related to people with learning disabilities. These were the National Development Group for the Mentally Handicapped, the Development Team for the Mentally Handicapped and the Independent Development Council for People with Mental Handicap (IDC) (Ayer, 1997). The IDC published principles for local services that included valuing people with a mental handicap as citizens with rights, who were to be consulted about their needs and the plans to meet those needs, irrespective of the degree of handicap experienced by the individual (Independent Development Council, 1981).

A 1988 report on community care arrangements stated that the service should be more sensitive to the needs of its users and establish means to consult with them (Griffiths, 1988). The 1989 White Paper *Caring for People* (Department of Health and Social Security, 1989) espoused the central principle that users and carers should be actively consulted on the planning, provision and evaluation of services. The subsequent National Health Service and Community Care Act (NHSCCA) (Department of Health, 1990; Mercer, 2004) reinforced this principle and established both political and legislative drives within the public sector to identify and act upon the needs and preferences of people accessing health and social services.

Fisher (1992) noted that the new language of social care embodied in both *Community Care: An Agenda for Action* (Griffiths, 1988) and *Caring for People* (Department of Health and Social Security, 1989, 1998) emphasised voluntary access to services by users, following their own definition of need, and parallels between the users of social services and consumers of goods and services. The model of user involvement that accompanied the health and social care reforms of the 1990s was that of the 'sovereign consumer' (Jones and Tucker, 2000) whereby individuals could participate in choices between a range of services in a hypothetical marketplace (Rea, 1998). Within this model the consumer is assumed to hold the power, can choose to go elsewhere for services and the role of the service is to satisfy the demands of its consumers (Symonds, 1998b). Prior to this the existence of standardised products and centralised hierarchies within health services were identified as creating inflexible, remote and unresponsive services. Services were also poorly attuned to the variety of needs of users (Barnes and Wistow, 1992). Hence a key feature of the community care reforms of the decade, alongside factors such as efficiency, value for money, competition, effectiveness, quality and customer care (Reed and Gilleard, 1995; Butcher, 2000), has been the emphasis on the user as central to both policy and practice (Beresford et al, 2000). At the same time a body of work emerged that supported the view that consumers should not be seen simply as passive recipients of services, with some right to comment on the quality of the service delivered, but as active participants in decision-making and priority setting around their needs (NHSME, 1990; Hogg, 1991; McIver, 1991).

This view of the patient as an involved partner, either individually or collectively, was detailed within *Patient and Public Involvement in the New NHS* (Department of Health, 1999). The NHS was urged to listen to local communities, to create an organisation and culture that promoted a consumer/user focus and to make patients partners in decision-making processes. However, The *NHS Plan* (Department of Health, 2000) noted that the NHS was not sufficiently attuned to the voice of patients and that patients had too little influence at any level within the NHS. The notion of a patient-centred NHS was carried forward by the Department of Health with policy guidance aimed at active patient/user involvement in the planning and delivery of services (Department of Health, 2002). Suggested measures included patient advocacy and liaison services (PALS), user representation within strategic health authorities, and patient forums within NHS trusts. User representatives have been involved in the development of National Service Frameworks (NSF) within healthcare and national user surveys. However, Styring and Grant (2005) argue that while people with learning disabilities are getting involved in developments aimed to improve quality of care, including PALS, service user councils and service reviews undertaken by the Commission for Health Improvement (an independent health services inspection and review body), much more needs to be done to include people with limited communication skills and people with profound disabilities.

In 2001 the Department of Health published *Valuing People*, the first White Paper specifically about people with learning disabilities to be released since *Better Services* (Department of Health and Social Security, 1971). The White Paper contained a section on choice and control for people with learning disabilities within which it was stated that 'people with learning disabilities have little involvement in decision making' and that 'people with learning disabilities and their families are not central to the planning process' (Department of Health, 2001: 44). A number of challenges for public services in giving people with learning disabilities more control are noted, including 'fully involving them in decisions affecting their lives', 'developing a person-centred approach to planning services' and 'improving information and communication with people with learning disabilities' (Department of Health, 2001: 45). The White Paper also noted the need to involve people with learning disabilities in decision making that affected their lives at all levels and as active partners in services. 'This applies to decisions on day to day matters, such as choice of activities, operational matters, such as staff selection, and strategic matters, such as changes to eligibility criteria' (Department of Health, 2001: 51). The principles of rights, independence, choice, and inclusion that are the foundations of *Valuing People* may be seen as the finale of policy movement toward participation and control by people with intellectual disabilities (Ramcharan and Grant, 2001).

In January 2003 Section 11 of the Health and Social Care Act 2001 came into force. This places a duty on NHS organisations to consult with, and involve, patients and the public in developing and planning proposals for major change and in the ongoing planning and operation of services. Braye (2000) notes the incorporation into UK law of the European Convention on Human Rights and Fundamental Freedoms as an important development in the legal mandate for participation. This legal mandate, enacted within the Human Rights Act 1998, may enable service users to challenge agency and professional decisions made without their participation and may also thus promote rights-based provision.

It may be ascertained from this overview of policy and legislative development that the involvement of users within health services has increasingly been seen as a priority for action. In addition a central theme within contemporary health care is that of empowerment, accompanied by the belief that professionals should be working in partnership with service users (Wright, 1995). Empowerment concerns approaches that support people with learning disabilities to cope with disabling environments and to develop valued social roles. It emphasises the requirement of service staff to facilitate user-defined services and to avoid using approaches that unduly control service users. Finlay (2000) argues the need for professionals to surrender their 'expert' status and to value the expertise of users, with respect to their own needs, in order to develop empowering relationships. McClimens (2005) adds that the dominance of professional knowledge may be countered through user involvement and thus the creation of new social knowledge that enhances user control and agency. However, people with learning disabilities will also want involvement in different ways, as befits their diversity, and thus any strategy for user involvement will be required to have many different strands and should be able to operate at a number of levels (Simons, 1995). Services cannot rely solely on internal processes to promote the empowerment of service users, they must be open to external, independent elements such as self-advocacy, citizen advocacy and circles of support (supportive networks of people for the person with a learning disability) (Simons, 1995).

Similarly in order for people with learning disabilities to be involved in nursing curricula a variety of approaches and levels of involvement may be required. It is important in a modern context that the nursing profession takes account of the views and concerns of service users within nurse education and thus in the preparation of future practitioners (Rush and Cook, 2006). Research into user involvement in education indicates that students who benefited from such an approach were less likely to use jargon; were more able to empathise with client's experiences of distress; were less likely to distance themselves from clients; were more likely to take an individualised approach to assessment and interventions; demonstrated positive changes in attitude; and positively evaluated user involvement in the curriculum (Wood and Wilson-Barnett, 1999; Happeli and Roper, 2003; and Cook et al, 1995; all cited in Rush and Barker, 2006). Users themselves may also benefit from increases in self-confidence, the development of a valued social role, the provision of an income, and a new awareness among professionals of their competence (Felton and Stickley, 2004).

A number of factors need to be considered though in order to ensure the effectiveness of user involvement within nursing curricula and to make the experience a positive one for both students and people with learning disabilities. These include the creation of the right size of student group to facilitate involvement; facilitators who are experienced in working with users and in teaching methods; and the creation of the necessary preparation, delivery and review time for users (Laverty et al, 2005; Rush and Barker, 2006). This latter element does have implications for the resourcing of sessions which may be in excess of that normally required to deliver the curriculum through other means.

In addition, user involvement inevitably involves financial expenditure through elements such as teaching or consultation fees and/or payment of expenses. The payment of fees has a particular context for people with learning disabilities and often is limited by the potential impact on other benefit payments received by the individual. Consequently fee payments may be of nominal amounts leading to accusations of tokenism. A further issue arises in the potential for role confusion among students working with people with learning disabilities who may be both service users and teachers. As Laverty et al (2005) note service users appreciated the opportunity to be involved in curriculum development and the idea that they may be of help to students in their practice. They also appreciated the recognition of their views and the notion that they may be viewed as experts in their own right. These are, however, facets of the teaching role that may be absent in practice wherein the student may become a carer and the person with a learning disability, who may still be a user of services, the cared for. As such the social identity of both the person with a learning disability and the student changes and it may be the case that neither the student nor the service user recognises or understands how this also changes their relationship with each other and their respective roles. There are also issues here about the transition of power between students and service users and Felton and Stickley (2004) note how user involvement may similarly challenge the power of educators that is derived from their position as experts within education systems. This may mean that people with learning disabilities are involved in curricula only on the terms of educators or the institutions that employ them and thus involvement may be 'characterised by tokenism rather than partnership' (Felton and Stickley, 2004: 91).

However, despite these difficulties, involving people with learning disabilities does ensure that they are part of the learning process for future practitioners; promotes the opportunity for nursing curricula and clinical practice to be aligned with the needs of service users; and provides the opportunity for the development of new valued social identities and competencies.

A standardised curriculum

Experienced practitioners and educators in England and Wales will remember a point in history when the pre-registration learning disability nursing programme was based on a single syllabus proscribed centrally by the General Nursing Council (GNC), which was the forerunner of both the United Kingdom Central Council for Nursing, Midwifery and Health Visiting (UKCC) and the Nursing and Midwifery Council (NMC). The 1982 *Training Syllabus for Nurses Caring for People with Mental Handicap* (GNC, 1982) detailed the skills and knowledge to be achieved by students to enable registration; set standard placement experiences; standardised curriculum structures and assessment processes within England and Wales; and was founded on a single validation body in the form of the GNC. The syllabus was designed to emphasise principles of normalisation and to promote practice within community and domiciliary settings rather than hospitals (Norman, 1998a). This may come as some surprise to readers familiar with the current national picture of a plethora of programmes designed, provided and validated by a range of higher education establishments across the UK. It may also come as a surprise to know that this syllabus detailed skills and knowledge that were specific to learning disability nursing as opposed to the generic outcomes currently used to assess students in practice. Prior to *Project 2000* (UKCC, 1986) educational curricula highlighted the unique contribution of learning disability nurses and distanced them from general (adult) nursing (Norman, 1998a). *Project 2000*, however, emphasised commonalities within the fields of nursing and led to the establishment of an 18 month common foundation programme which is now more usually 12 months in length. While the aim of this was to raise standards, criticism was levelled at the emphasis on general nursing within such curricula which was at the expense of the specialities (White et al, 1993). This may have been a reflection of the service world where Norman (1998b: 440) reported in his research of the 'lukewarm attitude of other nursing specialisms towards learning disability nursing and the lip service given by some professional bodies to its unique identity'. However, Norman (1998b) also felt that education programmes could be expected to mature into unique programmes that responded to the needs of educational purchasers and users of new learning disability nursing services. It is, though, debatable as to whether such a transition has actually taken place in nursing curricula that are dominated by shared learning, that are largely composed of content that reflects the concerns of branches of nursing other than learning disability, and that are inconsistently supported by central guidance and specific outcomes for learning disability nurses.

While the latter point may be indicative of provision in England, developments in Scotland, where NHS Education for Scotland (NES) launched a national framework for learning disability nurse education in 2005, offer a more promising future. The framework defines the value base of learning disability nursing; sets out principles from which higher education institutions (HEIs) may develop programmes, set assessments, establish practice placements and develop mentorship arrangements; defines branch programme content; and sets learning outcomes specific to learning disability nursing (Mathieson, 2005). The framework was developed in consultation with people with learning disabilities, carers, service providers, educators and students. It arguably enables the nursing curriculum in Scotland to be more pragmatically aligned with relevant learning disability policy than curricula elsewhere in the UK that do not benefit from such a degree of central direction. Curricula are also potentially more visible to student nurse candidates who can more easily ascertain what learning disability nursing is about and what outcomes they can expect from a learning disability nursing programme anywhere in the country. The framework, aligned with supportive policy as it is, sends a clear message that there is both a need for learning disability nurses and that curricula can be designed to deliver nursing services that meet the requirements of people with learning disabilities (Mathieson, 2005).

Prior to the publication of the national framework for learning disability,

NES published *Getting it Right Together* (NES, 2004). This document examined how knowledge about the health needs of people with learning disabilities may be strengthened within all nursing programmes. In particular it detailed outcomes for common foundation programme learning related to people with learning disabilities as well as outcomes to be incorporated within child branch programmes. As such it potentially addresses some of the concerns that emerged in England following the publication of *Valuing People* (Department of Health, 2001). Roberts (2002) noted the emerging policy drive to strengthen the role of mainstream services in meeting the health needs of people with learning disabilities. In order for this to happen though he argued that it would be important to ensure that nurses in mainstream health settings possessed the necessary competencies to work with people with learning disabilities before any change in role was contemplated for specialist services. This in turn posed new challenges for nurse education in that it would be necessary to ensure that all student nurses received both appropriate knowledge and meaningful experiences to develop their awareness of learning disability. Students would also benefit from greater experience in order to be able to communicate with people with learning disabilities and to work effectively with families, carers and support networks. The use of agreed learning outcomes within Scottish nursing programmes will certainly go some way towards addressing these concerns while elsewhere learning disability nurse educators may have to continue to rely on their powers of persuasion to access the curricula, the common foundation programme and of all branches of nursing.

Norman (1998a) argued that we need to rein in the dominant influence of general nursing within curricula in order that the learning disability specialism may flourish. Otherwise learning disability nurses will not have the opportunity to develop the specialist knowledge and skills valued by service managers. The presence of a defined learning disability curriculum may serve to re-establish the existence of specialist skills in learning disability nursing and thus counteract a belief within other nursing specialisms that such skills are simply variants used by all nurses. In addition some central guidance with respect to learning disability content within nursing curricula would help to better achieve contemporary healthcare policy and to better prepare nurses in all fields for delivering nursing care to, and with, people with learning disabilities.

The recent disquiet surrounding practice within both learning disabilities and mainstream health services (Disability Rights Commission, 2006; Healthcare Commission, 2007; Mencap, 2007; Michael, 2008) has led to some movement toward this aim. A vision for learning disability nursing (Northway et al, 2006) and benchmarks for good practice for learning disability nurses (Department of Health, 2007) provide a foundation for curriculum planners and it is to be hoped that the current Nursing and Midwifery Council (NMC) review of pre-registration nurse education in England (NMC, 2009) will stimulate new debate around curricula designed to support the healthcare needs of people with learning disabilities and the knowledge, understanding and competence of the learning disability nurse.

This chapter has sought to explore some of the current challenges within nurse education for learning disability curricula. Inevitably readers may feel that other concerns and issues have been ignored including the wider debates about genericism and specialism; unidisciplinary and multidisciplinary education and training; work-based and university-based learning; vocational and academic modes of training; and the appropriateness of education commissioning processes and their relationship to workforce models. It is hoped though that the challenges that are addressed here have resonance with the experiences and concerns of learning disability educators and practitioners elsewhere.

References

Ayer S (1997) Services for people with learning disabilities in the UK. In: Gates B, Beacock C (eds.) *Dimensions of Learning Disability*. Bailliere Tindall, London

Barnes M, Harrison S, Mort M, Shardlow P (1999) *Unequal Partners: User groups and community care*. The Policy Press, Bristol

Barnes M, Wistow G (1992) Understanding user involvement. In: Barnes M, Wistow G (eds.) *Researching User Involvement*. Nuffield Institute for Health Service Studies, Leeds

Booth T, Booth W (1998) Risk, resilience and competence: Parents with learning difficulties and their children. In: Jenkins R (ed.) *Questions of Competence – Culture, Classification and Intellectual Disability*. University Press, Cambridge

Beresford P, Croft S, Evans C, Harding T (2000) Quality in personal social services: The developing role of user involvement in the UK. In: Davies C, Finlay L, Bullman A (eds.) *Changing Practice in Health and Social Care*. Sage Publications/Open University, London

Braye S (2000) Participation and involvement in social care. In: Kemshall H, Littlechild R (eds.) *User Involvement and Participation in Social Care*. Jessica Kingsley Publishers, London

Brown H (2000) Challenges from service users. In: Brechin A, Brown H, Eby MA (eds.) *Critical Practice in Health and Social Care*. Sage Publications, London

Butcher T (2000) The public administration model of welfare delivery. In:

Davies C, Finlay L, Bullman A (eds.) *Changing Practice in Health and Social Care*. Sage Publications/Open University, London

Department of Health (1990) *The NHS and Community Care Act*. HMSO, London

Department of Health (1997) *The New NHS – Modern, Dependable*. The Stationary Office, London

Department of Health (1999) *Patient and Public Involvement in the New NHS*. The Stationary Office, London

Department of Health (2000) *The NHS Plan: A Plan for Investment, a Plan for Reform*. The Stationary Office, London

Department of Health (2001) *Valuing People: A Strategy for Learning Disability for the 21st Century*. HMSO, London

Department of Health (2002) *Involving Patients and the Public in Health Care*. The Stationary Office, London

Department of Health (2007) *Good Practice in Learning Disability Nursing*. Department of Health, London

Department of Health and Social Security (1971) *Better Services for the Mentally Handicapped*. HMSO, London

Department of Health and Social Security (1976) The Report of the Committee of Enquiry into Mental Handicap Nursing and Care. HMSO, London

Department of Health and Social Security (1989) *Caring for People - Community Care in the Next Decade and Beyond*. HMSO, London

Disability Rights Commission (2006) *Equal Treatment: Closing the Gap*. Disability Rights Commission, London

Drake RF (1998) Professionals and the voluntary sector. In: Symonds A, Kelly A (eds.) *The Social Construction of Community Care*. Macmillan Press Ltd, London

Felton A, Stickley T (2004) Pedagogy, power and service user involvement. *Journal of Psychiatric and Mental Health Nursing 11*: 89–98

Finlay L (2000) The challenge of professionalism. In: Brechin A, Brown H, Eby MA (eds.) *Critical Practice in Health and Social Care*. Sage Publications, London

Fisher M (1992) Users experiences of agreements in social care. In Barnes, M, Wistow G (eds.) *Researching User Involvement*. Nuffield Institute for Health Service Studies, Leeds.

GNC (1982) *Training Syllabus for Nurses Caring for People with Mental*

Handicap. The General Nursing Council for England and Wales, London

Griffiths R (1988) *Community Care: An Agenda for Action*. HMSO, London

Healthcare Commission (2007) *A Life Like No Other - A national audit of specialist inpatient healthcare services for people with learning difficulties in England*. Commission for Healthcare Audit and Inspection, London

Hogg C (1991) *Involving the Community: Guidelines for Health Service Managers*. National Consumer Council, London

Independent Development Council for People with Mental Handicap (1981) *Statement of Core Principles*. IDC, London

Jenkins R (1998) Culture, classification and (in)competence. In: Jenkins R (ed.) *Questions of Competence – Culture, Classification and Intellectual Disability*. University Press, Cambridge

Jones J, Tucker S (2000) Exploring continuity and change. In: Brechin A, Brown H, Eby MA (eds.) *Critical Practice in Health and Social Care*. Sage Publications/Open University. London

Kelly A (1998) Concepts of professions and professionalism. In: Symonds A, Kelly A (eds.) *The Social Construction of Community Care*. Macmillan Press Ltd, London

Laverty H, Challis PJ, Easters S, Smitheringale E, Thompson P (2005) Build a nurse! *Learning Disability Practice* **8**(2): 32–4

Mathieson A (2005) The real deal. *Learning Disability Practice* **8**(8): 6–7

Matthews D (2006) Endless evolution: How patterns of care shift over time. *Learning Disability Practice* **9**(5): 30–4

McIver S (1991) *An Introduction to Obtaining the Views of Users of Health Services*. Kings Fund Centre, London

McClimens A (2005) From vagabonds to Victorian values. In: Grant G, Goward P, Richardson M, Ramcharan P (eds.) *Learning Disability – A life Cycle Approach to Valuing People*. Open University Press, Maidenhead

Mencap (2007) *Death by Indifference - Following Up the Treat Me Right Report*. Mencap, London

Mercer G (2004) User-led organisations: Facilitating independent living. In: Swain J, French S, Barnes C, Thomas C (eds.) *Disabling Barriers – Enabling Environments*. 2nd edn. Sage Publications, London

Michael J (2008) *Report of the Independent Inquiry into access to Healthcare for People with Learning Disabilities*. London

NHS Education for Scotland (2004) *Getting It Right Together – The Implementation of Recommendations 16, 17 and 20 from Promoting Health, Supporting Inclusion*. NES, Edinburgh

NHS Education for Scotland (2005) *The Right Preparation. The Framework for Learning Disability* Nurse Education in Scotland. NES, Edinburgh

NHSME (1990) *Consultation and Involving the Consumer*. Department of Health, London

Norman IJ (1998a) The changing emphasis of mental health and learning disability nurse education in the UK and ideal models of its future development. *Journal of Psychiatric and Mental Health Nursing* **5**: 41–51

Norman IJ (1998b) Priorities for mental health and learning disability nurse education in the UK: A case study. *Journal of Clinical Nursing* **7**: 433–41

Northway R, Hutchinson C, Kingdon A (eds.) (2006) *Shaping the Future: A Vision for Learning Disability Nursing*. UK Learning Disability Consultant Nurse Network, London

Nursing and Midwifery Council (2009) *Review of Pre-Registration Nursing Education - Phase 2: Join our Field Working Groups* Available from: http://www.nmc-uk.org/aArticle.aspx?ArticleID=3566 [Last accessed 7 April 2009]

Nuttall M (1998) States and categories: Indigenous models of personhood in Northwest Greenland. In: Jenkins R (ed.) *Questions of Competence – Culture, Classification and Intellectual Disability*. University Press, Cambridge

O'Brien L, Tyne A (1974) *The Principles of Normalisation*. CMH Publications, London

Oliver M (2004) 'If I Had a Hammer: The Social Model in Action' in Swain J, French S, Barnes C, Thomas C (eds.) *Disabling Barriers – Enabling Environments*. 2nd Edn. Sage Publications, London

Øvretveit J (1996) How patient power and client participation affects relations between professions. In: Øvretveit J, Mathias P, Thompson T (eds.) *Interprofessional Working for Health and Social Care*. Macmillan, London

Ramcharan P, Grant G (2001) Views and experiences of people with intellectual disabilities and their families. (1) The user perspective. *Journal of Applied Research in Intellectual Disabilities* **14**: 348–63

Rea D (1998) The myth of the market in the organisation of community care. In: Symonds A, Kelly A (eds.) *The Social Construction of Community Care*. MacMillan Press Ltd, Basingstoke

Reed R, Gilleard C (1995) Elderly patients' satisfaction with a community nursing service. In: Wilson G (ed.) *Community Care: Asking the Users*. Chapman and Hall, London

Richardson A (1983) *Participation*. Routledge and Kegan Paul, London

Richardson M (2005) Critiques of segregation and eugenics. In: Grant G, Goward P, Richardson M, Ramcharan P (eds.) *Learning Disability – A Life Cycle Approach to Valuing People*. Open University Press, Maidenhead

Roberts S (2002) Challenging times. *Learning Disability Practice* **5**(4): 6

Rush B, Barker JH (2006) Involving mental health service users in nurse education through enquiry-based learning. *Nurse Education in Practice* **6**: 254–60

Rush B, Cook J (2006) What makes a good nurse? Views of patients and carers. *British Journal of Nursing* **15**(7): 382–5

Sang B (1999) The customer is sometimes right. *Health Service Journal* **Aug**: 22–3

Simons K (1995) Empowerment and advocacy. In: Malin N (ed.) *Services for People with Learning Disabilities*. Routledge, London

Styring L, Grant G (2005) Maintaining a commitment to quality. In: Grant G, Goward P, Richardson M, Ramcharan P (eds.) *Learning Disability – A Life Cycle Approach to Valuing People*. Open University Press, Maidenhead

Symonds A (1998a) Social construction and the concept of 'community'. In: Symonds A, Kelly A (eds.) The Social Construction of Community Care. Macmillan Press Ltd, London

Symonds A (1998b) Care for the community: inmates, patients, consumers and citizens. In: Symonds A, Kelly A (eds.) *The Social Construction of Community Care*. Macmillan Press Ltd, London

Thomas C (2004) Disability and impairment. In: Swain J, French S, Barnes C, Thomas C (eds.) *Disabling Barriers – Enabling Environments* 2nd edn. Sage Publications, London

Thompson C (1997) Political dimensions of learning disability. In: Gates B, Beacock C (eds.) *Dimensions of Learning Disability*. Bailliere Tindall, London

Truman C, Raine P (2002) Experience and meaning of user involvement: Some explorations from a community mental health project. Health and *Social Care in the Community* **10**(1): 136–43

United Kingdom Central Council for Nursing, Midwifery and Health Visiting (1986) *Project 2000: A New Preparation for Practice*. UKCC, London

UPIAS (1976) *Fundamental Principles of Disability*. Union of the Physically Impaired Against Segregation, London

Walmsley J (2005) Research and emancipation – prospects and problems. In: Grant G, Goward P, Richardson M, Ramcharan P (eds.) *Learning Disability – A Life Cycle Approach to Valuing People*. Open University Press, Maidenhead

White E, Riley E, Davies S, Twinn S (1993) *A Detailed Study of the Relationship between Teaching, Support, Supervision and Role Modelling in Clinical Areas within the context of Project 2000 Courses*. Report to the English National Board for Nursing, Midwifery and Health Visiting (ENB), Kings College London and University of Manchester

Wright S (1995) *We Thought We Knew…Involving Patients in Nursing Practice – Executive Summary*. Kings Fund, London

CHAPTER 16

Inter-professional education

Martin Bollard

Introduction

Today, the need for collaborative practice between healthcare professionals and agencies is probably more important than ever before (Norman, 2005). New service concepts, such as the one stop health and social care services, and the co-location of primary healthcare and social care staff (Department of Health, 2000) will demand greater collaborative working. Yet, there is still little sound evidence of how best to teach and construct inter-professional learning and therefore appropriately develop the health and social care practitioners of the future (Mattick and Bligh, 2003).

Despite many national and international inter-professional learning models and strategies emerging over the last three decades (Barr et al, 2000), many inter-professional educational issues still need to be addressed around the type of learning, the context for that learning and the evaluation methods best suited to this form of educational preparation. It is now widely acknowledged, however, that inter-professional education (IPE) is a potentially effective approach for enhancing collaborative practice between health and social care professionals. This educational approach creates opportunities for professionals and those in training to learn with and about each other, whereas uni-professional education does not provide this opportunity (Norman, 2005).

IPE can be seen to originate from the World Health Organisation's (WHO) report in 1988, *Learning Together to Work Together for Health*. This report encouraged the development of IPE approaches across the world to promote effective teamwork. In the UK, many policy drivers over the last three decades, most notably with the NHS and Community Care Act (1990), emphasised providing healthcare in the community, which led to a number of collaborative service models (Oandasan and Reeves, 2005a). The Centre for the Advancement of Inter-professional Education (CAIPE) was founded in 1987 to provide a central resource to assist health professional educators to exchange ideas, and discuss and create new IPE initiatives. Government policies have sought to promote the value of collaboration among professionals which has precipitated the need for 'shared learning'.

Integrated care for patients will rely on models of training and education that give staff a clear understanding of how their own roles fit with those of others within both the health and social care professions (Department of Health, 1997: 46).

The *NHS Plan* (Department of Health, 2000: 86) goes further than solely learning about each others roles, stating:

> *There will be new joint training across the professions in communications skills… they will form part of a new core curriculum for all education programmes for NHS staff.*

Finch (2000) argues that the implications of these policies for students are that they should:

- Know about the roles of other professionals.
- Be able to work with them in the context of teams where each member has a clearly defined role.
- Substitute for roles traditionally played by other professionals, when this may be more effective.
- Switch training pathways to enhance career progression.

It is clear then that, as Finch (2000) highlights, universities will require a clear perspective upon what inter-professional working would really mean, before curricula and IPE activities can be developed.

More recently, the Department of Health (2005) launched its strategy for creating an inter-professional workforce with a number of examples of best IPE practice cited on its website, many of which include its pilot projects hosted at the following institutions:

- Newcastle University: http://commonlearning.ncl.ac.uk.
- University of Southampton: http://www.mhbs.soton.ac.uk/ newgeneration.
- Sheffield Hallam University: http://shu.ac.uk/schools/hsc/ modernisation/summary.html.
- Coventry University: http://www.coventry.ac.uk/cipl, which focus on e-Learning.
- Kings College, London: http://www.kcl.ac.uk/ipe/intro/index.html.

These universities have been charged with developing what the Department of Health are referring to as common learning and IPE with a commitment to:

- Develop common learning programmes for all staff and professionals and core curricula in communications, NHS principles and organisation.

- Change workforce practices and develop new ways of working.
- Break down professional and organisational barriers to learning and work together through closer integration of health professional programmes.

Pietroni (1992) discussed that one of the difficulties around developing effective inter-professional working was that professions needed to be conversant with a range of different languages (professional terminology) and the way in which different professions communicate with each other. More than a decade on from that, information technology would be added to this discourse. Information sharing through the different information technology media available is an important contemporary issue within health and social care practice. Sharing information remains a source of tension for professionals, for while there is a need to protect confidentiality and personal information, this needs to be balanced with the necessity to share personal information across professional boundaries (Richardson and Asthana, 2006).

Changing terminology

As part of the modernisation of health and social care, organisational re-configurations have become the norm. As such, this has placed an unequivocal attention on inter-organisational working, that has not been equally matched with the attention upon inter-professional relationships (Hudson, 2002). Hudson (2002) departs from the pessimistic sociological literature on inter-professional working stating that it is hindered by difficulties with professional identity, status and accountability, and proposes a more optimistic model of inter-professionality, through a number of different hypotheses. These are based upon some of his research (Hudson, 2002) and work by Guy (1986) that not only provide a platform for further investigation in this area but in addition a clarity with which to consider inter-professional working. These researchers consider that:

- Members of one profession may have more in common with members of a different profession than with members of their own.
- The promotion of professional values of trust can form the basis of inter-professional partnership.
- Socialisation to an immediate work group can provide professional and hierarchical differences among staff.
- Professionals and bureaucracies can join forces in a collective effort to achieve goals.
- Effective inter-professional working can lead to more effective service delivery and user outcomes.

D'Amour and Oandasan (2005) believe the concept of inter-professionality is an attempt to bridge the gap in understanding between IPE and inter-professional practice, a project that is long overdue and should assist the evaluation and analysis of IPE. Gilbert (2005) argues that it has become impossible to evaluate IPE with the semantic implications around the term inter-professional. Although the prefixes, multi, inter and trans, are clear, it can be seen that in the context of inter-professional education and patient-centred care, differences in understanding and usage are clear barriers to useful evaluation of IPE (Gilbert, 2005).

Professionals come from different disciplines, work in different organisations and carry with them different conceptualisations of service users and their needs along with different responses to service users' complex situations. One of the challenges for inter-professional educators is to develop a common language for their students that can help make sense of such complex situations, in addition to offering a mix of experience that covers hospital settings and community settings (Barr et al, 2005).

Inter-professionality is defined as (D'Amour and Oandasan, 2005: 9):

The development of a cohesive practice between professionals from different disciplines. It is the process by which professionals reflect and develop ways of practising that provides an integrated and cohesive answer to the needs of the service user/family/population. Inter-professionality comes from the preoccupation of professionals to reconcile their differences and their sometimes opposing views, involving continuous interaction and knowledge sharing between professionals, organised to solve or explore a variety of education and care issues all while seeking to optimise service user participation.

D'Amour and Oandasan (2005) advocate that inter-professionality implies a better understanding of the determinants and processes that influence IPE and inter-professional practice.

Emerging from the literature is not necessarily another new concept but a framework that can help crystallise an understanding of inter-professional working. Gordon and Walsh (2005) put forward the inter-professional capability framework that focuses upon collaborative practice where the service user is central to guide students towards inter-professional capability. Drawn from the capable practitioner document (Sainsbury Centre for Mental Health, 2001), the framework attempts to acknowledge the complexity of inter-professional working by moving away from competency-based models of education to capability-focused learning. Given that an emphasis on capability is concerned with the extent to which individuals can apply, adapt and synthesise new knowledge in different settings (Fraser and Greenhalgh, 2001), this approach is suitable to the context of IPE.

The framework arose from an analysis of Quality Assurance Agency documentation eliciting four domains for the inter-professional capability framework:

- Knowledge in practice.
- Ethical practice.
- Inter-professional working.
- Reflection.

The capabilities within each domain are broken down with different learning achievement levels attached (see Gordon and Walsh, 2005, and Combined Universities Inter-professional Unit, University of Sheffield Medical School). An adapted example relating to learning disabilities has been developed and is shown in *Table 16.1*.

Underpinning inter-professional education

Colyer et al (2005), in an occasional paper for the Higher Education Academy, review a number of papers offering a theoretical underpinning to IPE. There is clear potential in these papers to contribute to the development

Table 16.1. An adapted inter-professional capability for learning disability practice

Capability	Domain: Knowledge in practice learning achievement level
The inter-professional team member interacts within the health and social care practice community consistently to promote and support patient/ user participation and autonomy on the basis of informed decision making and exercise of choice	Level 1: Person-centred approaches are recognised placing service users at the centre of the care and decision making process Level 2: Service users are supported through the development of effective communication systems to take part in inter-disciplinary care reviews Level 3: Inter-professional team assessment and involvement is made accessible through clear multi-professional planning that directly involves the user

of an epistemology to support IPE. However, the intention here is to revert back to two key concepts, collaboration and partnership, as the main drivers that can underpin this educational approach.

Most practitioners and educators would support an endeavour that strives to prepare health and social care professionals to work together effectively, respect each others' skills, values and knowledge with the ultimate goal of a smoother less frustrating experience for the patient/service user. This, in effect, is the goal of IPE. However, as many readers will be aware, there are many barriers to achieving effective IPE. These will be eluded to later in the chapter.

One of the main purposes of IPE is to promote early team-working skills and understanding of teams within different student groups. Collaboration is sometimes perceived as being synonymous with teamwork. However, Barr et al (2005) believe that all teamwork is collaboration, but all collaboration is not teamwork.

The notions of collaboration and partnership drive IPE (Gilbert, 2005) and therefore are worthy of closer attention as key concepts that can underpin any IPE strategy.

Put simply, collaboration is about working together. Meads and Ashcroft (2005) argue that the term collaboration implies both difference (it is something less than complete integration or unification) and commonality (there is some shared goal or activity that is the focus of collaboration. Collaboration therefore is also about relationships, working together and not just working alongside. It implies more than activities that overlap or interact in some way, and would usually involve some deliberate interaction between parties to achieve a common goal (Meads and Ashcroft, 2005). Building up an educational understanding of

Table 16.2. A taxonomy of collaboration

Aspects of collaboration	Examples of their expression
Goal	Functional or transformational
Level	Strategic, executive, operational, technical
Process	Co-operation, co-ordination, exchange, sharing
Structure	Networks, teams, pathways, partnerships, area-based activities, merged organisations
Power and influence	Participation, empowerment, co-option and control, infiltration and subversion
Proximity	In time and/or space
Duration	Temporary tasks focused or longer-term strategy
Complexity	Bipolar or multi-polar

collaboration is necessary, as it can then be translated into learning outcomes which can guide the planning and delivery of IPE. *Table 16.2* is a taxonomy of collaboration that can support that process (Huxham, 1996).

Collaboration is often put forward as a rational objective to achieve certain goals. It is important to note that the process of collaboration can change as can be clearly witnessed within the learning disability field. Numerous examples exist of collaborative tensions, from shifting professional priorities over the planning of care, to inter-agency collaboration as organisations reconfigure, and intricacies surrounding one-to-one consultations between practitioner and individual.

Inter-professional working is the axis around which collaboration within and between organisations and with service users, carers and communities revolves (Meads and Barr, 2005). IPE should therefore be trying to offer many different examples of collaboration through classroom activities and the practice setting.

Depicting the sequence of interactions that make up a partnership between a practitioner and a person with learning disabilities is difficult. Yet, everyday practice for many professionals, not just nurses, will rely upon some form of partnership to facilitate their work (Bollard, 2003). As people with learning disabilities often have complex needs, this, in the reality of practice, requires that partnerships are not only formed with people with learning disabilities but also with other professional groups (Bollard, 2003). Learning disability, as a case example, provides rich opportunities for inter-professional learning and can provide useful scenario and discussion points through an array of different media to highlight different professional roles. Meads and Ashcroft (2005) argue that professionals have a 'duty of partnership' within a new collaborative culture and the list below can help students and practitioners frame where their professional relationships (partnerships) can be:

- With own profession (nowadays with more differentiated roles and different terms of employment).
- With other professions (with shared referrals and procedures, larger multi-specialist teams and new skills mixes).
- With new partners (external consultancy and education, hybrid organisations, different accountabilities including voluntary and private agencies.
- With policy actors (links to political units, decision making on healthcare options and priorities and participative forums).
- With public (locally elected representatives with health-related roles, independent regulators of the public interest).
- With service users/patients (informed consumers and citizens, team-based care, incorporation of social care into holistic concept of health, advocates, care managers and carers).

Delivering IPE within higher education

For IPE to succeed it needs to be embraced as a worthy educational strategy by all staff. This should not imply that IPE is a panacea to all educational problems, but to make explicit that where IPE is dependent upon a few enthusiasts, it encounters problems (Freeth, 2001).

Although previous wisdom was that IPE was better introduced at a post-qualification level (Norman, 2005), this chapter will focus upon pre-registration training, as the more recent trend is to deliver IPE at a pre-registration level, in order to overcome the risk that separate or uni-professional programmes would reinforce tribalism and negative stereotyping of other professional groups. This would then hinder inter-professional working (Norman, 2005).

The purpose of this part of the chapter is not to review the various models of IPE that exist; the reader can review them by following the internet links given earlier in the chapter. Instead it is to present a clear purpose for IPE, what can make IPE effective, with a particular focus upon service user involvement, and to highlight some of the barriers to IPE.

The purpose of IPE

IPE should have one or more of the following aims/foci (Barr et al, 2005):

- Preparing individuals for collaboration: This focuses upon establishing knowledge bases, acquisition of skills and the modification of attitudes and perceptions by individuals to pave the way for collaborative practice between professions, within and between organisations and with clients, their caregivers and their communities.
- Cultivating collaboration in groups or teams: This focuses on how to collaborate as a group or team-based activity, either directly between parties (practitioners in the workplace) or by proxy (students during the course).
- Improving services and the quality of the care: This focuses on purposeful collective action to effect change and to improve the quality of services for clients, which becomes inter-professional education, if and when learning is built in between professions.

Although these foci overlap, working towards achieving them will be dependent upon whether the learning is before or after qualification, where the learning is taking place (classroom or practice-based) and the teaching methods that are being utilised to support the overall purpose.

Towards effective IPE

The end point of most health and social care training is the ability of such professionals to perform their roles as part of a team in the care of the different respective service user groups (D'Oen, 2005). This demands taking the students through an effective inter-professional learning strategy. To ascertain whether IPE is effective is difficult. However, Barr (2002) suggests a number of pre-requisites for effective IPE. IPE must:

- Put service users at the centre: This should involve service users, at the least, in designing, teaching, participating and assessing programmes.
- Promote collaboration: Applying what is learned to collaborative practice during practice placements, work-based assignments, collaboration within professions, within and between organisations and with communities, service users and carers.
- Reconcile competing objectives: Ensure that these principles are protected as the essential qualities of IPE while ensuring that they are compatible with other objectives and their implications for programme design, content and learning methods.
- Reinforce collaborative competence: Reach beyond modification of attitudes and secure common knowledge bases to reinforce collaborative competencies that are necessary to cope with contemporary practice.
- Incorporate inter-professional values: This could include, for example, inclusion, equality, openness, humility, mutuality, generosity and reciprocity.
- Include common and comparative learning: Treat comparative content as essential to inform learning from and about each other, to enhance understanding about respective roles and responsibilities and intelligent co-working.
- Employ a repertoire of interactive learning methods. There should not be too much reliance upon one method.
- Count towards qualifications: IPE is valued more when it counts towards qualifications.
- Assess and evaluate programmes: IPE is also valued more when programmes are approved and, where feasible, evaluated.
- Disseminate findings: To inform, stimulate and support wider development of IPE.

This latter list may appear daunting but can only be achieved if there is a willingness to integrate curricula. Barnett (1999) believes that integrating curricula is vital for the cognitive development of students who are required to respond flexibly to the needs of individuals, families and communities. A number of endeavours in UK universities have attempted to integrate related curricula, such as learning disability nursing and social work (Fagan and Plant, 2003). There is potential with these types of models to relate learning to real-life situations; create a context for new kinds of thinking; expose students to a wider range of teaching strategies, create supra-rationality, and develop capacity to challenge suppositions (Barnett, 1999). However, in the case of the joint training between nursing and social work no systematic evidence or evaluation exists to determine the real benefit of such an approach.

IPE should not be seen as a threat to uni-professional training. Moreover, it should complement separate professional training programmes. It should enhance practice within professions, respect the integrity and contribution of each profession and increase professional satisfaction by fostering mutual professional support (Barr et al, 2005).

One of the ways this can be realised is through acquiring common knowledge through mutual understanding of topics that overlap many health and social care professions. At a pre-registration level core topics such as ethics can ensure that the learning will be truly inter-professional (Aveyard et al, 2005).

In their study, Aveyard et al (2005) gained the viewpoints through workshops from all nursing branches, occupational therapy and physiotherapy tutors. Although a small study, it revealed seven core topics applicable across the respective professions: professional duty of care, codes of practice and accountability, informed consent and patient refusal, confidentiality, vulnerability, research ethics, and rationing. The authors did acknowledge however that caution should be taken when trying to integrate shared ethical decisions in an inter-professional approach, as not all ethical dilemmas are the same across all professions.

Other topics could be added to this which can help develop common knowledge bases for collaborative practice, but again with a similar warning label of ensuring applicability to similar professions:

- Risk
- Values
- Child protection
- Assessment.

IPE has adopted a range of different teaching methods. There is not the scope here to discuss each teaching method in turn and how it has been amalgamated into an inter-professional learning approach. Furthermore no one method is preferable as teachers decide upon a method dependent upon the students' learning needs (Barr et al, 2005). Barr et al (2000) reviewed the learning and teaching approaches utilised within IPE, which are:

- E-Learning and blended learning.
- Exchange (e.g. seminar and workshop discussions).
- Guideline development.
- Observation (e.g. work shadowing or site visits).
- Practice learning.
- Problem-based learning (PBL or problem solving activities).
- Received (lectures or presentations).
- Simulation (role play).

Most effective IPE is grounded in adult learning principles, that are aligned to problem solving approaches (Knowles, 1975). Given this, the learner is perceived as a self-directed and autonomous learner, where teachers are facilitators. The experience of the learner is important, learning is active and relevant, and the learner needs to be receptive and ready to learn (Brookfield, 1986). This places a heavy load on teachers involved in IPE, with the varying learning needs and diversity of inter-professional student groups, the necessity to challenge perceptions, and to show relevance of the learning to individuals (Barr et al, 2005).

Barriers to IPE

There is no doubt that there are barriers to delivering effective IPE within higher education. The amount of time and costs spent on developing and delivering curricula can be expensive and significant, with large numbers of staff and instructors involved. The organisation of cross-curricular activities is challenging with the need to understand and deliver different teaching methods (Gilbert, 2005). Different faculties will have different priorities for their budgets with some not placing a priority on the curriculum development required for IPE.

For students, IPE must be seen as part of the evaluation and assessment of their learning or IPE has no currency or value.

A further complication can be the different regulation of the health professions. The varying laws and responsibilities of care that relate to different professions can present hierarchies that affect clinical and practice education (Gilbert, 2005).

A key barrier to further adoption of IPE, despite its political emphasis, is the lack of systematic evidence of its effectiveness on improving patient/user outcomes (Zwarenstein et al, 2001). There clearly is a need to develop evaluations of the programmes themselves and evaluation of the assessment of student learning, knowledge, skills and attitudes developed through IPE activities (Oandasan and Reeves, 2005b).

Service user involvement and IPE

Service user and patient contribution to education is not new, with many individuals participating in health and social care teaching sessions or demonstrations for many years. Teaching methods that promote user involvement and encourage their real-life experiences, can show students the importance of working inter-profesionally with other disciplines and agencies, to provide care that is truly focused on people and their needs (Gordon and Walsh, 2005). Indeed, Glasby and Beresford (2006) explain that recognising the 'lived' experience of service users and the practice wisdom of practitioners is just as valid a way of knowing the world as research.

For IPE to be effective, it must put service users at the centre of its activities (Barr, 2002). For social work training, it is now a requirement that service user involvement takes place within all parts of the social work degree (Department of Health, 2000).

There are a number of generally agreed areas that service user involvement in education can take place (Le Var, 2002). These are:

● Curriculum development, planning and evaluation.
● Curriculum delivery: the teaching and training.
● Assessment of students during courses.

However, achieving involvement in all of these, thereby demonstrating 'inclusiveness', is challenging (see *Table 16.3*).

Principles of involvement

Before considering these areas, it is important to think about the key issues around service user involvement in education. Here, lessons can be learnt from social work education (Beresford and Page, 1994) and a number of key messages put forward in Beresford and Page's paper, are still very pertinent today and have relevance to involving people with learning disabilities in educational activities. These include:

● The service user experience and perspective should have equal standing with other expert perspectives.
● The educational environment must be accessible.
● Service users must be seen as educators. This experience must be validated and supported. The interests of the service users must be a distinct concern.
● Service users must be paid at the same rate as specialist or visiting

Table 16.3. Inclusive involvement in education (based upon the Learning Disability Nursing Course at Coventry University)

Area of involvement	Inclusive dimension
Commissioning of courses	The development and commissioning of courses are driven and involve the aspirations and desires of service users through effective consultation
Marketing and publicity	Service users are willingly and positively involved to endorse and market courses
Recruitment and admissions	Planned recruitment of staff and students takes place. Service users become key parts of interviewing panels and the decision making process.
User strategy	Service users are involved in the development of the faculty-wide service-user strategy and represent the widest possible diversity within the population group
Curriculum development	Service users help plan and evaluate the course through workshops and videoed input
Curriculum delivery	Service users are involved in teaching of students through initial 'getting to know you' sessions to 'sharing knowledge about health' sessions
Assessment	Service users are involved in the practice assessment of students, through poster evaluations and the students' ability to assess different aspects of health and communication
Evaluation	Individual debriefing to evaluate specific sessions are planned through to more formal end-of-year feedback sessions

lecturers. Payment should be in an appropriate form and cover all support required.

- A range of supports should be provided to help service users make the most effective contribution. This should involve the context for their contribution, the amount, how often, type, training and support required.
- Lecturers and staff may require training to ensure they respond positively to service user involvement.

- Involvement should be planned.
- Addressing involvement and partnership should be embedded into the curricula for students, to enable them to locate the value and importance of user involvement.

It is also necessary to have a strategy for user involvement that sits alongside or is informed by such principles. Le Var's (2002) review of the involvement of patients and service users in the education of nurses in England summarises some of the strategic issues that need to be addressed. Le Var (2002) highlights that patient/service user involvement should be incorporated into the infrastructure of the curriculum and supported by a comprehensive strategy, with a committee to oversee the implementation of that strategy.

The promotion of user involvement is now part of the mainstream policy agenda in health and social care sectors (Hodge, 2006). In healthcare education, more and more ways are being found to involve the patient/ service user voice. For a number of years the involvement of service users/ patients has been a requirement in the education of nurses, midwives and health visitors (UKCC, 2000). Yet establishing comprehensive involvement of the service user throughout all educational activities is still not achieved (English National Board for Nursing, Midwifery and Health Visiting (ENB), 2000). Developing a clear, coherent and inclusive model of service user involvement in healthcare education is demanding and the ENB's (2000) message still rings true nine years on. Establishing inclusive models of involvement that visibly move away from claims of 'tokenism' and populism (Beresford, 2001) are difficult.

The next part of the chapter puts forward a model being developed with people with learning disabilities at Coventry University, that strives to be inclusive (See *Table 16.3*).

Coventry University model

At Coventry University, the Learning Disability Team have sought to involve people with learning disabilities incrementally within the teaching aspects of the curriculum delivery. This has involved a 'getting to know you session' within the first term aimed at developing the student's ability to communicate. A group of six people with learning disabilities were involved, each acting as facilitators to assess the student's communication ability. The students were divided into groups of five to six with the service users facilitating one group at a time. The service users had varied levels of functioning, all being able to articulate themselves and field most questions. Some were supported by an advocate or keyworker. Feedback from the service users was conducted by myself and the advocate. This has been summarised as positive or negative.

Both the negative and positive user feedback is presented below.

Positive feedback

- All service users felt they were treated with respect.
- All service users felt they were listened to and their viewpoints valued.
- Service users felt that the questions started easy (getting to know you questions) through to more detailed personal questions that were asked sensitively and were agreed areas to discuss.
- Service users enjoyed the range of topics that were fielded.
- When a description of a personal turmoil/difficulty was disclosed by the service user, some students used praise and shared comparable experiences which demonstrated empathy and support. This was valued by the service uses and allowed a rapport to be built.
- In general the students took turns to ask questions.
- The exchange of information between both parties was valued.

Negative

- One service user felt that some students were quiet and this made them uncomfortable.
- Not all students asked questions.
- The room used with all the groups in was noisy.
- Not all students made sure that they understood what was being said by the service user.
- On some occasions the service user felt talked over (students deliberately made efforts to speak to and draw in the carer, not speaking directly to the service user).

The students involved were half way through their first year as part of their first theoretical learning disability module. The experience from both the students' and the service user perspective was largely positive. There are some learning points for future sessions. These include:

- Planning: Room size could have been larger or more rooms used to reduce noise and distractions.
- Support and preparation: Preparing the service users to strive to engage as many students as possible in the event.
- Preparation for students: For students to be confident to ask service users to repeat themselves when necessary.
- Clarity of ground rules: Ensure students seek clarification of issues via the service user not the carer/advocate.

The students on the learning disability course at Coventry University have also benefited from the strong inter-professional learning theme that runs through the course. The following comments are from a first year student and reflect the different ways that he has been assessed by people with learning disabilities and how learning disability, as an excellent learning exemplar, has been part of the IPE strategy for all health and social care students within the faculty.

We have been assessed in diverse ways from essay writing, to making posters, to having our practical skills assessed both in the skills lab and out on placement. One of the most interesting modules we have undertaken is the Inter-Professional Learning Pathway (IPLP). For this, we had to discuss a scenario involving a person with a learning disability with students on other courses such as occupational therapy, dietetics, psychology, social work and not forgetting medical students, online. This was a valuable tool, which enabled us to advocate the needs of people with learning disabilities and to promote the role of the RNLD in facilitating health. This module is due to carry on through out our training.

(Darren Orritt, first year learning disability nursing student)

It is worth considering the difficulties of involving service users and the bad practice that can arise. The Shaping our Lives National User Network, reported the following concerns to the Central Council for Education and Training in Social Work in 2000:

- User involvement is often an 'add on', rather than being properly planned throughout the curriculum.
- Users are just brought in to tell their 'life-stories' and give their personal views and experiences.
- Higher education institutions are negative about the idea of user involvement in relation to their courses and more generally in relation to practice.
- Training takes place in facilities that are not accessible.
- Users' contributions are not valued; users are often not paid for their time, sometimes not even receiving expenses.
- There is exclusion from the planning and the development of courses and the curriculum.
- There is exclusion from the assessment of students.

Despite the many challenges surrounding the involvement of service users in education, for service user involvement to have true 'added value' then an inclusive model must be pursued.

Conclusion

This chapter has sought to provide an overview of the contemporary importance of IPE and its potential for developing collaborative practice. The current political climate and the realities of health and social care practice still place a necessity on higher education institutions to develop different methods of common learning and IPE among health and social care students. Although the changing terminology associated with IPE has been a source of confusion in the past, the presentation of new terminology within the chapter is meant to add clarity to the IPE discourse.

Different teaching and learning models exist to help develop IPE, however it remains a challenging area to teach with a number of barriers that can affect the development of IPE initiatives.

Service user involvement should be integral to any IPE development. A learning disability exemplar has been presented here with the focus upon an inclusive educational approach that promotes involvement through all key educational activities. The learning disability experience provides rich learning opportunities for IPE. In summary:

- The need for health and social care professionals to work effectively together is more evident now than before.
- There is a greater demand for health and social care students to know and learn about other professional roles.
- IPE must be underpinned by the realities of inter-professional practice and the continual emphasis upon collaboration and partnership.
- Emerging terms of inter-professionality and inter-professional capability are meant to add clarity to the discourse around IPE not further complicate it with the addition of more terms.
- IPE is not a panacea to all educational problems but must be adopted by all staff, not just a few, for it to work.
- The end point of most health and social care training is the ability of such professionals to perform their roles as part of a team in the care of the different service user groups. IPE is now perceived as having the potential to achieve this.
- There should be acquisition of common knowledge through mutual understanding of topics (such as ethics, risk and values) that overlap many health and social care professions. This can enhance collaborative practice.
- There are many barriers to IPE including cost, lack of commitment and lack of sound evidence to promote this educational approach.
- User involvement in education must be underpinned by a set of principles and a faculty-wide strategy.

- An inclusive model of user involvement should be pursued to avoid labels of tokenism

References

Aveyard H, Edwards S, West S (2005) Core topics of healthcare ethics. The identification of core topics for interprofessional education. *Journal of Interprofessional Care* **19**(1): 63–9

Barnett R (1999) *The Idea of Higher Education*. Open University Press, Buckingham

Barr H (2002) *Interprofessional Education: Today, Yesterday and Tomorrow*. LTSN for Health Sciences Practice, Kings College, London

Barr H, Freeth D, Hammick M, Koppel I, Reeves S (2000) *Evaluations of Interprofessional Education: A United Kingdom Review for Health and Social Care*. BERA. CAIPE, London

Barr H, Koppel I, Reeves S, Hammick M, Freeth D (2005) *Effective Interprofessional Education: Argument, Assumption and Evidence*. Blackwell Publishing, Oxford

Beresford P (2001) Service users, social policy and the future of welfare. *Critical Social Policy* **21**(4): 494–512

Beresford P, Page L (1994) *Changing the Culture: Involving Service Users in Social Work Education*. CCETSW Paper 32.2. Central Council for Education and Training in Social Work, London

Bollard M (2003) Inter-professional working: Its relevance and importance to learning disability practice. In: Jukes M, Bollard M (eds.) *Contemporary Learning Disability Practice*. Chapter 2. Quay Books, Salisbury: 20–30

Brookfield SD (1986) *Understanding and Facilitating Adult Learning: A Comprehensive Analysis of Principles and Effective Practices*. Open University Press, Milton Keynes

Colyer H, Heleme M, Jones I (2005) *The Theory Practice Relationship in Inter-professional Education*. Occassional Paper No 7. Higher Education Education Academy, London

D'Amour D, Oandasan I (2005) Interprofessionality as the field of interprofessional practice and interprofessional education: An emerging concept. *Journal of Interprofessional Care* **1**: 8–20

D'eon M (2005) A blueprint for inter professional learning. *Journal of Interprofessional Care* **1**: 49–59

Department of Health (1997) *The New NHS: Modern and Dependable*. HMSO, London

Department of Health (2000) *The NHS Plan*. The Stationary Office, London

Department of Health (2005) *Creating an Inter-Professional Workforce: An Education and Training Framework for Health and Social Care in England*. Centre for Advancement of Interprofessional Education, Department of Health, London

English National Board for Nursing Midwifery and Health Visiting (2000) *Education in Focus: Strengthening Pre-Registration Nursing and Midwifery*. English National Board, London

Fagan N, Plant T (2003) Joint practitioners in health and social care. In: Jukes M, Bollard M (eds.) *Contemporary Learning Disability Practice*. Quay Books, Salisbury: 289–99

Finch J (2000) Interprofessional education and team working: A view from education providers. *British Medical Journal* **321**: 1138–40

Fraser SW, Greenhalgh T (2001) Coping with complexity: Educating for capability. *British Medical Journal* **323**(2201): 799–803

Gilbert JH (2005) Interprofessional learning in higher education structural barriers. *Journal of Interprofessional Care* **1**: 87–106

Glasby J, Beresford P (2006) Who knows best? Evidence based practice and the service user contribution. *Critical Social Policy* **26**(1): 268–84

Gordon F, Walsh C (2005) A framework for interprofessional capability: Developing students for health and social care as collaborative workers. *Journal of Integrated Care* **13**(3): 26–33

Guy EM (1986) *Professionals in Organisations: Debunking the Myth*. Praeger, New York

Hodge S (2006) Participation, discourse and power: A case study in service user involvement. *Critical Social Policy* **25**(2): 164–79

Hudson B (2002) Interprofessionality in health and social care: The Achilles heel of partnership? *Journal of Interprofessional Care* **16**(1): 7–17

Huxham C (ed.) (1996) *Creating Collaborative Advantage*. Sage, London: 1–18

Knowles M (1975) *Self-Directed Learning: A Guide for Learners and Teachers*. Follett, Chicago:

Le Var RMH (2002) Patient involvement in education for enhanced quality of care. *International Nursing Review* **49**: 215–25

Mattick E, Bligh J (2003) Interprofessional learning involving medical students or doctors. *Medical Education* **37**: 1008–11

Meads G, Ashcroft J (2005) *The Case for Inter-Professional Collaboration, in Health and Social Care*. Blackwell Publishing, Oxford

Meads G, Barr H (2005) The professional experience. In: Meads G, Ashcroft J (eds.) *The Case for Interprofessional Collaboration*. Blackwell Publishing: 121–35

Norman I (2005) Inter-professional education for pre-registration students in health professions: Recent developments in the UK and emerging lessons. *International Journal of Nursing Studies* **42:** 119–23

Oandasan I, Reeves S (2005a) Key elements for interprofessioal education. Part 1: The learner, the educator and the learning context. *Journal of Interprofessional Care* **1:** 21–8

Oandasan I, Reeves S (2005b) Key elements of interprofessional education. Part 2: Factors, processes and outcomes. *Journal of Interprofessional Care* **1:** 39–48

Piertroni PC (1992) Towards reflective practice – languages of health and social care. *Journal of Interprofessional Care* **6**(1): 7–16

Richardson S, Asthana S (2006) Interagency information sharing in health and social care services: The role of professional culture. *British Journal of Social Work* **36:** 657–69

Sainsbury Centre for Mental Health (2001) *The Capable Practitioner: A Framework for the Whole of the Mental Health Workforce*. Sainsbury Centre, London

United Kingdom Central Council for Nursing, Health Visiting and Midwifery (2000) *Registrars Letter 17/2000. Requirements for Pre-Registration Programmes*. UKCC, London

World Health Organisation (1988) *Learning Together to Work Together for Health. Report of a study group on multi-professional education of health personnel: The team approach*. WHO Technical Report Series No 769, Geneva

Zwarenstein M, Reeves S, Barr H, Hammick M, Koppel I, Atkins J (2001) Interprofessional Education: Effects on professional practice and healthcare outcomes. *The Cochrane Library*, Issue 3 Oxford

CHAPTER 17

Continuing practice development in learning disability nursing

Caron Thomas and Penny Pritchard

Introduction

The nature of continuing practice development in learning disability nursing within the UK has developed and evolved in response to the increasing influence of social models of care shaped by social and educational policy. This can be demonstrated by examining the influences on learning disability nursing practice from a historical perspective, and consideration of the changing nature of the health professions in modern health services. This includes the blurring of roles within the wider context of economic, technological, and organisational change, and throws up many challenges to the claims to legitimacy and the foundations of professions (Fournier, 2000).

Historical influences on practice development

Historically, the evolution of learning disability nursing practice within Europe was based on the influence and dominance of medical practice through the role of medical helper (Dent, 2003). This is reflected in the history of learning disability nursing which can be traced back to the asylums, with the role of attendants who were subordinate to doctors and worked within a custodial model of care. Throughout the last century, this subordination can be seen in all aspects of nurse education and practice. The 1919 Nurse Registration Act was a precursor to the setting up of the General Nursing Council (GNC) in the early 1920s, and although this saw learning disability nursing being included on the mental supplementary register (Mitchell, 1998, 2000), nurse training in this field was largely carried out by doctors within the institutional setting through the Royal Medico-Psychological Association (RMPA). Although the RMPA was a medical organisation which later became the Royal College of Psychiatrists, the association continued to play a leading role in the training of learning disability nurses until the GNC took sole control in 1951 (Mitchell, 1998, 2000). During this time nurse education took place in schools of nursing based in segregated hospital institutions with students being employed as part of the workforce with care practices isolated within the institutional setting.

The last three decades have seen major changes in the policies for services for people with learning disabilities. Following the recommendations contained in a series of reports, such as the report on Ely Hospital, Cardiff (Department of Health and Social Services, 1969), there was a move away from providing long-term care within an institutional medical model, to a social care model with the emphasis on living an 'ordinary life' (King's Fund, 1980). This changing emphasis from a medical to a social model of care meant that learning disability nursing was experiencing problems in defining itself. Justifying a role in the life of people with learning disabilities and their families was difficult due to the shadow cast over the association with the medical model of care and damning reports of poor practice. This was perhaps the nadir of learning disability nursing as a profession which was still perceived as being subordinate to the medical profession and associated with outdated institutional care.

Inevitably, new ways of thinking about the knowledge and skills required by the future workforce were identified and a series of reports including the Briggs Report (DHSS 1972), the Jay Report (DHSS 1979) and the seminal Griffiths Report (Griffiths 1988) supported the need for a new caring profession for 'mentally handicapped' people. Closer collaboration between health and social services was already in evidence in 1982 with a new nurse training curriculum which focused on joint training and education initiatives; this signalled a significant break away from a medical model to a social model of care (Fagan and Plant, 2003). These influential reports had far reaching consequences in relation to perceptions of learning disability nursing and nursing roles, but the introduction of the NHS and Community Care Act (Department of Health, 1990) and the creation of community nursing roles gave learning disability nurses the opportunity to demonstrate the flexibility, adaptability, and transferability of their knowledge and skills.

A major shift in the provision of nurse education also took place at this time with a move from schools of nursing, based in hospitals, into higher education establishments. The development of diploma and degree programmes through Project 2000 (UKCC, 1986) provided a more recognisable education-led base for practice and reinforced the claim to a professional identity based on a valued educational system. Project 2000 was seen to move further away from the biomedical model to a more holistic humanistic approach to care. Following on from community care initiatives, the future of the learning disability nursing profession in the UK was then the subject of a national consultation by the Department of Health in 1993 which saw practitioners and nurse educators galvanised into action to influence the outcome and gain support for the continuation of learning disability nursing roles. These developments were then followed in 1995 by an endorsement of learning disabilities nursing roles by the Department of Health in the *Continuing the Commitment* publication (Department of Health, 1995).

Despite describing specialist learning disability practice, *Continuing the Commitment* did not go into sufficient detail regarding the dynamic and assertive nature of nursing practice in a way that clearly separates it out from other roles such as social work and management. Indeed, the term learning disability is a social and educational label which makes no representation of the range and type of health needs experienced by people with this label, such as people with syndrome-specific health needs (Corbett, 2007), and higher rates of respiratory diseases and early death (Disability Rights Commission, 2006), with a mortality rate reported to be 58 times higher than the non-disabled population to die before the age of 50 (Hollins et al, 1998). More recently, although nursing roles have embraced an individual person-centred model of care, commensurate with national policy and recognising the demographic changes within society affecting health, the only roles advocated for learning disability nurses following the publication of the *Valuing People* White Paper (Department of Health, 2001a) was the role of health facilitation and community nursing roles to support gaining access to mainstream services. According to Barr (2004), this is a central tenet of the role of the learning disability nurse. Having said that, these roles alone are arguably not reflective of the complex direct care interventions carried out with this client group. Overall, the White Paper was essentially an excellent social chapter based on individuals being able to exercise their rights, live an independent life, make life choices, and be socially included. Disappointingly, the White Paper did not really emphasise in any detail the need for development of specialist roles to meet complex healthcare needs, for example, mental impairment, multiple and profound disabilities, working with sex offenders and people with forensic needs, through to a range of care and treatment programmes including psychological therapies and physical health needs.

The influence of the market environment

The market environment, or enterprise culture, has resulted in the boundaries between public service and private sector gradually being eradicated (Bolton, 2000). Learning disability nurses working within health service organisations are now required to work within multifunctional, integrated teams, in a flexible way (Department of Health, 2007b). This involves working within a mixed economy of care influenced by market forces, with their healthcare activities being defined by the State as a third party mediator (Malin, 2000) and being managerially led rather than professionally led. Within the National

Health Service and public sector, another major paradigm shift which occurred following the introduction of the quasi market economies was the primacy of the consumer. The concept of the expert patient (Department of Health, 2000) and informed choice has meant that consumerism has changed and continues to change the whole dynamics of the professions and the boundaries that surround them. Fournier (2000) suggested that what is being witnessed here is the 'unmaking of the professions' and the dismantling of three boundaries essential to the making of the professions: the dismantling of the independent and self-contained knowledge, dismantling of profession/ market barriers, and dismantling of profession/client barriers.

Workforce trends within modern health services have shown a move away from profession-determined education to employer-led education, making it vital to break down role demarcation which was seen as impeding client care (Nally and Steele, 1998). In the future, a review of workforce needs within the health service may demonstrate that fewer nurses will be required to provide basic care and support. It is against this backdrop that learning disability nursing needs to consider how it will continue to evolve to ensure that practice is 'fit for purpose'. This requires articulation and demonstration of specialist therapeutic skills and the extension of roles into domains previously seen as being medical, such as prescribing (Department of Health, 2001b), and the 'responsible clinician' role within the Mental Health Act 2007, and incorporating this into nursing practice. This is coupled with an increasing focus on specific areas of nursing practice carried out by teams supported by clinical nurse specialists, advanced practitioners and nurse consultants. The spotlight is on the concept of advanced clinical practice which requires nurses to be involved in assessment, diagnosis, and treatment in nurse-led clinics (Nursing and Midwifery Council, 2006). This signals a significant encroachment of traditional areas of practice historically provided by the medical and psychology professions.

These developments are reflected in a framework identified by the International Council of Nurses as far back as 1992 (*Table 17.1*). This framework articulates the external forces and forces from within the nursing profession which drive the creation of nursing specialties and helps to capture the dynamic nature of learning disability nursing practice.

External forces affecting learning disability nursing

The concept of segmentation differentiates between sub-groups within nursing (Dent and Burtney, 1997; Dent, 2003). Learning disability nursing is located within the 'family of nursing' and as such can be considered to be at the very least a professional segment of that family which draws on multiple sources of knowledge. New technologies, such as new drug therapies and computer-based therapies covered by guidance published by the National Institute for Health and Clinical Excellence (2009), and the advent of computer-based therapy programmes will play a significant role in care practices in the future. The complexity of need demonstrated by people with learning disabilities is reflected in the knowledge, skills and experience required to understand multiple disabilities and the impact of co-morbid conditions when assessing need and planning strategies to manage care.

It is essential that learning disability nurses have an understanding of health policy, population needs and trends, health surveillance, health promotion, and health education programmes. Some learning disability nurses have focused their skills and developed their practice through specialising in one area of care, gaining in depth expert knowledge, experience, and skills and working with people who share a specific characteristic or diagnosis (UK Learning Disability Consultant Nurse Network 2006). Other external forces impacting upon learning disability nursing practice include lobby groups such as Mencap (2004, 2007), who have raised the issue not only of inequalities in health experienced by people with learning disabilities, but also have influenced national guidance requiring knowledge of the range of health needs and skilled intervention (Department of Health, 2007a,b), and independent inquiries (Michael, 2008).

Table 17.1. Forces driving the creation of nursing specialties

External forces	Forces within the profession
• Increased complexity of healthcare	• Development of nursing science, knowledge and research
• Changing health needs, e.g. demographic changes, epidemiology of disease	• Extension of boundaries of nursing, e.g. assessment, diagnosis and treatment
• Health policy decisions Structural changes in health care, e.g. nurse-led clinics	• Development of post-registration curricula
• New technologies	• Search for improved career progression, e.g. career pathways
• Delegation by medical profession, e.g. nurse prescribing	• Search for recognition through better financial reward and authority and status
• Advances in medical practice and creation of new medical specialties	• Servicing or working in parallel to medical specialities as an autonomous practitioner
• Resources	• Affiliation movements
• Consumer demand	
• Political interests, e.g. lobbying by special interest groups	
• Product merchandising	

Forces within the profession

Specialist practice in learning disability nursing has evolved in terms of the care and treatment of epilepsy, mental health, profound and multiple physical disabilities, behavioural and psychological therapies, forensic nursing, and care of the elderly, particularly dementia care. Within the UK, pre-registration nurse education is university based and ensures a professional nurse qualification as well as an academic award (Barr, 2004) from higher education-based diploma and degree courses. This provides a sound basis for practice on which to build further knowledge and skills in the specialisms.

Although new nursing roles have enabled learning disability nurses to assess and treat certain conditions including continence, epilepsy, challenging behaviours, and mental health problems, the main criticisms to the claim of learning disability nursing being a profession, are that learning disability nurses do not exercise the same level of autonomy as doctors. Neither has it ever really been comfortably placed as a single exclusive entity in terms of a body of knowledge and skills. It has been reliant on taking its lead from psychiatry and psychology in terms of discourse, labels, and terminology. However, drawing on multiple sources of knowledge, and adapting terminology and discourse to the particular needs of the individual, enables people with learning disabilities to exercise their rights to care as valued citizens (Barr, 2004), and to develop knowledge and skills to live as independently as possible and lead fulfilling lives. Advanced practice nurses can also adapt to providing and influencing healthcare provision to an increasingly diverse population, taking into account the cost-effectiveness of interventions and the critical evaluation of outcomes of care on an individual as well as a population-wide basis. In the UK, the advanced practice role is seen as encompassing not only clinical assessment skills, but also the diagnosis and treatment of healthcare needs. This is a radical shift away from traditional nursing roles and demonstrates the versatility of nursing roles in managing entire processes of care and treatment, including prescribing medication where necessary (Nursing and Midwifery Council, 2006). Learning disability nurses have demonstrated over time that they are well equipped to adapt to the changing demographics of workforce needs, and there is scope to develop advanced practice in long-term conditions, age-related disorders and other areas of practice previously identified within this text to meet complex health needs.

This has to be matched with critical analysis skills in terms of understanding and articulating the evidence base for practice. In order to inform future practice it is essential that learning disability nurses are involved in research activity that informs changes to the way care is delivered.

Evidence-based healthcare

As stated by Giddens (1989), specialist knowledge and education are crucial to the identity of a profession. Within health services in the UK, the notion of clinical expertise has become increasingly dependent on the evidence-based medicine or practice (EBP) movement which is dominated by positivist 'gold standard' research frameworks such as randomised control trials (RCTs), systematic reviews, meta-analyses, and mega-trials (Colyer and Kamath, 1999). However, it has been recognised that there is a place for theory and knowledge which may not fit into positivist or post-positivist views of reality (Wolfer, 1993), which reflect a cultural bias towards 'scientism'. Clinical expertise in a given area incorporates not only knowledge, but also ways of knowing (McCormack, 2003), and is a term used to describe proficiency and professional judgement acquired by practitioners through professional education and clinical experience (Colyer and Kamath, 1999). These ways of knowing include subjective elements of private judgement informed by the interaction between practitioner and patient, as well as the evidence base for practice, recognising that neither is sufficient alone (Sackett et al, 1997). The subjective nature of professional judgement reflects the difficulties experienced by learning disability nurses in articulating the almost intuitive decision making processes in the course of their everyday practice. McCormack and Titchen (2001) suggest that this is because nurses think 'holistically' rather than in a linear task-orientated fashion. Expertise can be identified through professional artistry involving rapid interplay and a balance of intuition and rationality when engaged in practice, characterised by the complex harmonisation of the domains of professional craft knowledge and theoretical knowledge (Titchen, 2000). The depth and breadth of learning disability nursing practice is therefore difficult to quantify, especially the micro skills that help to develop intuitive practice which are not visible to the 'naked eye' so to speak. On the other hand, task-orientated care is perhaps more easily measurable and recognisable to the target-driven world of healthcare services.

In order to articulate the nature of practice development in learning disability nursing, the real essence of practice must be understood and captured by placing practice within recognisable frameworks such as clinical governance (National Health Service Executive, 1999). Clinical governance requires nurses to have a service user and carer focus, be involved in research and audit activity, participate in training and development activity, base their practice on the most up-to-date evidence, and adhere to standards for care delivery. Evidence-based nursing practice mirrors the philosophy behind evidence-based medicine which has been described by Sackett et al (1977) as,

The conscientious, explicit, and judicious use of current best evidence in making decisions about the care of individual patients.

This evidence supports decision making processes and centres around direct care strategies and interventions carried out by the nurse with individuals or groups of people in a variety of care settings. Clinical governance facilitates the bringing together of the professions through standardised practice using guidance including National Service Frameworks (NSFs), National Institute for Health and Clinical Excellence guidance, Essence of Care standards, Codes of Conduct, clinical supervision and guidance from professional associations. The standardisation of processes and clinical pathways, coupled with a risk averse culture, has resulted in learning disability nurses having to embrace the principles of clinical governance, as well as accepting other professionals, and more recently service users, as equal partners in decision making processes (Department of Health, 2000). The primacy of the service user lies at the heart of clinical governance as well as being central to the concept of person-centred planning, the key framework from within which learning disability services (Department of Health, 2001a) engage with service users in planning to meet their needs.

This was supported by McCormack and Titchen (2001) who suggested that a person-centred philosophy demonstrated a deep respect for the autonomy of the individual as a person, transforming their experience of care by offering personal support and practical expertise, while enabling the individual to follow a path of their own choosing in their own way. Learning disability nurses use an enabling, facilitative style in engaging people with learning disabilities and their carers in complex healthcare interventions. This may involve a combination of psychological therapies, for example family therapy or cognitive behavioural therapy, with sensory interventions and perhaps medication. The emphasis of nurse prescribing and reviewing and monitoring the use of medication with an individual should be to move towards reducing reliance on medication and polytherapy for conditions such as epilepsy, mental health problems and, more contentiously, challenging behaviour. This helps to demonstrate the level of autonomy required to make changes based on a clinical assessment and knowledge of the social, emotional, biological, and psychological factors affecting the health of an individual.

Having undertaken post-registration education and training relevant to the speciality, learning disability nurses have opportunities to extend their boundaries of practice with increased autonomy as clinical nurse specialists, nurse consultants, and advanced practitioners, not to mention nurse prescribing and the responsible clinician role (Mental Health Act

2007), bringing with them increased status and remuneration. Research, audit, and evaluation are also integral to the development of these roles and influence changes in clinical practice offering the opportunity for clinical academic careers. This activity needs to focus on the effectiveness and outcomes of clinical interventions to inform future practice as well as measuring service user satisfaction with their healthcare experiences. Complex adaptive systems from biology to economics in healthcare form the basis of learning disability nursing practice, with research, education, and nursing theory as structures within this (Holden, 2005). This is supported by 'action learning' which is a continuous process of learning and reflection, supported by colleagues, with the intention of ensuring that real problems are worked out and that nurses reflect on their own experiences (McGill and Beaty, 2001). This applies to whatever setting learning disability nurses find themselves working in as their knowledge and skills are arguably transferable to a wide variety of settings and teams (Department of Health, 2007b). The following two case studies attempt to demonstrate the flexibility of knowledge and skills of the learning disabilities nurse in specialist and advanced practice roles.

Case study 1

Background

Following the implementation of the Changing Workforce Programme, (Department of Health, 2001c) within the Developmental Neurosciences and Learning Disabilities Directorate, a post was developed specifically to work with older people with learning disabilities. The remit of this role was to support the implementation of the Older Person's National Service Framework (NSF) (Department of Health, 2001d) and subsequently supported the NSF for Long-Term Conditions (Department of Health, 2005). The nurse's role has been specifically to focus on the health needs of people with Down syndrome and dementia, and older people with learning disabilities who have age-related conditions. The role has enabled development of a multi-disciplinary approach to meeting the needs of people with Down syndrome and dementia. Nurses, psychologists, psychiatrists, and occupational therapists are developing a specific care pathway to support this client group.

The following case study outlines how the older person's facilitator shaped and co-ordinated the assessment of a client referred for a possible diagnosis of dementia. This brief resume demonstrates how learning disabilities nurses have developed specialist skills in order to respond to the healthcare needs of older people with learning disabilities

'Susan'

A young lady with Down syndrome, 'Susan', who had recently moved into her own flat, was referred to the community learning disabilities team due to concerns that she was exhibiting signs of dementia. Following discussion by the multidisciplinary team, Susan was invited to attend a clinic appointment with the older person's health facilitator (a registered learning disabilities nurse) which she subsequently attended accompanied by her mother and social worker.

A full past history was taken and further appointments were made to carry out detailed baseline assessments by the team. The baseline assessments included:

- A broadscreen assessment of observed changes (developed by the older person's health facilitator).
- Mum was instructed by the nurse on the completion of the Assessment for Adults with Developmental Disabilities (McQuillan et al, 2001), Hampshire Social Services Staff Support Levels Assessment, and the Dementia Questionnaire for Retarded Persons (Evenhuis et al, 1990) to complete at home.
- Psychological assessments were arranged at the day services.
- An assessment of motor processing skills (AMPS).

The broadscreen assessment involves the nurse undertaking a detailed health screen and identifies any subsequent need for investigations which may be useful in excluding other underlying health needs that could mask and give a false clinical picture, e.g. urine infection, thyroid function, epilepsy, depression, stroke. This also involves the nurse liaising with the general practitioner and the primary care team to facilitate completion of investigations.

Each assessment was given a timescale for completion so that all assessments were completed by a proposed date for the next appointment. Susan and her family were invited back for a second clinic appointment to discuss the outcomes.

The assessments identified that Susan was not exhibiting signs of dementia, which was a great relief to Susan and her family. The process undertaken and led by the nurse highlights how specialist clinical knowledge and skills used in an effective and efficient way can improve the outcomes for service users and their families. As well as working with the team in undertaking the baseline assessment, the nurse co-ordinated the care pathway to ensure the service was timely and efficient in responding to concerns. This outcome was achieved in under six weeks from the first clinic appointment.

There is now a detailed baseline assessment of Susan's needs and her skill levels and abilities which will prove invaluable should she be referred back to the service in the future.

Case study 2

Background

Over the last five years South Staffordshire and Shropshire Healthcare NHS Foundation Trust's learning disabilities service changed its focus to incorporate the developmental neurosciences. This led to the opportunity for development of advanced practitioner roles. These roles were identified within specific areas, to develop clinical expertise in key areas of practice. An advanced practitioner in epilepsy was subsequently appointed, with extensive expertise in supplementary nurse prescribing and post-registration education in managing epilepsy with people with learning disabilities. The advanced practitioner role is one of expert practitioner, educator and facilitator.

'Enid'

Following an initial referral to the Community Learning Disabilities Team, the advanced practitioner accepted a referral for a woman with learning disabilities and unstable epilepsy, 'Enid'. Enid was living at home with her elderly mother who also has learning disabilities and there was a mutual caring arrangement in the home.

Initial contact was made through a clinic appointment, and information gathered in the form of the epilepsy care pathway documentation. Gaining a description of seizures was difficult due to Enid and her mother's learning disabilities, and their problems with comprehension and communication. It was also identified that administration of medication was chaotic at times, and there were difficulties due to interactions of medicines used to control Enid's epilepsy.

Enid was seen by the neuropsychiatrist and together with the advanced practitioner a clinical management plan was devised to support gaining control of her unstable condition. The advanced practitioner continued to see Enid at her nurse-led clinics and work to the clinical management plan. Titration of medication was involved at this stage. Enid developed a relationship during this time, and her new partner was able to give a good description of seizures; this enabled the advanced practitioner to gain a much better picture, and support the neuropsychiatrist to inform the clinical management plan. However, there were still problems in taking her anti-convulsant medication, and this led to an increase of seizures which required a hospital admission. During the hospital stay Enid's medication was changed and was no longer concordant with her clinical management plan. Enid was subsequently discharged from hospital but was still experiencing seizures. The advanced practitioner liaised with the hospital and Enid's general practitioner to determine a stable medication regime. The Community Learning Disabilities Team was informed and a social worker was engaged in addressing Enid and her mother's vulnerability. The team has also played a key role in supporting Enid to take prescribed medication through the use of blister packs, and education in how to use these properly.

The advanced practitioner has taken a lead role in this facilitation; using a combination of:

- Extensive community nursing experience in addressing healthcare needs.
- Specialist knowledge and skills in epilepsy management.
- Supplementary nurse prescribing skills.
- Leadership skills and multi-disciplinary working.
- Education and training skills in facilitating learning.

Enid's epilepsy management has been difficult. However, through the use of specialist knowledge and skills, and interagency and multidisciplinary approaches to meeting her healthcare needs effectively, Enid has been supported to remain in her own home and to manage her epilepsy more effectively. This has meant that she has been supported to manage her own healthcare needs while maintaining significant social relationships with her partner and her family.

This case study highlights the advantages of extending nursing roles and new ways of working, and supports nurses working in a 'hands on' way in clinical and social settings to meet complex life-long conditions.

A statistical analysis of the Nursing and Midwifery Council (2005) register identified that of the 784 959 nurses qualified to practise on the register, 24 604 are learning disability nurses. However not all of these nurses are actually practising in a 'hands on' way. They work in a variety of settings including the private and voluntary sector, within NHS and social services departments, and in managerial, research and education posts. This begins to demonstrate the transferability of skills and different practice models that learning disability nurses are working within. The evolution of the knowledge and skills of the learning disability nurse has allowed them to rise to demographic challenges within the environment, and they continue to evolve and make a significant impact on the health needs of people with learning disabilities from a variety of perspectives.

Paradoxically, learning disability nurses often find that they are devalued and possibly marginalised by other professions because they work with people with learning disabilities; creating a shared experience of parallel stigma (Mitchell, 2000). Abbott (1995) argued that professional status is achieved by constructing boundaries which isolate professionals from service users, allowing them to maintain high status without compromising the purity of their scientific knowledge. The nature and validity of this scientific knowledge however, has come under increasing scrutiny within the NHS since the introduction of the evidence-based healthcare concept over the last decade. It is perhaps more useful to view practice development as a dynamic process, with professional dominance always being susceptible to new threats and challenges.

Conclusion

Although it could be argued that learning disability nursing is a segment of the wider nursing profession rather than a profession in its own right (Dent, 2003), learning disability nurses have demonstrated their breadth of knowledge and skills in a range of care activities which amount to a specialist body of knowledge practised by a critical mass of practitioners.

Learning disability nurses are well placed to respond to the continuing challenges of evolving and maintaining a professional identity, through continuing education, advancing practice, influencing health and social care policy, and ensuring that health needs are better met through evidence-based practice. New knowledge and practice development is generated through research and evaluative processes with clinical supervision and reflective practice also playing a significant role in this process. Learning disability nurses have demonstrated the ability to adapt and change their practice to any care environment, recognising the need to accept that the role is constantly evolving in response to changing demographics, technologies, and needs. However, as with other professions it is acknowledged that professional status for learning disability nursing is State mediated, and therefore subject to the influence of external forces. Through expediency and State-mediated intervention, the blurring of professional boundaries in areas such as prescribing and other inter-professional practices may mean that learning disability nurses are increasingly being educated alongside other professionals. The key outcome to this will be the impact of the changing professions on the health needs of people with learning disabilities and how these needs are met. This will affect the 'credentialism' currently awarded to the professions in terms of theory underpinning practice, training and education, professional accreditation, ethical codes, access to professionals, and control over the supply of practitioners (Berman Brown and McCartney,

2000). The very nature of what is understood by practice development will continue to evolve and we may see the emergence of new 'hybrid' professions in the care of people with learning disabilities in response to the external forces identified by the International Council of Nurses (1992) (*Table 17.1*). What is clear is that learning disability nursing practice is a complex combination of theory, practice, and 'ways of knowing' through experience and intuition, with person-centred approaches and clinical governance as frameworks for practice. This is underpinned by knowledge and skills in research, audit, education and development and standards for practice, coupled with a fundamental commitment to working with people with learning disabilities and their families in recognising and meeting a range of healthcare needs.

References

Abbott A (1995) Boundaries of social work or social work boundaries? *Social Service Review* **Dec:** 547–62

Barr O (2004) Nurses for people with learning disabilities within the United Kingdom: An overview and some challenges for the future. *International Journal of Nursing in Intellectual and Developmental Disabilities* **1**(1): 5

Berman Brown R, McCartney S (2000) Professionalism definitions in 'managing' health services: Perspectives on the differeng views of clinicans and general managers in an NHS Trust. In Malin N (ed) *Professionalism, Boundaries, and the Workplace*. Routledge, London

Bolton S (2000) Mixed feelings: Emotion management in a caring profession. In: Malin N (ed.) *Professionalism, Boundaries, and the Workplace*. Routledge, London

Colyer H, Kamath P (1999) Evidence-based practice. A philosophical and political analysis: Some matters for consideration by professional practitioners. *Journal of Advanced Nursing* **29**(1): 188–93

Corbett J (2007) *Healthcare Provision and People with Learning Disabilities: A Guide for Health Professionals*. Wiley, Chichester

Dent M (2003) *Remodelling Hospitals and Health Professions in Europe: Medicine, Nursing, and the State*. Palgrave MacMillan, Basingstoke

Dent M (2005) *Changing Jurisdictions within the Health Professions? Autonomy, Accountability, and Evidence Based Practice*. 4th International Critical Management Studies Conference, Cambridge University

Dent M, Burtney E (1997) Changes in Practice Nursing: Professionalism,

Segmentation, and Sponsorship. *Journal of Clinical Nursing* **6**(5): 355–63

Department of Health (1990) *NHS and Community Care Act*. HMSO, London

Department of Health (1995) *Continuing the Commitment. The Report of the Learning Disability Nursing Project*. Department of Health, London

Department of Health (1999) *Saving Lives – Our Healthier Nation*. HMSO, London

Department of Health (2000) *The NHS Plan: A Plan for Investment, a Plan for Reform*. HMSO, London

Department of Health (2001a) *Valuing People: A New Strategy for Learning Disability in the 21st Century*. HMSO, London

Department of Health (2001b) *National Prescribing Centre 'Maintaining Competency in Prescribing: An Outline Framework to Help Nurse Prescribers'*, 1st edn. NHS Prescribing Centre, Liverpool

Department of Health (2001c) *Changing Workforce Programme Toolkit*. Department of Health, London

Department of Health (2001d) *National Service Framework for Older People*. Department of Health, London

Department of Health (2005) *National Service Framework for Long Term Conditions*. Department of Health, London

Department of Health (2007a) *Commissioning Specialist Adult Learning Disability Health Services; Good Practice Guidance*. Department of Health, London

Department of Health (2007b) *Good Practice in Learning disability Nursing*, Department of Health, London

Department of Health and Social Security (1969) *Report of the Committee of Inquiry into Allegations of Ill Treatment of Patients and other Irregularities at the Ely Hospital, Cardiff*, Cmnd 3975, HMSO, London

Department of Health and Social Security (1971) *Better Services for the Mentally Handicapped*. Cmnd 4683, HMSO, London

Department of Health and Social Security (1972) *Report of the Committee on Nursing (Briggs Report)*, Cmnd 5115. HMSO, London

Department of Health and Social Security (1979) *Report of the Committee of Enquiry into Mental Handicap Nursing and Care (Jay Report)* Cmnd 7468, HMSO, London

Disability Rights Commission (2006) *Equal treatment: Closing the Gap*,

Disability Rights Commission, London

Evenhuis H, Kangene MMF, and Eurlings HAL (1990) *Dementia Questionnaire for Mentally Retarded Persons*. Erasmus University, Rotterdam, The Netherlands

Fagan N, Plant T (2003) Joint practitioners in health and social care. In Jukes M, Bollard M (eds.) *Contemporary Learning Disability Practice*. Quay books, Salisbury

Fournier V (2000) Boundary work and the (un)making of the professions. In: Malin N (ed.) *Professionalism, Boundaries, and the Workplace*. Routledge, London

Giddens A (1989) *Sociology*. Polity Press, Cambridge, in association with Basil Blackwell, Oxford

Griffiths R (1988) *Community Care: Agenda for Action*. HMSO, London

Holden LM (2005) Complex adaptive systems: Concept analysis. *Journal of Advanced Nursing* 52(6): 651–7

Hollins S, Attard MT, von Fraunhofer N, Sedgwick P (1998) Mortality in people with learning disability: Risks, causes, and death certification findings in London. *Developmental Medicine and Child Neurology* 40: 50–6

International Council of Nurses (1992) *Guidelines on Specialisation in Nursing*. ICN, Geneva

King's Fund (1980) *An Ordinary Life*. Project Paper Number 24, King's Fund Centre, London

Malin N (ed.) (2000) *Professionalism, Boundaries, and the Workplace*. Routledge, London

McCormack B (2003) Knowing and acting – A strategic practitioner focused approach to nursing research and practice development. *Nursing Times Research* 8(2): 86–99

McCormack B, Titchen A (2001) Patient-centred practice: An emerging focus for nursing expertise. In: Higgs J, Titchen A (eds.) *Practice Knowledge and Expertise in the Health Professions*. Butterworth Heineman, Oxford

McGill I, Beaty L (2001) *Action Learning: A Guide for Professional, Management, and Educational Development*. Revised 2nd edn. Kogan Page, London

McQuillan S, Kalsy S, Oliver C, Hall S (2001) *Assessment for Adults with Developmental Disabilities*. School of Psychology, University of Birmingham, UK

Mencap (2004) *Treat Me Right, Better Healthcare for People with a Learning Disability*. Mencap, London

Mencap (2007) *Death by Indifference; Following up the Treat me right! Report*. Mencap, London

Michael J (2008) *Healthcare for All; Report of the Independent Inquiry into Access to Healthcare for People with Learning Disabilities*. Independent Inquiry into Access to Healthcare for People with Learning Disabilities, London

Mitchell D (1996) Learning disability in the post-War period. *International History of Nursing Journal* 1(4): 20–33

Mitchell D (1998) Learning Disability Nursing: Reflections on History. *Journal of Learning Disability Nursing, Health, and Social Care* 2(1): 45–9

Mitchell D (2000) Parallel stigma? Nurses and people with learning disabilities. *British Journal of Learning Disabilities* **28:** 78–81

Nally B, Steele J (1998) Policy, organisation and practice in the provision of community services for people with intellectual disability. In: Thompson T, Matthias P (eds.) *Standards and Mental Handicap* 2nd edn. Bailliere Tindall, London

National Institute for Health and Clinical Excellence (2009) guidelines. Available from: www.nice.org.uk [accessed 2 April 2009]

National Health Service Executive (1999) *Clinical Governance and Quality in the NHS*. NHSE, Leeds

Nursing and Midwifery Council (2005) *Guidelines for Records and Record Keeping* (Update on previous publication 2004) NMC, London

Nursing and Midwifery Council (2005) *Statistical Analysis of the Register*. NMC, London

Nursing and Midwifery Council (2006) *Advanced Nursing Practice*. NMC, London

Sackett D, Richardson WS, Rosenberg W, Haynes RB (1997) *Evidence-Based Medicine: How to Practice and Teach EBM*. Churchill Livingstone, London

Titchen A (2000) *Professional Craft Knowledge in Patient Centred Nursing and the Facilitation of its Development*. DPhil Thesis, University of Oxford; Ashdale Press, Oxford

United Kingdom Central Council for Nursing Midwifery and Health Visiting (1986) *Project 2000: A New Preparation for Practice*. UKCC, London

UK Consultant Nurse Network (2006) *Shaping the Future: A Vision for*

Learning Disability Nursing. UK Learning Disability Consultant Nurse Network, UK

Wolfer J (1993) Aspects of 'reality' and ways of knowing in nursing: In search of an integrating paradigm. *IMAGE Journal of Nursing Scholarship* 25(2): 141–6

Index